Contemporary Systems Thinking

Series Editor
Robert L. Flood
Maastricht School of Management
The Netherlands

Contemporary Systems Thinking is a series of texts, each of which deals comparatively and/or critically with different aspects of holistic thinking at the frontiers of the discipline. Traditionally, writings by systems thinkers have been concerned with single theme propositions like General Systems Theory, Cybernetics, Operations Research, System Dynamics, Soft Systems Methodology and many others. Recently there have been attempts to fulfill a different yet equally important role by comparative analyses of viewpoints and approaches, each addressing disparate areas of study such as: modeling and simulation, measurement, management, 'problem solving' methods, international relations, social theory and last, but not exhaustively or least, philosophy.

Bringing together many sources yields several achievements, among which is showing a great diversity of approaches, ideas and application areas that systems thinking contributes to (although, often with difficulties unresolved). There is a need for a series of books, each focusing in detail on the study areas mentioned above. While modeling and simulation are served well in the scientific literature, this is not the case for systems thinking in management, 'problem solving' methods, social theory, or philosophy to name a handful. Each book in this series makes a contribution by concentrating on one of these topics.

More information about this series at http://www.springer.com/series/5807

Janet McIntyre-Mills

Transformation from Wall Street to Wellbeing

Joining Up the Dots Through Participatory Democracy and Governance to Mitigate the Causes and Adapt to the Effects of Climate Change

Springer

Janet McIntyre-Mills
Flinders University
Adelaide
South Australia
Australia

ISSN 1568-2846
ISBN 978-1-4899-7465-5 ISBN 978-1-4899-7466-2 (eBook)
DOI 10.1007/978-1-4899-7466-2
Springer Boston Heidelberg New York Dordrecht London

Library of Congress Control Number: 2014940066

Printed on acid-free paper

Springer is part of Springer Science+Business Media (www.springer.com)

Dedication and Remembering

To the displaced and hungry
To my mother who taught me to question
To George Thompson on whom the light of day might shine[1] *I dedicate this book.*

Hua Hu Ching's 77th lesson

" ... it will be from the misuse and partial development of intelligence that a time of confusion will arise and grow progressively worse. People will lose their appreciation for a healthy life of plainness after being attracted to and entrapped by all kinds of accumulated bad habits. Slavery will pervade human life and all human relationships under different names and reasons. If one is not a slave of social under development, he will be the slave of all kinds of emotional entrapment; if not the slave of his desires; then the slave of his ego ...Most people become slaves to natural demands, fashionable luxuries, social power, artificial religion or ideology, destiny, and most of all, psychological excuses. All kinds of unnecessary conflict will be brought about, aggravating turmoil and creating unprecedented calamity on a large scale ... "

(tr. Hua-Ching 1989, p. 201)

Perhaps we need a simpler approach, namely a recognition that what we do to others and to the environment, we do to ourselves. My hope is that we will be able to re-evaluate our lives and relationships with others.

[1] Travels and Adventures in Southern Africa, by George Thompson edited by Vernon, S. Forbes, with poems by Thomas Pringle. Thompson relates his journey to map out some of the interior of South Africa and was described by the Baralong as one "on whom the light of day might shine".

Acknowledgements

My thanks to Peter Turner who lives in Alice Springs for his mentoring and friendship since 1997 when we met in Alice Springs and for all the conversations[1] since the International Systems Sciences Conference in Brisbane entitled "Making Liveable, Sustainable Systems Unremarkable" (12–17th July, University of Queensland).

My thanks to Local Government for the funding that made this research possible and for the generous support by those who participated in the research, in particular David Hope, John Mugabushaka, Adib Muhammad Shomad and Bevin Wilson. My thanks also to the University of Indonesia for the opportunities over the years to develop a regional sense of the potential for overlapping biospheres that could be protected through local stewardship rather than through local exploitation.

I also acknowledge and thank Norma Romm for commenting on sections of this manuscript.

I thank Systems Research and Behavioural Science for allowing me to include sections of material published as two articles, entitled:

McIntyre-Mills, J and de Vries, D. 2012b. 'Transformation from Wall Street to Well-being' Syst. Research and Behavioural Science First published online: 10 Oct 2012 doi: 10.1002/sres.2133

I acknowledge that sections have been presented at the following conferences and that abstracts appear in the proceedings or on the conference websites:

McIntyre-Mills, J. 2013. Binchai, N and Hope, D. Engagement to address the policy and governance challenges of climate change mitigation. Local Government Researchers Forum, University of Adelaide, 7th July, abstract in conference proceedings.

McIntyre-Mills, J. with Binchai, N. 2013. 'Being, having, doing and interacting': towards ethical democracy, governance and stewardship International Systems Sciences Conference, 13–19th July Haiphong Paper, User Guide and abstract accepted and double blind refereed Conference website ISBN number 978-1-906740-11-5.

All photos in this publication were taken by this author.

[1] Conversations recorded on Sunday 20th and Sunday 27 Feb and Tuesday the 13th April which are the basis of this introduction.

This is the first of two volumes comprised of a series of essays that can be read separately and in any order or as chapters on a common theme, namely how should we live? The first aim is to explore ways to achieve wellbeing (whilst addressing the challenges for mitigation and adaptation to climate change). The second aim is to invite participation in sustainable and ethical governance. Read together the overlapping chapters deepen an understanding of governance, democracy and ethics applied to this area of concern. Read separately each chapter stands alone in developing an argument.The book strives to provide a resource to help address this concern by enabling current and future policy makers, managers and researchers to work across professional and organizational boundaries. Gibbons et al. (1994) argue that the ability to work across boundaries is vital for 'The new production of knowledge' and vital for *'the dynamics of research' to address current complex challenges.* A core capability will be to transcend disciplinary boundaries, synthesize diverse perspectives and critically analyse the role of science in public policy. The capabilities required to contribute effectively to the exploration and resolution of significant social and policy issues are vital (Increasingly those working at the interfaces of policy, science and society are turning to systemic participatory approaches and 'multiple methods' to address the challenges of complexity, integration, participation and improved communication in addressing issues that span disciplinary boundaries. Managers, policy makers, scientists and technologists have been drawn into increasingly visible policy struggles and debates on scientific interpretation, as well as moral, ethical, and value based uncertainties about the applications of new technologies).

Contents

About the Authors

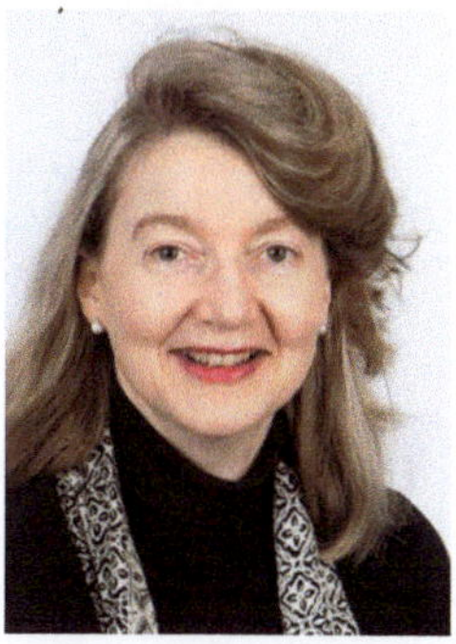

Janet McIntyre-Mills is an Associate Professor at Flinders University and an Adjunct Professor at the University of Indonesia. Her books address social and environmental justice concerns and include, for example: 'Global Citizenship and Social Movements', Harwood, McMillan, 'Critical Systemic Praxis for Social and Environmental Justice', Springer; 'Systemic Governance and Accountability: Working and Re-working the Conceptual and Spatial Boundaries', Springer; 'User Centric Policy Design to Address Complex Need's, Nova Science. Emergence has recently published 'Identity, Democracy and Sustainability'. It proposes a new architecture for governance.

Her research addresses wellbeing, consciousness and cosmopolitan ethics associated with the design and transformation of governance and democracy. It focuses on excessive social, economic and environmental consumption and suggests ways to mitigate the worst impacts of climate change through protecting cultural ecosystems. She is a board member of several journals, including the *Journal of Globalization Studies, Systems Research and Behavioural Science*, for example. She is an elected board member of Research Committee 10 on Participation and Organizational Transformation of the International Sociological Association, and has participated in Research Committee 51 of Socio-cybernetics. She is also a member of the International Systems Sciences and the Action Learning and Action Association.

Denise de Vries is a lecturer in the School of Computer Science Engineering and Mathematics at Flinders University. Her research interests focus on complex data modeling using methods, such as mesodata modeling, as well as other issues relevant to metadata modeling related to data mining, knowledge management, schema evolution and data semantics. De Vries developed this sophisticated software system to capture both tangible and non-tangible factors relating to complex social problems, which allows quantitative and qualitative analysis of information gathered. The interrelationships between issues as well as the perceived priorities are also acquired enabling informed decision making to take place.

Natasan Binchai is a Flinders University BSc graduate. Since early 2012 he has been the software developer for this Pathway to Wellbeing Project. He revised the user interface developed by Denise de Vries, expanded the database and helped to prepare the user guide and training video for the project.

Chapter 1
Introduction and Overview

Towards Ethical Democracy, Governance and Stewardship

1.1 Introduction: Being, Having, Doing and Interacting

The research project is based on previous research on social inclusion with First Australians (McIntyre-Mills 2010), in order to protect the global commons and the public good (Eder 1996).[1] The philosophy underpinning the approach grew out of the research in Alice Springs and in the Southern Region with Aboriginal Australians who stressed that 'we are the land'. Olive Veverbrants, an Arrernte Australian, stressed 'the earth is our mother' and we depend on it for our survival.

The weaving together of stories of what works and why shapes the approach. Participants are invited to reflect on their lives in terms of what they *already have* and what *they still need* in order to enhance their wellbeing. They are asked to consider what they would be prepared to add to their 'in baskets' and what they would be prepared to discard to their 'out baskets'. These are metaphors for thinking that were used to design the software—not just in the sense of managing our lives—but more poetically, they are Murray River grasses woven into baskets that symbolize our connections to one another and to the land. River grasses remove the salinity from the soil. They symbolize a renewable resource and a source of renewing.

[1] Initially, the concept of global commons was narrowly defined as 'assets outside the national frontiers such as oceans, space and the Antarctic' OECD definition http://stats.oecd.org/glossary/search.asp. Our area of concern is the extent to which resilience could be achieved through attitudinal and behavioural change fostered through participatory democracy and systemic governance that incorporates structured 'if then considerations' (Christakis and Bausch 2006, McIntyre-Mills and De Vries 2011) to develop clear priorities as to how to respond to contextual challenges (Ng 2011).The theme of global stewardship, democracy and governance frameworks to support wellbeing is addressed in this program of research by asking questions guided by a Design of Inquiring Systems (DIS; adapted from the work of West Churchman (1979, 1982) (McIntyre-Mills 2006a, b, c, 2010, McIntyre-Mills and De Vries 2011). The DIS refers to addressing an area of concern by 'unfolding' human values and 'sweeping in' contextual considerations and many domains of knowledge spanning logic, empiricism, idealism, the dialectic and pragmatism before making any decision.

J. McIntyre-Mills, *Transformation from Wall Street to Wellbeing*,
Contemporary Systems Thinking, DOI 10.1007/978-1-4899-7466-2_1,

The more we weave together strands of experience and respect the other—including the land—the more chance we have to achieve wellbeing.[2] This is the assumption of the project that builds on a previously funded ARC linkage project with the SA Dept. of Health and Neporendi to address complex needs by making better decisions to match services and to enhance wellbeing. It is also informed by the work of Thinker in Residence Susan Greenfield, a neuroscientist. The more we are able to 'join up the dots' by making more neural connections the more conscious or aware we become. The approach aims to make a contribution to the literature on ethics, kindness and a new architecture for governance and policymaking that is based on enhancing the capability of members of the public to think in terms of larger assemblages of ideas spanning many kinds of knowledge.

The plasticity of the brain is such that it shapes the environment and it in turn is shaped by the environment (Bateson 1972; Beer 1994; Greenfield 2000; Von Foerster 1995). The research addresses discourses, habits and a range of behaviours (Hogget 2010) shaping dualistic attitudes towards rights and responsibilities and the denial of responsibility for unsustainable consumerist culture.

The book makes a case for recognizing the need to contain capitalism. Our so-called containment anxiety cannot be addressed by living a schizophrenic existence where we see ourselves as benefitting at the expense of other people, the voiceless and future generations of life. Mamphela (2012) stresses the need for local conversations to weave together stories of forgiveness, resilience and hope that are based on what local people have to offer to one another, in order to develop their local communities.

Instead of assuming that people have nothing, each person should be asked to consider what they can offer. It may be a story of survival, time to help another with their household chores or some food that they are able to share with a neighbour. It may be sympathy, a greeting or encouragement. These local gifts of a material and non-material nature are the basis of building reciprocity.

Mamphela's community project resonates with the findings of the research approach practiced at Neporendi in South Australia. It is this philosophy that underpins the approach to wellbeing. The findings also resonate with the work of Stiglitz et al. (2010) whose book: *Mismeasuring Our Lives* stresses the need to value a web of factors that together provide the basis for a life worth living. Learning to save by not wasting resources could help people to be more generous to one another, and to be more generous to themselves, by allowing them time to connect with their surroundings.

The risk to personal health and to future generations of life is ignored by politicians, but also by the majority of research projects that do not 'join up the dots',

[2] This is the assumption of the project that builds on a previously funded ARC linkage project with the SA Dept. of Health and Neporendi to address complex needs by making better decisions to match services and to enhance wellbeing. It is also informed by the work of Baroness Professor Susan Greenfield, a neuroscientist who was South Australian 'Thinker in Residence' as part of the Premier's Dept. The more we are able to 'join up the dots' by making more neural connections the more conscious or aware we become. Human beings tend to engage in conflict to limit the size of territory.

because the terms of reference are defined too narrowly. By compartmentalizing our areas of concern to 'the social', the economic and the environmental, we cut up the fabric of life on which we depend. As a result, this approach to academic endeavour is complicit in placing our lives and the lives of future generations at risk.

All people need is to show leadership and to take time to build communities and to share their resources—time being one of the most valuable resources. This is difficult when people base their lives on the notion, 'time is money'.

The commodification of people, animals and the environment is at the heart of the problem. If humanity continues to ignore the value of the environment, if we lose species to pollinate plants, if the soil degrades as a result of monoculture and diverse organic matter, then we will face a grim future. The prospect of a Dubai-type urban landscape where the elites can afford to live in luxury in digitally controlled, secure gated communities and the rest live outside in the artificial environment in the desert or wastelands is already on the horizon—unless we re-consider how *we ought to live.*

The potential of vertical cities based on ensuring carbon-neutral lifestyles (powered by solar energy and reliant on recycling resources) is modelled (in part) by the Burj Khalifa towers. But the potential needs to be extended to prefigure sustainable, vertical agriculture (rather than pleasure gardens).

It builds on the work of cosmopolitans and stresses that we have responsibilities to others not only because we are now part of one global institution—as a result of the interconnectedness of the economy and our complicity in it—but also because our actions have an impact across space and time that cannot be limited to a single generation or nation state. The multilayered and multidimensional implications for democracy and governance are the starting point for this research.

Human rights underpin all relationships within the nation state and within the wider region. This has implications for social and environmental justice. Gro Brundtland (1989) and Mary Kaldor (in Held 2005, p. 177) have stressed that human security rests on creating a peaceful world, enshrined in rights expressed in the United Nations Charter (Article 55, 56) and in the constitution of the European Union. As stressed below (see McIntyre-Mills 2011), rising living costs led to food riots and the so-called Arab Spring, culminating in the Occupy Wall Street movement. Unfortunately, the human rights commissioner could not complete her term, because lobbyists complained about her support for Palestine.[3] Even though she was supported by Bishop Tutu, the wider lobby group did not support her.

The move towards re-membering and re-connecting with the land echoes the voices of Indigenous First national movements and the implications for the way we live, our relationships, our sense of identity and for new forms of governance and democracy.

The book suggests a way to decolonise our minds as a precursor to helping us to value others and the environment on which we depend.[4]

---

[3] Interview on One Plus One, ABC News. Accessed 6/01/2013.

[4] The ideas of Mathews (1991, 2010) and Rose Bird (1996, 2004) and Donna Haraway help to shape the agenda.

This has implications for the way in which we live and it has specific implications for democracy, governance and ethics.

According to Butler (2011):

> Occupations are about bodies; bodies "being" and bodies staying and claiming space and change. Self and collective selves are the site for protest; bodies create the material happening of public protest as a means to bring forward some kind of desired transformation.

The occupation of Wall Street along with the occupation of public spaces in Europe, Turkey, Egypt and the Ukraine, for example, are attempts to transform society. Butler (2011) goes on to say:

> 'This continual struggle for and claim over public space is accompanied by a struggle "over those basic ways in which we are, as bodies, supported in the world—a struggle against disenfranchisement, effacement, and abandonment" .... The body is political and it is guided by changing ideas and a consciousness about self and the world and "our" place in this world. The "occupation" of a limited number of spaces/bodies is changing our collective conversation about how we understand capitalism to work. "1 % of the population owns 60 % of the wealth...there is no sense in trying to live the American dream" (OWS 2011). The very clear realization that "the people are oppressed" became the front line of shaping the meaning of OWS.... But this lack of a "realistic message" is seen as mirroring the true nature of finance: "OWS is being portrayed as incoherent and Wall Street as coherent; there is nothing coherent about Wall Street since the firms of finance are often in conflict and have interests that are in conflict with each other (Facebook post 1 2011)...." (Žižek 2011)' (Cobbett and Germain 2012, p. 110).

We already have regional conflicts fuelled by energy shortages and competition for the last of the non-renewables. Satellite monitoring from above seems to be more of a priority at the moment by the USA than space travel. Digital communications are already widely used, but their potential is under-tapped (as a means to sustain wellbeing and ethics) as stressed in this chapter and other research on wellbeing, representation, accountability and sustainability (McIntyre-Mills and de Vries 2011).

- How can engagement be enhanced so that the Orwellian future is avoided?
- How can designs reframe technology in ways that (a) re-claim designs from below and (b) drive policy so that they inform the final decisions?
- How can elected leaders be held to account on the basis of the lived experiences of the electorate as well as by those who are so-called discipline experts?
- How can policy decisions be made by the elected representatives in ways that balance individual and collective interests—rather that the interests of elites. The challenge is that individualism has been taken too far as a result of the power associated with capital. It is possible that the low carbon footprint could be decreed from above as necessary for human survival, but that the elites will exempt themselves from the low carbon lifestyle. This could become increasingly likely if the media (print and digital) are owned by elites. This is why it is vital that cosmopolitan citizens hold elites to account.[5]

[5] Cosmopolitan rights and responsibilities have been stressed upon by David Held and Ulrich Beck who stress the 'boomerang effect' of poverty, pollution and a carbon-based economy on this

The argument builds on the liberative potential of Anna Florini's work in the *Coming New Democracy* on the way in which the Aarhus convention could be scaled up in post-national federations (see McIntyre-Mills 2011) that place human rights above citizenship rights. Nussbaum (2006) has stressed the need to consider the ethical rights of the voiceless young people, the disabled and the rights of all sentient creatures (who have the right to quality of life in which they can achieve their animal capabilities, just as human beings achieve their human animal capabilities) in her book *Beyond the Frontiers of Justice*.[6]

If national constitutions were 'imprinted with global social conditions' that 'stress the discourse of human rights' (Beck et al. 2012, p. 483), then the rights of asylum seekers, young people and sentients who are not protected as citizens could be addressed.

1.2 The Challenge of Poverty and Climate Change

The rationale for this book and its companion volume is that we face risks that could undermine quality of life and our capacity to achieve wellbeing, resilience and a sustainable future.

Droughts, floods and storm surges are regional concerns that affect human security. Many of these risks are the result of climate change. The challenge is to address ways to balance social, economic and environmental rights and responsibilities to this generation and the next. The research addresses the ethical challenge to think about the policy consequences for the majority in this generation and the next whose life chances are sacrificed by a sociopolitical system (and associated culture) that no longer supports a sustainable future.

The research creates, tests and discusses a stewardship process to enable a greater understanding of what Australians value, why and how it relates to their perceived sense of wellbeing and resilience to natural weather events associated with climate change.

The engagement process has the potential to manage consumption and to protect biodiversity, thereby promoting cultural transformation towards stewardship and an appreciation of our rights and our responsibilities to current and future generations.

The research tries to answer the question: What water, energy and food resources (amongst others) are consumed, why and how? An exploration of the perceived implications for wellbeing, resilience and the stewardship of biospheres are dis-

generation of life and the next. Sir Nicholas Stern has stressed that we need to make changes now to reframing economics.

[6] Hybridity and the potential of digital futures (Elliot 2010; Fukuyama 2002) pose some dangers. Policymakers also need to consider the ethical issues associated with human–machine and human–animal engineering (Greenfield 2003, 2008; Haraway 1991, 1992, 2010) as human beings become more reliant on biotechnology. Even more importantly, the implications for hybridisation would need to be addressed internationally as they impact human and environmental rights.

cussed. The research aims to enable policy to address the consequences in the short, medium and long term.

Climate change is a significant problem in Australia country. There is little doubt that accelerated climate change will adversely affect wellbeing and sustainability in Australia (Flannery 2005; Pretty 2013; Stiglitz et al. 2010)—particularly if we continue to consume at current rates (Davies and World Institute 2008)—resulting in devastation and profound implications for the life chances of many species. The impact of climate change has been underestimated (Lovelock 2009; Rockström et al. 2009) and local solutions have been overlooked. Aboriginal cultures teach us about stewardship and relationships with the land, but these relationships have been lost by many in non-Aboriginal cultures. As Major Sumner, a Ngarrindjeri Aboriginal elder from the periodically drought-ravaged lower Murray River in South Australia and custodian of the river stresses, *we are the land and the land is us*. Re-establishing relationships with the land is at the heart of effective ecosystem management (see http://www.mdba.gov.au/what-we-do/working-with-others/aboriginal-communities/ringbalin).

There is evidence that many non-Aboriginal people desire more environmentally sustainable lives, but little is known about the influences on choices around land, water and food that affect the environment. Government response to human wellbeing is often based on economic development, which inadvertently increases consumerism, resulting in greater environmental degradation.

We know that environmental sustainability and human wellbeing are intimately linked, but there is little knowledge about how this linkage can be built upon to improve both areas. Attempts to address climate change are often based on policy information that is not grounded in citizen experiences and fails to address what we do know about human behaviour or choices. How can we increase engagement in the environment that balances individual and collective wellbeing and simultaneously protects the environment when we know little about the vital nature of these connections?

Existential risk has implications for representation, accountability and sustainability. Consumption is very unequal and the gaps between rich and poor become wider and wider. The root cause of consumption is power without responsibility—so whoever comes to power needs to be held to account through mechanisms to main social, economic and environmental indicators that secure the 'wellbeing stocks' for the future.

The decisions taken at the local level on how we live have an impact on the way others live. So when personal decisions are made on what food, energy or water resources to use, why and how, it has public implications for others as well as the environment.

Thus, the research enables the development of a personal decision tree in response to basic scenarios linked with a scorecard to manage social, economic and environmental decisions. Wicked problems have many interrelated variables with diverse value dimensions. Developing responses to wicked problems involves enhancing our capability to work across disciplines and with many diverse interest groups. We will need to co-create shared narratives that recognize the areas of overlap.

Ethically, we will need to consider the consequences of our decisions for ourselves, others and the environment in this generation and the next. Sustainable futures rest on careful stewardship of the appropriate management of cultural ecosystems that support our wellbeing. Thus, economics needs to be reframed and supported by new forms of monitory democracy and governance.

This book makes the case that decisions need to be informed by connecting many kinds of knowledge and through appreciation of many ways of knowing. If people make conceptual connections through thinking through scenarios it could enable those of us who are not physicists to think about the big picture.

Our wellbeing depends on the wellbeing of the planet. Our home or sense of place is thus both local and global. The following definition of wellbeing is developed on the basis of research firstly in the Northern Territory with Aboriginal Australians and then in South Australia in the southern region of Adelaide on complex needs. The relevance of this definition is that the Northern Territory and South Australia are, respectively, one of the hottest and driest parts of Australia and thus most affected by climate change. Furthermore, sustainability thinking is now more relevant than ever for planetary wellbeing.

Most importantly it is relevant, because it is likely that the sorts of challenges faced by the poorest on the planet—are the sorts of conditions that humanity as a whole will face in the future—if we continue our addiction to consumption of resources. The Max Neef Human Sustainability Index (1991) *of being, having doing and interacting* shapes the design and analysis of the research and illustrates the need to be the change through rethinking the way in which we place human beings above our responsibility for the land. Our sense of identity as citizens of nation states needs to be transformed to take into account the needs of our neighbours and future generations of life.

This research explores the narratives on wellbeing and stories about how we ought to live, in order to develop a bridge between the thinking underpinning cosmopolitan ethics to the practice that needs to underpin cosmopolitan governance. The idea is to find ways to support greater awareness and willingness to live ethically and elegantly using cultural designs for living that support quality of life. The research spans the five core domains that have emerged from the research on:

- Home safety (personal safety—social indicators and physical indicators, physical safety of the home and environs)
- Physical and mental health (Wilkinson and Pickett 2009).
- Sense of purpose (indicators of satisfaction with employment).
- Connection/belonging to healthy community and healthy environment (people and land or place), and that this requires time to connect with others, including sentient beings.
- Self-respect and confidence to speak out. These are seen as overlapping needs which need to be addressed (McIntyre-Mills and De Vries 2008, p. 307).[7]

[7] This is currently under threat. The management of so-called introduced species', such as a fox, rabbit or cane toads (Taylor, 2013:113) needs to be conducted along humane lines if we are to

Empirical data on more than 300 pathways have been collected and analysed based on the themes that are indicative of wellbeing (https://wellbeing.csem.flinders.edu.au/).

The ex-head of the World Bank, Stiglitz (2010), along with his colleagues has adopted similar ideas based on his experiences in response to an invitation from Sarkozy to address the poverty, and global financial issues facing Europe. It recognizes the convergent social, economic and environmental challenges and the need to develop 'wellbeing stocks'.

Interestingly, the work of Stiglitz et al. (2011, p. 15) uses a multidimensional measure of wellbeing spanning:

> 1. Material living standards (income, consumption and wealth), 2. Health, 3. Education, 4. Personal activities including work, 5. Political voice and governance, 6. Social connections and relationships, 7. Environment (present and future conditions), 8. Insecurity, of an economy as well as a physical nature.

According to Stiglitz et al. (2010), the essence of the commission's findings is that wealth needs to include stocks for the future. The decisions taken at the local level on how we live have an impact on the way others live. So when personal decisions are made to use food, energy or water resources, it has public implications for others as well as the environment. Thus, the research enables the development of a personal scorecard to manage social, economic and environmental decisions. The cumulative, de-identified data provide the basis for making evidence-based policy to enable sustainable living.

1.3 Building Wellbeing Stocks for Future Generations of Life

The concept 'Wall Street' is used to symbolise economic rationalism and 'wellbeing' to symbolise a reframed approach to 'being interconnected' and through treading lightly. The software provides a way to enable people to explore the question, how should we live and what constitutes wellbeing? Participants are invited to consider what have, they need, what their turning points are for the better or the worse and what the barriers are. Services that help them meet their needs are detailed as well. The software updates as it is used.

The IPPC formula suggests that the privileged lives of some could lead to existential risk for people and the planet. The research responds to the possible

evolve into a more compassionate society. People want to spend more time exercising, working in gardens, walking, saving money through living simply and slowly, but many who strive for middle and upper middle class lives work long hours and cannot afford to take time out of work. The cost to their own physical and mental health, the environment and future generations is the subject of this book. The 'wounding of the spirit' (Ramphela 2012) is central as people strive to have more material resources, rather than being fully human through their relationships with others and the environment. The glossy life of luxury at the expense of the environment is unsustainable.

existential risks[8] (Bostrom 2011) posed by denial. This has implications for the way we live and the need to change our way of life through living sustainably.

Representation, accountability and sustainability challenges need to be met through addressing consumption choices that are currently very unequal. The gaps between rich and poor become wider and wider.

1.3.1 Addressing Complicity Through Subsidiarity, Sustainable Governance and Regionalism

To sum up, the research explores people's perceptions of what works why and how, but also strives to assess whether the process of engagement enables them to move from denial towards making changes towards a more sustainable future. The research also explores the viability of multilevel and multiagency approaches to support social and environmental justice.[9]

No community can be expected to transform from a high-carbon lifestyle (or aspiring to this lifestyle) without feeling part of the design process and owning the decisions as to how resources should be used.[10]

---

[8] Cultural values transformation rests on behavioural change prompted by laws. Just as laws for wearing seat belts and laws preventing smoking in public places have influenced behaviour and achieved public health outcomes, laws to fine people for parking in disabled parking bays raises awareness and leads to values transformation. Laws and rules can lead to values transformation as people learn to conform to laws that will uphold rights and responsibilities. Regional scorecards can be developed that respond to social, economic and environmental needs and to the rankings people achieve along a continuum from business as usual to small changes to living in ways that support wellbeing now and in the future. Sustainability cannot be allowed to fall under the limitations of competitive nation states. The sovereign nation state has treated the planet as zero sum—when in fact the notion of externalities is quite wrong. Kantian personal ethics, public ethics (interstate) and cosmopolitan ethics need to be applied in overlapping regions that override zero-sum approaches.

[9] A sustainable local community is determined by a sustainable region in which food, energy and water supplies are considered as major determinants for wellbeing. Rights to consume need to be balanced by responsibility to consume in ways that impact the life chances of others (including future generations of life). Thus, the rule of law needs to be post national and global supported by a covenant to protect all life. This needs to be secured by overlapping federations of biospheres buttressed in law and supported by a judicial system. Hence, the axiom for expanding pragmatism—human beings the can be free and diverse to the extent that our freedom and diversity do not undermine the rights of others or future generations of life.

[10] The root cause of consumption is power without responsibility—so whoever comes to power needs to be held to account through mechanisms to develop social, economic and environmental indicators that secure the wellbeing stocks for the future. This research emphasizes the creation of multiple paths to form webs to wellbeing through critical, systemic engagement to ensure that local people get to know about local resources (that are listed in directories created by both service users and providers) and that their identity is protected. They are able to see the typical scenarios of what people have, need, are prepared to add or discard from their lives and what they think are turning points for the better and worse.

1.3.2 Wellbeing and Relationships Underpin Systemic Approaches to Economics

The ability to make and re-make connections in the brain—neurogenesis—has been raised by Baroness Professor Susan Greenfield (2000, 2008). Thinking in small compartments and stress stunts creativity.[11] But more importantly, it could leave us disadvantaged in the evolutionary stakes. This book responds to the research by Greenfield that stresses the plasticity of the human brain and its ability to respond systemically and creatively to challenges. The *will to change* is the stumbling block.

Wellbeing requires seeing ourselves as one of many species in biospheres. This has implications for identity, ethics and governance. Nation states face social, economic and environmental challenges. Protecting the global commons at the local and regional level is the focus of an ongoing research program in public policy and public administration, which has implications for education and the transformation of organizations spanning the state, market and nongovernment. The fact that this planet is overpopulated and that the minority live at the expense of the minority is the elephant in the room. The fact that the planet's population is mostly located in urban areas requires urgent cultural transformation to address food security.

Cities need to become green and green areas should not be urbanized. Innovative buildings could become food producers. Rooftops and walls could be terraces for food.

Mitigation policies that address rights and responsibilities in all areas of life need to help us limit overconsumption at the personal, local, state, national and international level whilst adaption politics need to enable us to deal with the consequences of overconsumptions through enabling them to consider the implications of different scenarios.

The book makes the case that to address existential risk we need to (a) rethink our values and our relationships with others and the environment and (b) reframe the state, market and civil society by extending the social contract to include biospheres, so that food security for current and future generations can be protected. This requires identifying with and co-operating with others, rather than merely competing with others, based on the zero-sum/us–them approach. It makes a case

---

[11] We need to be mindful of Arthur Koestler's comment (1978) that we have created a sick civilization. Koestler (1967) developed an argument in 'Ghost in the Machine', that human evolution of the brain has retained the basic drives which override reason. So emotion and desire for power can lead to irrational decisions. '…evolution superimposed a new superior structure onto an old one, with purely overlapping functions, and without providing the new with a clear-cut, hierarchic control over the old- thus inviting confusion and conflict…. The limbic system may be compared to a primitive television screen which combines, and often confuses, projections from the internal, visceral environment with the external environment…But Nature in her frugality did not discard the old screen. Since it seemed adequate for smelling, tasting and feeling what is going on inside the body, she has kept the filaments in the tube of the old screen glowing night and day…' (Koestler 1967, p. 283).

for engagement to help people to consider the potential consequences of their choices. These approaches span narrative (to explore complexity and to enable a creative flow of ideas), dialogue and questioning to reformulate boundaries. Scenarios were also explored spanning 'business as usual', 'small steps towards a sustainable future' and achieving a sustainable future through building up 'wellbeing stocks' (Stiglitz et al. 2010).

Wellbeing today does not need to cost the planet. So many people say that they want to be the change, but how can we achieve monitory democracy?

The book develops an argument for developing new cosmopolitan approaches for systemic governance and democracy. The cosmopolitan age is based on caring for others. It requires the private world of caring within the household or the home and extending solidarity outwards to the community. It requires choosing appropriate responses to addressing problems and more than a critical ability—it requires an ability to think in terms of responses to areas of concern. The building of solidarity and networks needs to be local in the first instance and then scaled up progressively. The concerns raised by naysayers that the carbon-controlled nightmare of big brother dictating carbon allowances needs to be closely unpacked.

We do not need to polarize 'tribal trading' versus 'regional warlordism' as suggested by Urry (2007, p. 289) in a chapter entitled 'Systems and Dark Futures'. It is possible to enlarge our capacity to understand through engagement and through a range of monitory approaches that enable cosmopolitan global citizens to have a say: the notion that the female domain is local and the male domain is global.

Compassion on a global scale needs to draw on the principle of subsidiarity—in which each local group has an effect on local decisions and are free to make decisions to the extent that they do not undermine the rights of others or the environment or the next generation of life. This participatory approach extends humanist ethics to caring for the environment.

The problem with the Western enlightenment thinking is that it identified ethics with human rights—whilst forgetting that human rights are in turn determined by our relationships with others. So although we do not want to lose our capacity to care compassionately for others—we do need to find ways to moderate our human passions—shaped by 'religion, morality politics and aesthetics' (West Churchman 1979). These values comprise the so-called enemies within, which West Churchman stresses need to be carefully examined.

We can do this by learning to think about our thinking and learning that emotions and values prompt us to be human—which includes both passionate and compassionate behaviour. The point is that a scorecard approach is only a starting point for 'being the change'. We need to be able to shape the thinking system to reflect the diverse viewpoints of a range of participants.

The elegance of the design is that people are able (in real time and on a regular basis) to update how they feel about social, economic and environmental dimensions of their lives. These dimensions are seen as overlapping and not mutually exclusive. Furthermore, those who do not like computers (I include myself in this category) are able to engage in other ways—such as through narrative and telling others who can load their ideas directly onto the web for them.

According to data cited from World Bank,[12] 3 billion people live on US$ 2.50 per day. The will to make a difference is the challenge.[13]

The Sydney Peace Prize winner Vandana Shiva[14] sums up the challenge for this century as one of preventing the commodification of life. Multinational companies and the WTO have made it possible to patent the conditions of life thereby causing almost a quarter of a million suicides by Indian farmers who cannot afford to purchase the seeds and the pesticides that are needed (despite the claims by the manufacturers). Furthermore, the attempt to criminalize farmers who store old varieties of seed could lead to very vulnerable monocultures of foods. The idea that the very basis for life—seeds and genes can be patented is part of the process of commodifying people, animals and the fabric of life.

The open democracy forum was the starting point for research in response to David Held's proposal that the core challenge of the day is to address the vast differences in standard of living between rich and poor through reforming world trade and using the market to address global warming by means of a global covenant that prevents unilateral interventions. In response to his critics, he claims that the resources exist for a reformed United Nations (UN) to make a difference, if there was a will. The UN according to Scruton (2005, pp. 47–48) is corrupt, the bureaucrats are overpaid and he argues that national sovereignty is the only way to make a difference through controlling corruption.[15]

[12] http://www.globalissues.org/article/26/poverty-facts-and-stats#fact2.

[13] Held, 2005: (33–34): 'We may lack the will but it cannot be said that we lack the means. A few telling examples make the point. The UN budget is $ 1.25 billion plus the necessary finance for peace keeping per annum. Against this, US citizens spend over $ 8 billion per annum on cosmetics, 27 billion per annum on confectionery, 70 billion per annum on alcohol and over 560 billion per annum on cars…. Or take the European Union: its citizens spend 11 billion per annum on ice cream 150 billion on cigarettes and alcohol; while the EU and the US together spend over 17 billion per annum on pet food…What do we require to make a substantial difference to the basic wellbeing of the world's poorest? Again the statistics are available. Required would be 6 billion per annum on basic education, 9 billion per annum for water and sanitation, 12 billion per annum for the reproductive health of women, 13 billion per annum for basic health nutrition…These figures are substantial, but when judged against the major consumption expenditure in the US and EU they are not beyond our reach. Moreover if all the OECD agricultural subsidies were removed and spent on the world's poorest peoples this would release some 300 billion per annum…. In addition a small shift between military and aid budgets- 900 billion and 50 billion a year globally would make a marked difference to the human security agenda….'

[14] http://www.youtube.com/watch?v=UOfM7QD7-kk.
http://www.navdanya.org/news/229-awesome.
http://www.vandanashiva.org/

[15] But the challenges facing nation states go beyond what nation states can do on their own. This is why a 'new sword' is needed according to Barber (2005, p. 97) and that this needs to be based on social networks, not just a new world order. Bond agrees arguing more social movements from below are needed, as a result of his experience with the trade union movement in South Africa. He stresses that the TRIPS laws were only addressed in SA through marches and not by the state.

The market failures Held anticipated fall short of what has actually occurred. The problem is not only concerning externalities that are not factored into calculations of the degradation to the environment, it also involves shifting the extraction of profit to where labour is cheaper and where governments and citizens are less likely to complain about degradation of environment and short-term profits at the expense of future generations. This undermines—not only the conditions of employment so that full-time employment becomes less available—but also the very fabric of life on which all economic development depends. This is aided by the lack of control of the market and the movement funds (see McIntyre-Mills and De Vries 2011).

Ironically, Aarhus (Denmark)—despite being the place where the convention on local participation and freedom of information was framed—has become a site for right-wing groups to organize in the wake of the Toulouse shootings by Mohamed Merah (ABC news 1 April, 2012, 7pm TV news) in France. It illustrates the point made by Anthony Giddens (2009) and David Held (2005) that social networks do not always support social or environmental justice.[16] We need to find ways to balance individual and collective needs in increasingly diverse nation states.

The book explores some of the issues discussed above and addresses the hypothesis: The greater the level of participation at a local level in discussing the policy and governance implications of our food, water and energy use, the greater the level of understanding of our responsibility to others to use, reuse and manage these resources sustainably and the greater the level of our wellbeing and resilience outcomes.[17]

Desai (London School of Economics) argues for post-statist social democracy based on governance from below, based on the: 'erosion of state sovereignty and the strengthening of human rights independently of nation states. The days when statism was any sort of answer to humanity's problems are past. Certainly not global statism!' (Desai 2005, p. 69).

[16] Malley, N. 2012 One fatal shot echoes across a divided US *The Saturday Age March 31.* More or less at the same time, a Brazilian was tasered in Australia and a young black man was shot in America by a white neighbourhood watch patroller. Zimmerman was white, the boy was black. Obama spoke out about this saying his own child would look like this child. Republicans say this is not the point.

[17] Resilience is defined as the adaptive capacity of the physical environment, of an individual or of a group. It concerns factors such as the capacity of members of a community to act together and to be able to modify or even transform existing ways of life (Rose 2005; Hulme 2009) and thus personal, community or regional resilience, measured by a human sustainability footprint that will be developed based on an adaptation of the Max Neef (1991) Human Sustainability Scale, the Tuvalu test (Murray et al. 2007) and West Churchman's (1971) Design of Inquiring Systems Approach that strives to enrich the testing of ideas through 'sweeping in' variables and 'unfolding the values' of diverse stakeholders. Arendt (1963) criticized the systems approach for imposing change through simplistic scenarios that pose a false dichotomy or an oversimplification of options and then encourages a compromise. Whilst the criticism is apt for closed systems and operations research, it does not apply to the work of critical heuristics or systemic intervention (Midgley 2000) that builds on the critical tradition of the Frankfurt School.

Chapter 2
Vulnerability and Risk: Towards Stewardship of a Post-Carbon Economy

2.1 Participatory Democracy and Governance to Mitigate and Adapt to Climate Change

The research aims to establish if it is possible for cultural transformation to enable a shift from denial to ambivalence to sustainable cosmopolitanism.[1] It strives to

[1] *Firstly,* the aim is to develop a participatory democracy and governance cybernetics approach to support sustainable approaches to living well in geographically and socially diverse communities and contribute to developing the research capability on democracy, governance and sustainability in Australia. The research will provide greater insight of how diverse residents perceive their rights and responsibilities to mitigate the causes of climate change and adapt to the effects. *Secondly,* the research aims to discover whether participation enhances awareness of the need to live sustainably and whether this translates into measurable social changes indicated by the resilience scorecard based on the West Churchman's design of inquiring systems approach and an adapted form of Max–Neef's Human Sustainability Index. *Thirdly,* we will find out how socio-demographic, cultural characteristics and geographic location impact on consumer decisions about the way they live. It addresses the question of how to 'reconcile universalistic principles of human rights, autonomy, and freedom' with our identity 'as members of certain human communities divided by language, ethnicity or religion' (Benhabib 2007). It explores the extent to which cultural stewardship and concern for future generations plays a role in the way people choose to live and the extent that engagement leads to greater understanding of sustainable living, wellbeing and resilience. *Thirdly,* we explore which forms of engagement are most likely to have an impact on decision making and to what extent participants change their attitudes as a result of engaging with others and thinking about the consequences of their choices. The results based on measures are adapted from the Max–Neef Human Scale Sustainability Index (1991). It details: (a) what kinds of interactive processes help residents to think through the consumption choices they would like to make at the local level and the implications in terms of costs (social, economic and environmental); (b) the relevance of participation for rights and responsibilities; (c) an appreciation of an extended sense of space and time; and (d) the implications for consumption, policy and administration. These qualitative and quantitative data could provide valuable evidence for policy and planning on what works, why and how in order to enhance the wellbeing, sustainability and resilience of local communities. It will contribute to the theory on democratic engagement and how to address sustainable living through governance. It is always necessary to have standards and monitoring of standards. But what should these standards be? Excellence needs to be measured in terms of wellbeing and sustainability, not the economic bottom line. So whilst I applaud these efforts, I think we need to find ways to build

J. McIntyre-Mills, *Transformation from Wall Street to Wellbeing,*
Contemporary Systems Thinking, DOI 10.1007/978-1-4899-7466-2_2,

enable a greater awareness of consciousness of our rights and responsibilities as global citizens.[2]

This chapter discusses a participatory action research project in a place I will call 'Middleville' in South Australia.[3] The chapter aims to:

- Address the challenge posed by Stiglitz (2010) to the Australian Productivity Commission, namely to foster an understanding that the wellbeing of humanity is dependent on the global commons. It makes the case that an Orwellian future of digital top-down controls or a breakdown of essential services in ungoverned regions is already a reality that needs to be controlled and reversed through balancing individual and collective needs.
- Explore the potential for participatory democracy and governance to (a) monitor, (b) match services to need and (c) blow the whistle on injustice. It makes the case that the following are amongst the greatest challenges facing humanity and that they potentially pose an 'existential risk': (a) representation of the increasingly diverse populations within nation states; (b) accountability to ensure that resources are used fairly and equitably and sustainably and (c) engagement to enhance the capability of people to understand that attitudes towards consumption have profound implications for social and environmental justice issues. The area

---

in ongoing evaluation to environmental concerns, and not the market. According to Stiglitz et al. (2011, p 15), building 'wellbeing stocks' for the future requires reframing our thinking, practice and our relationships to one another and the land.

[2] It is practical in that it attempts to acknowledge that localized, slow lives that are sustainable could lapse into the Orwellian nightmare of control from above—without surveillance from below to hold the elites to account. It is for this reason that the future needs to be shaped not only by the state military complex but also by members of the public—protected by a scaled-up version of the Aarhus Convention that gives residents within post-national regions the right to access information and the right to be heard by the state (1998, see McIntyre-Mills 2011).

[3] The research has been funded by the Centre for Research into Aboriginal Health (CRCAH) Australian Local Government Association and is currently in progress (McIntyre-Mills and de Vries 2011). The transdisciplinary team comprises: Janet McIntyre (Social and Policy studies) to conceptualise and implement the project with Dr. Denise de Vries (Informatics, Flinders University) with the assistance of Sun Binchai (Hons. graduate, Informatics, Flinders University), Ivantia Mokoginta (PhD student, Economics and Public Policy), Adib Mohamned Shomad (PhD student, Public policy and management), Barbara Dickson (MA student, Public Policy and engagement specialist for an urban renewal department, public sector, Adelaide), Dr. John Mugabushaka (PhD student and public policy and youth justice officer, public sector, Adelaide) and David Hope (accountant and risk management consultant for local government). Details can be found at: and an earlier version at http://www.socsci.flinders.edu.au/av/pathways/binder.php. Application for local government: https://socsci.flinders.edu.au/fippm/pathways_lg/. https://wellbeing.csem.flinders.edu.au/. The log in is user name=test, code=test.

The chapter needs to acknowledge the following publications on this research: McIntyre-Mills and De Vries, 2012, *Wellbeing and existential risk: engagement to address the policy and governance challenges of mitigation and accountability*, McIntyre, J. (School of Social and Policy Studies, Flinders University, janet.mcintyre@flinders.edu.au presenting author, De Vries, D. (Computer Science, Engineering and informatics, Flinders University, denise.devries@flinders.edu.au, paper delivered at CASS Research Conference *Sustainable Environmental Policy and Global Governance*, Beijing, China, 18–19 September 2012 and submitted to the journal of convergence, China Permission to publish UKSS paper.

of concern is to take into account social, economic and environmental factors that make a difference to wellbeing and our ability to mitigate or adapt to climate change and to develop climate change policy and actions, using a participatory process with local residents to inform policy makers and service providers.

The research on representation, accountability and engagement strives to prefigure[4] another way to engage the public to adapt to and mitigate the extent of the risks posed by climate change. The research tests the principle of subsidiarity and Ashby's rule of requisite variety (1956) to establish ways to enhance representation, accountability and engagement.

In the resource-rich cities of the world, mobile people spend their time rushing from one appointment to another. They use mobile technology in ways that can make life frenetic. But digital technology could be used in different ways—not to constantly reschedule meetings but to enable life to be lived at a slower pace. It can be used to enable people to think about alternative ways of living and to 'join up the dots'. The containment of anxiety has been stressed as one of the main reasons for using digital technology by many very mobile workers. Containment anxiety is felt increasingly by overwrought people living very fast-paced lives (Elliot 2010, p 21) and so digital technology tends to be used to address isolation and rescheduling—but it can be used for transformation. The chapter suggests a different way of using technology, in order to support being rooted in one particular place. Mobility is greater than it has ever been in the past. Powerful decision makers live lives that are mobile and information rich, because they have wide networks. The current research with a local community in South Australia indicates an increasing awareness of the need to live sustainably.

The mobile hunter-gatherer is as normal as the localized cultivator of the earth in human history. Archaeological history and anthropology have also demonstrated that food security is not achieved only by the hunter-gatherers (who forage beyond the immediate neighbourhood) but also through localized agriculture, that needs to be sustainable, or it will lead to the sort of collapse that occurred at Chichen Itza, Mexico, or on Easter Island. Living locally and eating locally could become the norm in the event of a collapse in the carbon economy and rising costs, but it will need the careful governance of resources.

It is likely that a greater balance will need to be achieved between individual and collective needs through emphasizing the determinants of wellbeing for this generation and the next. This requires a new approach to public education, democracy, governance and ethics that places food security at the centre of decisions. The role of local participation and governance thus becomes increasingly important. Our research strives to enable people to have a say about how scarce resources should be used, in order to inform elected representatives of their perceived social, economic and environmental needs.

It is hoped that by thinking about what they have and what they need and what they are prepared to change (by being prompted to consider the consequences of

[4] Thus, its emphasis is not merely to describe what the case is, but to design alternative praxis as a seed for transformation.

their choices for others and for the environment) thinking and practice will support local socio-environmental systems.[5] The notion of engagement in 'if-then scenarios' is helpful to enable people to develop sustainable social, economic and environmental decisions (McIntyre-Mills and De Vries 2011).

Local government is able to address policy and governance based on an analysis of their perceptions and choices. By considering the implications of three scenarios, the users of the interactive software program are inspired to think about social, economic and environmental choices. The scenarios range from 'business as usual' to 'small adjustments to green economies' to 'sustainability and wellbeing'.

The aim is to enhance their awareness and to help local government decision makers to understand the needs and perceptions of local voters. The software is populated by data on services that are available to enable greener choices. Thus, it aims to help with raising consciousness which can provide a step towards the creation of a new suburban culture.[6]

A digital future need not be Orwellian, based on skyscrapers such as the tallest building in the world in Dubai, controlled through digital means and top-down controls.[7] It could instead be based on a form of participatory democracy and governance aimed at balancing individual and collective needs (McIntyre-Mills and De Vries 2011). Local community resilience could be enhanced through engaging

---

[5] This research emphasizes the creation of multiple paths to form webs to wellbeing through critical, systemic engagement to ensure that local people get to know about local resources (that are listed in directories created by both service users and providers) and that their identity is protected. They are able to see the typical scenarios of what people have, need, are prepared to add or discard from their lives and what they think are turning points for better or worse. A sustainable local community is determined by a sustainable region in which food, energy and water supplies are considered as major determinants for wellbeing. No community can be expected to transform from a high-carbon lifestyle (or aspiring to this lifestyle) without feeling part of the design process and owning the decisions as to how resources should be used. The exercise of 'thinking about their thinking' is an attempt to build new neural pathways in the mind—to rehearse a different way of 'being in the world', based on thinking about the consequences for themselves, others and the environment.

[6] This research explores people's perceptions of what works why and how, but also assesses whether the process of engagement enables them to move from denial towards making changes towards a more sustainable future. Contradictions need to be identified and addressed by policy (supported by legal frameworks) at the local, national and post-national regional level to achieve transformation. The challenge is to enable people to become aware of the need for a cultural shift from a large carbon footprint created by 'business as usual' and to move towards making logical steps towards sustainable living, rather than making confused gestures at best, or making contradictory decisions in personal and public lives. But the point that is made in 'Identity, Democracy and Sustainability' (2011) is that a legal bipartisan agreement between the major emitters—USA, China and India—is vital. Good faith needs to be demonstrated by local networks that prefigure change on the ground and that link up with global networks, such as 350.org to make a change. '350.org is an international campaign dedicated to building a movement to unite the world around solutions to the climate crisis–the solutions that science and justice demand.www.350.org/en/node/3108', accessed 27/05/2012. Other social movements such as Avaaz or open democracy are examples of other online movements that can ask for responses, such as the following: 'We urge you to save the Earth Summit and the planet by delivering a real deal to end fossil fuel subsidies.'

[7] http://www.dubai-architecture.info/DUB-004.htm.

with people to decide on how scarce resources should be used, in order to avert a breakdown in governance and democracy.[8] Furthermore, monitory democracy and governance becomes increasingly relevant for adaptation to climate change, in order to mitigate the effects (greater extremes in temperatures, water shortages in droughts, inundations during floods or storm surges and greater risk of bush fires in summer). All these risks will become increasingly frequent. Wellbeing—not the economic bottom line—needs to be the focus of our attention for cultural transformation, according to Stiglitz et al. (2010). But this requires reconceptualising culture.

Wellbeing rests on mindfulness of our relationships with others and with the environment, not on status or ability to live 'high-carbon lifestyles' of our own choosing that are epitomized by mobility[9] for pleasure, maintaining family connections or for work purposes (Elliot 2012).

Our research (McIntyre-Mills and De Vries 2010, 2011) explores whether we can change the architecture of engagement to enable more inclusive and creative designs that balance individual and collective needs through participation—based

[8] Monitory democracy (Keane 2009) will need to support post-national governance (McIntyre-Mills 2012, in press). The aim is to pilot this approach at a local level and then to test it out at a subnational regional level and at a post-national regional level. A 'small is beautiful' (Schumacher 1973), post-carbon future in which energy alternatives are still at an early stage of redevelopment (sun-, wind- and ocean-powered tidal systems) may be a likely future. For this reason learning to live sustainably in smaller, slower and more localized communities could be an important way to adapt to climate change.

[9] Mobility that is enforced could become greater as a result of increased regional conflict as a result of resource scarcity, disaster or climate change. Whilst there is resistance to this scenario at the moment whilst many live according to the principles of conspicuous consumption, because carbon-based lives are still within the reach of the middle classes, it is likely that this will be increasingly the preserve of the super-rich elites. The monitoring of scarce resources will become increasingly important for the democracy project, in order to ensure that cynicism and distrust does not alienate electorates. This requires many kinds of engagement—ranging from face-to-face focus groups to community agoras with an 'online' link to regional parliaments. This could enable all those who live within a region to voice their opinions. Giving 'a voice to the mob' is regarded as fraught by liberals and neo-liberals—not only because majorities do not always uphold social and environmental justice but also because the current status quo could be overturned! But in a post-consumerist world, wealth would need to be re-evaluated and reconceptualised, because, to draw on, adapt and apply Einstein's well-known aphorism: We cannot solve the economic and environmental problems of today with the same ideas of *property and consumption* that created the problem of an *unsustainable* way of life. But to enable freedom of thought in science and democratic testing out of ideas requires a democratic state—but the problem is that the nation state has not acted in the interests of freedom and democracy as Keane (2009a, b) points out. Emotions run high as resources run out, but it is pointless to polarize emotional and rationalist responses to climate change. Our capability as human beings to think about our thinking requires reflexivity. The more we are able to think about our emotions and the emotions of others, the more likely we are to make decisions that are rational. At times of high risk, this becomes increasingly important for policy makers. The subjective, objective and intersubjective domains of knowledge are vital, and as Habermas has stressed it is the latter that require the most work in policy making. Reflexivity is both emotional and rational (see Holmes 2010).The recognition of the symbolic meanings people attribute to ideas needs to be given attention (Collins 2008, 2010). Human agency to respond to rising temperatures cannot be avoided and will require rational responses that take into account diverse emotions—particularly the outrage of the disenfranchised.

on the axiom that we can be free and diverse to the extent that freedom and diversity does not undermine the rights of others?

What does this mean for constructing and reconstructing the way in which we live?

As we face convergent social, economic and environmental challenges, complex, wicked choices are posed; these are changing society, changing the environment and changing ourselves. Social engineering has stared into the abyss of totalitarianist control and free market capitalism.

We face climate change challenges and market failure as starving people protest. The potential for adaptation to climate change poses suggestions that bioengineering and speciation that includes a post-human future has been raised and set aside as a choice that ought not to be made, even if it can be made (Fukuyama 2002, p 218). Liberal democracy as it is currently framed is considered better, by Fukuyama, because it protects our 'human essence', but the 'hopes, fears and struggles' of those who live wretched lives of exploitation are not necessarily understood by those who live privileged lives.

The research also explores whether face-to-face engagement processes as well as a computer-aided engagement could enhance data collection, analysis and ongoing awareness of complex social, economic and environmental issues associated with climate change.

The software is loaded onto the Flinders Website,[10] in the first instance, but has the potential for links with local governments elsewhere at a sub- and post-national level within the region.

Part of the rationale for trialling the software was to establish to what extent computing per se is a useful way to engage different interest groups and whether it could be useful to enable managing large, diverse data sets spanning many diverse interrelated variables about which residents have strong values. A diverse range of values, emotions and opinions are associated with wellbeing, quality of life and climate change. These can be regarded as a wicked problem, in the sense that it has many, diverse and interrelated variables that are viewed differently by people with different values (see the West Churchman Series 2006).

The process aims to enable people to think through the 'if-then' scenarios, not merely to 'unfreeze' habitual praxis (to cite Lewin's concept), but to work towards sustainable praxis, based on an understanding of our interrelatedness. This requires

[10] Until broadband is made widely available, the software will run less effectively at peak hours. Participation is thus effected by the lack of broadband. This point was made strongly by the Thinker in Residence, Genevieve Bell (2009), who was invited to review the potential for ICTs in South Australia in her report 'Getting connected, Staying Connected, Exploring South Australia's digital futures.' Another challenge was the migration of data from one part of the server to another and the right to obtain access to log into the data systems by both users and administrators. The next hurdle will be to link the Flinders website to the Local Government Association (LGA) website. It is currently linked as a demonstration to the ISA wiki site and also to Abdushomad Muhammad's website. As a senior public servant in the Ministry of Religion in Indonesia and my PhD student at Flinders University, he is well placed to assist.

ongoing changes to learning (Schein 1996), 'habitus' (Bourdieu 1977) or ways of 'being in the world' (Haraway 1991, 1992, 2010).

Local government is able to address policy and governance based on a study of the participant's perceptions and choices. By considering the implications of three scenarios, the users of the interactive software program are inspired to think about social, economic and environmental choices.

The scenarios range from 'business as usual' to 'small adjustments to green economies' to 'sustainability and wellbeing'. The aim is to enhance their awareness and to help local government decision makers to understand the needs and perceptions of local voters. The software is populated by data on services that are available to enable greener choices. The challenge is to enable people to become aware of the need for a cultural shift from a large carbon footprint created by 'business as usual' and to move towards making logical steps towards sustainable living, rather than making confused gestures at best, or making contradictory decisions in personal and public lives.[11] But the point that is made in 'Identity, Democracy and Sustainability' (2011) is that a legal bipartisan agreement across the major emitters—USA, China and India—is vital. Good faith needs to be demonstrated by local networks that prefigure change on the ground and that link up with global networks, such as 350. org to make a change.[12] A digital future need not be Orwellian.[13] It could instead be based on a form of participatory democracy and governance aimed at balancing individual and collective needs (McIntyre-Mills and De Vries 2011). Monitory democracy (Keane 2009) will need to support post-national governance (McIntyre-Mills 2012, in press).

The aim is to pilot this approach at a local level and then to test it out at a sub-national regional level and at a post-national regional level. A 'small is beautiful' (Schumacher 1973), post-carbon future in which energy alternatives are still at an early stage of redevelopment (sun, wind, and ocean powered tidal systems) may be a likely future. For this reason, learning to live sustainably in smaller, slower and more localized communities could be an important way to adapt to climate change. Local community resilience could be enhanced through engaging with people to decide on how scarce resources should be used, in order to avert a breakdown in governance and democracy. Furthermore, monitory democracy and governance

[11] Thus, it aims to help with raising consciousness which can provide a step towards the creation of a new suburban culture. The aim of this research is to explore people's perceptions of what works, why and how, but also to assess whether the process of engagement enables them to move from denial towards making changes towards a more sustainable future. Contradictions need to be identified and addressed by policy (supported by legal frameworks) at the local, national and post-national regional level to achieve transformation.

[12] '350.org is an international campaign dedicated to building a movement to unite the world around solutions to the climate crisis—the solutions that science and justice demand.www.350. org/en/node/3108', accessed 27/05/2012. Other social movements such as Avaaz or open democracy are examples of other online movements that can ask for responses, such as the following: 'We urge you to save the Earth Summit and the planet by delivering a real deal to end fossil fuel subsidies.'

[13] http://www.dubai-architecture.info/DUB-004.htm.

becomes increasingly relevant for adaptation to climate change, in order to mitigate the effects (greater extremes in temperatures, water shortages in droughts, inundations during floods or storm surges and greater risk of bush fires in summer). All these risks will become increasingly frequent.

Wellbeing—not the economic bottom line—needs to be the focus of our attention for cultural transformation, according to Stiglitz et al. (2010). But this requires reconceptualising culture. Participants are asked to think about their quality of life in terms of health, housing, employment, education and social inclusion within their communities and what they are prepared to change in terms of their thinking and practice, in order to adapt to the effects and to strive to address the causes through mitigation. The monitory democracy and governance scorecard does not merely rank the outcome of indicators in terms of business as usual, small changes and sustainable futures. It provides weightings of each of the individual choices and invites participants to consider the consequences of their choices.

The aim is to establish if it is possible for cultural transformation to enable a shift from denial to ambivalence to sustainable cosmopolitanism. It strives to enable a greater awareness of consciousness of our rights and responsibilities as global citizens. It is practical in that it attempts to acknowledge that localized, slow lives that are sustainable could lapse into the Orwellian nightmare of control from above—without surveillance from below to hold the elites to account. It is for this reason that the future needs to be shaped not only by the state military complex—but by those who wish to act as whistleblowers. Members of the public need to be protected by a scaled-up version of the Aarhus Convention that gives residents within post-national regions the right to access information and to the right to be heard by the state (1998; see McIntyre-Mills 2011); thus, this section: (a) discusses the theory of participatory democracy—based on the principles of subsidiarity and Ashby's rule of requisite variety—and (b) makes a case for new forms of accountability to support regional governance that is capable of extending the social contract beyond the nation state and thus to protect biospheres and the diversity within them. The governance decisions will need to be upheld by rule of law based on the axiom that we can be free and diverse to the extent that freedom and democracy is not undermined (McIntyre-Mills et al. 2006). The program of research makes the case for:

- Systemic matching of governance options in context through a range of engagement processes
- Social change to address wellbeing not merely being about productivity for profit
- Transdisciplinarity and a reframed approach to wellbeing

The 'small is beautiful' philosophy of Schumacher resonates with the notion of caretaking stressed by Aboriginal Australians. The conundrum I address is how to combine localism with a concern for the global commons. The case is made for scaling up subsidiarity, so that local people make local decisions within overlapping regional biospheres. As populations increase in size, compete for scarce resources and emphasize 'time is money' in a fast carbon-based economy, we are at risk of forgetting our dependency on the land.

2.2 Local Governance Process to Address Perceptions and Choices

The research is a practical attempt to develop an architecture for participatory democracy and governance guided by the axiom that wellbeing and happiness rest on the notion that we should be free and diverse to the extent that our freedom and diversity is not at the expense of others or future generations of life.

- How can subsidiarity be applied within and across increasingly large nation states that are made up of increasingly diverse people?
- How can cosmopolitan governance architecture protect the global commons without becoming a leviathan? The issue is that the nation state is no longer the only basis for identity. People are connected to one another as a result of cross cutting loyalties, by virtue of shared concerns. On the one hand, independence has been fiercely fought for by past colonies, or subsections of marginalised groups who wish to splinter away from dominant centralised control of authoritarian governments. The powerful economies of the world have been built upon exploitation and the lack of representation. It is no surprise that the old and new powers rule through state control. Access to controlling resources, military and/or economic might[14] is the basis for controlling others. The issue of national identity versus global identity has never been more important. The problem is that as people compete for scarce resources they fracture the shared identity that is so important for a sustainable world.

The implications are as follows:

- Extending digital technology could either enable us to achieve our potential which could, in the words used by John Man, turn us into 'cells in a planet-sized brain' (Florini 2003, p 195) or it could lead to our becoming increasingly disconnected and disengaged in face-to-face communication.
- Alternatively, the development of local versions of participatory democracy and governance platforms could help to enhance real-time responsiveness to local experiences. This needs to extend the process of engaging with one another face to face in real time that requires being able to connect emotionally with one another. The capability to communicate in many ways and to respond effectively and quickly to increased risks is the topic of this book.

By considering the implications of three scenarios, the users of the interactive software program are inspired to think about social, economic and environmental choices. This chapter addresses the scenarios that range from 'business as usual' to 'small adjustments to green economies' to 'sustainability and wellbeing'. The aim is to enhance their awareness and to help local government decision makers to

---

[14] http://databank.worldbank.org/databank/download/GDP_PPP.pdf World Bank Gross domestic product 2011, PPP, (millions of Ranking Economy international dollars): "(1) USA, 14,991,300, (2) China 11,290,911, (3) India 4,531,655 (4) Japan 4,303,352 (5) Germany 3,227,444 (6) Russian Federation 3,133,81".

understand the needs and perceptions of local voters. The software is populated by data on services that are available to enable greener choices. Thus, it aims to help with raising consciousness which can provide a step towards the creation of a new suburban culture.

The challenge is to enable people to become aware of the need for a cultural shift from a large carbon footprint created by 'business as usual' and to move towards making logical steps towards sustainable living, rather than making confused gestures at best, or making contradictory decisions in personal and public lives.

A legal agreement is needed between the major emitters—USA, China and India—as well as the demonstration of good faith by local networks that prefigure change on the ground and that link up with global networks. Cosmopolitan initiatives, such as 350.org, need to scale up their collaboration to make the difference.[15]

2.2.1 Learning Ethical Agency

How should wellbeing be defined? Should we follow a definition of wellbeing based on: 'contentment and experienced wellbeing, in a Benthamite hedonic utility sense? Or do we care about eudaimonia or life purpose, in an Aristotelian sense? Particular individuals will value one more than the other depending, in part, on what they are capable of. While scholars surely can measure both, from a societal and policy perspective, which dimension of happiness should policy aim to maximise?' (Graham 2011, p 121)

Wellbeing rests on mindfulness of our relationships with others and with the environment, not on status or ability to live 'high-carbon lifestyles' of our own choosing that are epitomized by mobility for pleasure, maintaining family connections or for work purposes (Elliot 2012). Mobility that is enforced could become greater as a result of increased regional conflict as a result of resource scarcity, disaster or climate change. Whilst there is resistance to this scenario at the moment whilst many live according to the principles of conspicuous consumption,[16] because

[15] '350.org is an international campaign dedicated to building a movement to unite the world around solutions to the climate crisis—the solutions that science and justice demand.www.350.org/en/node/3108', accessed 27/05/2012. Other social movements such as Avaaz or open democracy are examples of other online movements that can ask for responses, such as the following: 'We urge you to save the Earth Summit and the planet by delivering a real deal to end fossil fuel subsidies.'

[16] Originally, conspicuous consumption was possible only for the leisure class and now they are more widely emulated, in order to keep up appearances in capitalist society. 'Conspicuous consumption of valuable goods is a means of reputability to the gentleman of leisure. As wealth accumulates on his hands, his own unaided effort will not avail to sufficiently put his opulence in evidence by this method. The aid of friends and competitors is therefore brought in by resorting to the giving of valuable presents and expensive feasts and entertainments. Presents and feasts had probably another origin than that of naïve ostentation, but they acquired their utility for this purpose very early, and they have retained that character to the present; so that their utility in this respect has now long been the substantial ground on which these usages rest. Costly entertainments, such as the potlatch or the ball, are peculiarly adapted to serve this end. The competitor with whom

carbon-based lives are still within the reach of the middle classes, it is likely that this will be increasingly the preserve of the super-rich elites. The monitoring of scarce resources will become increasingly important for the democracy project, in order to ensure that cynicism and distrust do not alienate electorates. This requires many kinds of engagement—ranging from face-to-face focus groups to community agoras with an 'on-line' link to regional parliaments. This could enable all those who live within a region to voice their opinions. Giving 'a voice to the mob' is regarded as fraught by liberals and neo-liberals—not only because majorities do not always uphold social and environmental justice but also because the current status quo could be overturned! But in a post-consumerist world wealth would need to be re-evaluated and reconceptualised, because, to draw on, adapt and apply Einstein's well-known aphorism: We cannot solve the economic and environmental problems of today with the same ideas of *property and consumption* that created the problem of an *unsustainable* way of life. But to enable freedom of thought in science and democratic testing out of ideas requires a democratic state—but the problem is that the nation state has not acted in the interests of freedom and democracy as Keane (2009a, b) points out.

Emotions run high as resources run out, but it is pointless to polarize emotional and rationalist responses to climate change. Our capability as human beings to think about our thinking requires reflexivity. The more we are able to think about our emotions and the emotions of others, the more likely we are to make decisions that are rational[17].

Participants are first prompted to join up the dots by considering which of three possible scenarios they identify with. The software does not make the decisions; it enables people to address the convergent social, economic and environmental challenges and to consider how these challenges affect their wellbeing. It also helps them to consider the consequences of their ranked and weighted personal choices and to consider how closely their haves and needs are shaped by what they are prepared to change in their lives.

The focus of the research is on creating a decision-making tool to address social, economic and environmental factors that help to mitigate and adapt to climate

---

the entertainer wishes to institute a comparison is, by this method, made to serve as a means to the end. He consumes vicariously for his host at the same time that he is a witness to the consumption of that excess of good things.' Project Gutenberg's The Theory of the Leisure Class, by Thorstein Veblen's eBook or online at www.gutenberg.orgTitle. Accessed 25/06/2012.

[17] At times of high risk, this becomes increasingly important for policy makers. The subjective, objective and intersubjective domains of knowledge are vital, and as Habermas has stressed it is the latter that require the most work in policy making. Reflexivity is both emotional and rational (see Holmes 2010).The recognition of the symbolic meanings people attribute to ideas needs to be given attention (Collins 2008, 2010). Human agency to respond to rising temperatures cannot be avoided and will require rational responses that take into account diverse emotions—particularly the outrage of the disenfranchised. The participatory action research is based on the axiom that freedom and diversity ought to be fostered to support wellbeing and creativity, but only to the extent that the rights of others and the next generation of life are respected. Many researchers suggest that we make a difference to climate change through our choices and our impact on the carbon footprint, and create software to support engagement and complex decision making.

change. Denial is a problem; how do we address denial? How do we enhance engagement? Denial of the toxic effect of the way we live needs to be addressed. The addictive culture consumption is unsustainable and so enabling people to understand that decisions to support the mitigation and adaptation to climate change are rooted in enhancing wellbeing.

At the invitation of the Australian Productivity Commission, Stiglitz (past president of the World Bank) stressed in a lecture in 2010 that the bottom line is wellbeing. This requires building stocks for the future (see Stiglitz et al. 2010). Wellbeing is crucial to redesigning economics. Encouraging people to enjoy walking, making friends in their local community through community gardening and local sport help to support slower more locally based lives. The project responds to the possible existential risks (Bostrom 2011) posed by denial. It is rational to take policy precautions—whatever side of the scientific debate you are located

This requires wellbeing and sustainability decisions and reconsidering our democratic rights and responsibilities by using participatory engagement aimed to match services to needs—within limits—so that local communities make the best decisions that minimise social, economic and environmental risks and that shape 'policy from below' by enabling people to engage in a process of thinking about what *material and non-material* resources they have to support wellbeing; what they still need; what they are prepared *to do* to enhance their social, economic and environmental wellbeing; what they are prepared to discard; and then to consider what they personally consider to be the social, economic and environmental turning points for better or worse. They are also asked to consider the barriers that experience in achieving wellbeing. All their decisions are based on their own perceptions about material and non-material facets of their life. The software updates as they add their new ideas and these help to inform others who see only the list of de-identified social, economic and environmental factors and the particular local resources that are available to assist them to move from (a) business as usual to (b) making small changes and (c) sustainable wellbeing.

The planet is not a credit card to be used to benefit some, whilst others pick up the tab! The responsibility weighs differently on developed and less developed nations and also differently on the rich and poor, this generation and the next.

The more we engage in thinking about our thinking and engage in testing out ideas with others the closer we get to truth. The engagement process is to help achieve a change of heart and 'mindfulness' about our interconnectedness. It is guided by the ethical axiom for democracy and governance that 'we can be free and diverse to the extent that we do not undermine the rights of others or the next generation of life.'[18]

[18] The global commons and our relationship to it needs to be recognized as not merely entangled but codetermined. We need to understand that by identifying with others and with biodiversity (Lever-Tracey 2011) we extend the circle of those with whom we feel solidarity and compassion and redefine our identity without hubris—then we may be able to transform the culture (Hulme 2010, 2011) which shapes the planet on which we depend. This requires some space for diversity and freedom and a sense of irony (Rorty 1989).

By exploring detailed stories of the patterns of what works, why and how emerge across diverse socio-demographic and diverse geographical areas.

Participants are invited to reflect on their lives in terms of what they *already have* and what *they still need* in order to enhance their wellbeing. They are asked to consider what they would be prepared to add to their 'in baskets' and what they would be prepared to discard to their 'out baskets'. The river grasses in a free-flowing river remove salinity and need to be nurtured, not removed.[19] The health of people is dependent on the land and the water systems. Wellbeing is linked with the health of the environment.

The exercise of 'thinking about our thinking' is an attempt to build new neural pathways in the mind—to rehearse a different way of 'being in the world', based on thinking about the consequences for themselves, others and the environment. Our approach to design is an essential aspect of creating a livable planet. As tool makers, we have the potential to use technology in diverse ways:

- Designs that foster 'business as usual' and development along lines that polarize *planetary development* and *poverty reduction* or
- Designs that enable us to hold in mind multiple variables and to find a way through the thicket of tangled policies and practices, in order to adapt to and mitigate the worst effects of climate change *and*
- Designs that harmonise our desires, wants and needs, so that we develop new forms of solidarity based on an understanding that what we do to others, we do to ourselves and the next generation of life.[20] Design refers to the way in which we respond to challenges; the assumption is that engagement is fostered when people are invited to be the subjects and cocreators of decisions to address risks and to enable them to respond with resilience to risks associated with a high-carbon lifestyle.

Design refers to the way in which we respond to challenges; the assumption is that engagement is fostered when people are invited to be the subjects and cocreators of decisions to address risks and to enable them to respond with resilience to risks associated with a high-carbon lifestyle.

[19] The more we weave together strands of experience and respect the other—including the land—the more chance we have to achieve wellbeing (McIntyre-Mills 2008, User centric policy design to address complex needs, p 136; McIntyre-Mills and De Vries 2011, 'Identity, Democracy and Sustainability', pp 233–235).

[20] This approach to ethics is based on considering the implications—social, cultural, political, economic and environmental in the short, medium and long term for all forms of life. The ethical axiom or ideal on which the approach is based is that democracy and governance for a sustainable future needs to support freedom and diversity to the extent that freedom and diversity does not undermine the rights of others or the next generation of life. It requires a very different approach to framing representation and accountability (McIntyre-Mills, 2006, 2008, 2010, McIntyre-Mills and De Vries, 2011).

The focus of the research is on addressing social, economic and environmental factors that help to mitigate and adapt to climate change.[21] How do we address denial of the toxic effect of the way we live? The loss of species, such as bees, for example, needs to be understood to have wide-ranging implications for the future of food security, and taken together the loss of species could affect the very fabric of the ecosystem and our existence (Mathews 2010).

The Brundtland Report (1987) on our Common Future stressed our interconnectedness and the rights of future generations. Clarke (2000) stressed that the planet is a system, but all the policy documents and conferences to date have been limited by the containerist philosophy echoed by the rights of sovereign states (UN 1992, COP and Cancun) to make decisions on the use of resources—most particularly in connection with the carbon-based economy. If we are to balance the interests of the planet as well as ensure the rights of less developed nations to redress poverty, then we must find a way not only to innovate but also to limit the misuse of resources and to enable the fair distribution of rights and responsibilities to ensure food, energy, water supplies that underpin quality of life and wellbeing. The United Nations Declaration of Human Rights will remain rhetoric unless new forms of governance that respect diversity and freedom to the extent that the diversity and freedom of the next generation of life is not undermined. Anthropocentrism and humanism need to move towards respect for biodiversity (Nagoya Summit in Japan in 2010).[22]

---

[21] Joseph Stiglitz previously chief economist and senior vice president of the World Bank has stressed (at the invitation of the Australian Productivity Commission) that the bottom line is wellbeing—this requires building *stocks for the future* (Stiglitz et al. 2010). Wellbeing is crucial to redesigning economics. Encouraging people to enjoy walking, making friends in their local community through community gardening and local sport helps to support slower more locally based lives.

[22] The Brundtland Report (1987) on 'Our Common Future' stressed our interconnectedness and the rights of future generations. Clarke (2000) stressed that the planet is a system, but all the policy documents and conferences to date have been limited by the containerist philosophy echoed by the rights of sovereign states (UN 1992; Copenhagen 2010; Cancun 2011; and Johannesburg 2012) to make decisions on the use of resources—most particularly in connection with the carbon-based economy. If we are to balance the interests of the planet as well as ensure the rights of less developed nations to redress poverty, then we must find a way not only to innovate but also to limit the misuse of resources and to enable the fair distribution (Rawls 1999) of rights and responsibilities to ensure food, energy and water supplies that underpin quality of life and wellbeing. The planet is not a credit card to be used to benefit some, whilst others pick up the tab! The responsibility weighs differently on developed and less developed nations and also differently on the rich and poor, this generation and the next. The architecture of governance (Archibugi 2008) needs to respond to environmental needs that protect the wellbeing of global citizens (Haydon 2005). Consequently, sovereign nation states need to consider regional rights and responsibilities in a series of overlapping organizations that apply the rule of law to ensure equitable and fair distribution of rights and responsibilities for food, energy and water. The research is about developing post-national organizations to ensure human rights. Disaster management, movement of people fleeing disaster or injustice and securing food, energy and water are concerns that span boundaries (spatial, conceptual and temporal). We need to solve problems across generations across disciplines and across nation states to create good neighbourhoods. This requires trust and better communication so that we understand one another better.

2.3 The Max–Neef Human Sustainability Index

The Max–Neef Human Sustainability Index (199 *of being, having doing and interacting* shapes the design and analysis of the research and illustrates the need to be the change through rethinking the way in which we place human beings above our responsibility for the land. Our sense of identity as citizens of nation states needs to be transformed to take into account the needs of our neighbours and future generations of life.

2.4 Wellbeing and Existential Risk

The participatory democracy and governance scorecard aims to assist strategic planning and evidence-based policy to adapt to climate change and contribute to mitigation policy and practice.

2.4.1 The Implications of Transboundary Democracy and Governance for Accounting and Accountability

- Why should people save resources so that others can squander them?
- How can we ensure that everyone has a fair share?

The program of research strives to develop an alternative way of engaging in governance through monitory democracy (McIntyre–Mills and De Vries 2010, 2011). The software program enables choices to be made based on considering the consequences. Then individuals make a contract to set particular targets for themselves. Local government can monitor what people have chosen to do to adapt to climate change. This may include using public transport or creating a vegetable garden.

Local government is able to follow their choices. By considering the implications of three scenarios—ranging from business as usual to 'small adjustments' to 'green economies for sustainability'—the users of the interactive software program are inspired to think about social, economic and environmental choices. The aim is to enhance their awareness and to help local government decision makers to understand the needs and perceptions of local voters.

The software is populated by data on services that are available to enable greener choices. Thus, it aims to help with the creation of a new culture.

We need to restore the narrative 'from below' about what works socially, economically and environmentally. This expanded pragmatism of considering the consequences for others and the environment fits well with a range of thinkers from the Buddhists, Hindus, indigenous healers in Africa, South America and Central Australia to green activists and now mainstream economists such as Joseph Stiglitz.

The elephant in the room is that overcrowding is an issue for the planet and not just for one nation state. Once our governance and democracy designs are robust we will understand that space ship earth requires protection—not one nation state versus another. One biosphere made of many overlapping regions is the responsibility of all nations and all governments and global citizens. We cannot profit at the expense of others, because the fiction of externalities will return to haunt us in the form of rising temperatures, rising fuel and energy costs and rising conflict.

The recent revelation about the Fukushima disaster highlights the importance of monitory democracy and the need to think systemically.[23]

2.5 Policy Context and Options for Social Democracy

The decisions taken at the local level on how we live have an impact on the way others live. So when personal decisions are made to use food, energy or water resources, it has public implications for others as well as the environment. Thus, the research enables the development of a personal scorecard to manage social, economic and environmental decisions. Triple-bottom-line (TBL) accounting and accountability is applied through United Nations Local Agenda 21 at the local level. This is a macro-policy that has been applied by local governments in Australia. The challenge is to develop more systemic indicators that are meaningful for residents, who need to understand the links across personal choices and the implications these could have for adapting to climate change and mitigating the worst effects. Furthermore, it provides the means to achieve scoring personal choices to enable people to consider what they have, what they need to achieve wellbeing, what changes they are prepared to take through adding actions or adding changes in their attitudes towards others or the environment and through discarding certain taken-for-granted ideas.

The sticking point is that weak cosmopolitanism argues for equality of all human beings—without realizing that recognition of human rights requires securing the basic conditions for life. Today, the understanding of carbon-based cultures and economies is relevant to climate change. So the starting point is a recognition that economically wellbeing needs to be the outcome of economic choices—not merely productivity.[24] So how can we address the issue of rights and responsibilities at a

[23] The Fukushima reactor could have been abandoned by the company and this could have released a chain of nuclear reactions. The governance directive for the company to take control and for workers to be sent in to maintain the reactor has resulted in containment. But the margin for error was so close that the lesson is not that the nuclear power option is safe. Alternative measures are preferable—even if the nuclear power option is used very cautiously to buy time for green economies and green technology to be implemented widely.

[24] These public interests include environmental considerations. Today, the decision to, for example, to use energy selfishly and excessively has implications for other communities who may be more affected by extreme weather events as a result of our choices. For example, we may choose to drive a sport utility vehicle (SUV) when it is unnecessary or when it is possible to walk to meet

local level? Could this be the basis for scaling up management of our social, economic and environmental choices at a regional level? Florini (2003) suggests the potential of the Aarhus convention (1998).

Thus, this participatory action research grasps the nettle to: 'address the challenge posed by the Earth Charter: "Everyone shares responsibility for the present and future wellbeing of the human family and the larger living world"' (cited by Hayden, 368).

The challenge is to move beyond the rhetoric of cosmopolitan citizenship and to address both justice and sovereignty. The nation state needs to be held to account by an Earth Charter that is supported by overlapping regional institutions (supported by inclusive regional research institutions, policies, the rule of law including parliaments and courts).

2.6 Area of Concern: Adaptation to the Effects and mitigation of the Causes of Climate Change

The greatest challenges are the consequences of inaction that will potentially pose an existential risk to humanity.[25] The research made use of many forms of engagement to help participants to consider the potential consequences of their choices. These approaches span narrative (to explore complexity and to enable a creative flow of ideas), dialogue and questioning to reformulate boundaries. Scenarios were also explored spanning 'business as usual', 'small steps towards a sustainable future' and achieving a sustainable future through building up 'wellbeing stocks' (Stiglitz et al. 2010).

The section considers the potential for a digital scorecard to address social, economic and environmental factors that support or undermine adaptation and mitigation of climate change. It evaluates the extent to which the approach enables the community to consider their perceived assets and risks and the implications of their consumption choices.

While enabling individual citizens to manage their pathways, the software enables analysis of the responses to inform and assist local government in matching service outcomes to the perceived needs of service users. It is conceived as an

our friends. We may use water excessively for forms of agriculture that will have a downstream risk to other communities needs to be governed by laws that protect the common good. Furthermore, complex decisions need to be informed by those who will be affected by the decisions and Ashby's rule of requisite variety (1956) to establish ways to enhance representation, accountability and engagement.

[25] These challenges include representation of the increasingly diverse populations within nation states along with accountability to ensure that resources (e.g., water, food, and energy) are used fairly, equitably and sustainably in local and regional biospheres. Better forms of engagement are needed to enhance the capability of people to understand that attitudes towards consumption have profound implications for social and environmental justice.

online process to work out where to 'draw the line' based on inclusive testing of ideas with those who are to be affected by the decisions.

It also enables comparisons across the different pathways taken from the three core scenarios to establish not only how the pathways differ but also how they overlap—and therefore to find common ground with regard to their views—their concerns, values, priorities and approaches to how they want to live their lives. The chapter considers the potential for a digital scorecard to address social, economic and environmental factors that support or undermine adaptation to the challenges and mitigation of the effects of climate change. It evaluates the extent to which the approach enables the community to consider their perceived assets and risks and the implications of their consumption choices for developing *wellbeing stocks*.

The focus of the research is on addressing social, economic and environmental factors that help to mitigate and adapt to climate change. Joseph Stiglitz, past president of the World Bank, has stressed (at the invitation of the Australian Productivity Commission) that the bottom line is wellbeing—this requires building *stocks for the future* (Stiglitz et al. 2010). Wellbeing is crucial to redesigning economics.

We face increased risks associated with droughts, fire and floods and thus need to become more resilient to the convergent social, economic and environmental challenges. Energy, food and water supply will impact on human health. Engagement with those who are to be affected by policy decisions helps to enhance attachment to policy and thus helps to increase the extent to which people understand and support the governance processes. Quality of life will be affected by the changes to heat and air quality, water supply and water quality, bush fires, inundation and erosion in coastal areas according to the Wentworth group of concerned scientists. Participants are asked to think about their quality of life in terms of health, housing, employment, education and social inclusion within their communities and what they are prepared to change in terms of their thinking and practice, in order to adapt to the effects and to strive to address the causes through mitigation. The scorecard does not merely rank the outcome of indicators in terms of business as usual, small changes and sustainable futures. It provides weightings of each of the individual choices and invites participants to consider the consequences of their choices.

2.7 Wellbeing, Monitory Democracy and Ethical Governance to Protect the Biosphere

Food and energy are the bases for human wellbeing and security (Kaldor 2004) that need to be protected by means of social and environmental justice. Urry highlights the implications of living in a world where the majority are urban based and reliant on the carbon economy for cooling and the transport of their food to the city. This raises the prospect of 'failed city states' (Urry 2010). In the USA, the top 1 % own 40 % of the wealth (Flannery 2010). Lavish consumption and measuring the values that make life worth living by opulence are 'unrealistic aspirations' which are 'toxic' (Bauman 2011, p 8) to wellbeing. Religion and addiction to consumption are the two opiates which need to be addressed through an acknowledgement of both emotional and rational dimensions. Mass rioting indicates that the standard of living in Europe is deteriorating or 'going South' (Comaroff 2011; Judt 2010), and it could be argued that America has also headed South as indicated by its loss of a triple AAA rating from Standard and Poor's on 6 August 2011 and broad class protests on Wall Street. The time for change—perhaps the great transformation, predicted by many but ignored by most—has arrived.[26]

In order to foster wellbeing and a social demographic transition, new forms of monitory democracy are needed within post-national regions to support food energy and water supplies in Europe, Africa, the Middle East and Asia. The poverty in rural China, rural North Korea and Africa as crops fail has already led to protests, but it remains an open question as to how the situation will unfold. The burden of debt needs to be borne by the wealthy nations and not by future generations or the poor of this generation.

National identity and solidarity are regionalist concerns not only for Europe (Gould 2007) but also for the Asia Pacific region of which Australia is a part.

The outrage felt by the disenfranchised in this planet of seven billion people could find expression through politics and/or religion. The poor from Tunisia have sought refuge from drought in Paris. The refugees from unrest in PNG or East Timor, or from further afield (Afghanistan, Sri Lanka or Iran), arrive in Australia. The prospect of climate change refugees is also likely as sea levels rise in Bangladesh, Tuvalu and Samoa, for example. The devastating tsunami that affected much of the region (Sri Lanka, India, Thailand and in particular Ache, Indonesia) on 26 December 2004 provides an example of the scale of disaster and the need to plan for post-national regionalist responses. For example, the radiation seeping from the Fukushima nuclear reactor as a result of a tsunami that hit the coast of Japan has been detected in the ocean and in food supplies.[27] The risk of contamination is unseen, but felt by those outside the widening containment zones.

The potential for the United Nations Educational, Scientific and Cultural Organization (UNESCO) biospheres[28] approach and related efforts to protect specific habitats (Nguyen et al. 2011) has the policy potential to be extended, reframed and scaled up to address the need for sustainable forms of governance which is developed in this paper. The fluidity and 'flow-on' effects of social, political and economic policy choices cannot be denied in sustainable designs for the future. Water will become the new gold over which wars are waged (Hulme 2009) and needs to be valued along with laws to support sustainable regions that can support the production of food and limit the misuse of agriculture. Is it more important to mine uranium in South Australia than to consider the long-term social, economic and environmental

[26] We face ongoing social, economic and environmental challenges that are unprecedented. The global economic meltdown needs to be used as an opportunity to change direction.

[27] ABC news March 31, 2011.

[28] http://portal.unesco.org/science/en/ev.php-URL_ID=4793&URL_DO=DO_TOPIC&URL_SECTION=201.html accessed 10/01/2012.

implications (McIntyre-Mills 2008) of selling uranium to our neighbours (including those who do not have signatory to the nuclear non-proliferation treaty)?

The next decade requires decisive socio-economic intervention (Stern 2006; Lovelock 2006, 2009). Greed, zero-sum competition for resources and the commodification of the powerless, the voiceless and the environment is the area of concern. The multidisciplinary research begins with questions about social, economic and environmental sustainability. It explores post-materialism and engagement to establish whether it is possible to move beyond being ambivalent cosmopolitans and to raise awareness on what or resilience entails for everyday life choices as well as policy and governance choices (McIntyre-Mills and De Vries 2011). The praxis undertaken in South Australia and detailed in Chaps. 1 and 2 draws on the work of Murray et al., but remains focused on human agency:

> Those groups in society who spend considerably more than the average time on earth and in doing so, wittingly or unwittingly, diminish the time that others have to spend, could be said to be acting unfairly… there is a biological base for human ethics…. (2006, p 16)

If we are to respond to the Stern Review (2006) on the economics of climate change, then dramatic changes (Rockström et al. 2009) in what we value need to be modelled through markets that are guided by overarching covenants to ensure that the size of the carbon footprint is indeed addressed. For this reason, Stiglitz (2010) reframes the nature of rights and responsibilities to protect the collective good and the global commons. When making policy to address climate change and to protect the global commons, we need to address emotions and rationality. If people do not feel a sense of connection to policy and the law, then they will resist them. Policy needs to grow out of public dialogue and the law needs to be made meaningful and accessible. Productivity through genetically modified foods and increased use of nuclear power are technocratic 'solutions' that could also have disastrous side effects.

TBL accounting is applied through United Nations Local Agenda 21. This is a macro-policy that has been applied by local governments in Australia. The challenge is to develop indicators that are meaningful for residents, who need to understand the links across personal choices and the implications these could have for adapting to climate change and mitigating the worst effects. Furthermore, it provides the means to achieve scoring personal choices to enable people to consider what they have, what they need to achieve wellbeing, what praxis they are prepared to take through adding actions or adding changes in their attitudes towards others or the environment and through discarding certain taken for granted ideas. The sticking point is that weak cosmopolitanism argues for equality of all human beings without realising that recognition of human rights requires securing the basic conditions for life. Today, the understanding of carbon-based cultures and economies are relevant to climate change. So the starting point is a recognition that economically wellbeing needs to be the outcome of economic choices—not merely productivity.

The past president of the World Bank, Professor Joseph Stiglitz links wellbeing with economics in a recent address to the Australian Productivity Commission. He has published a book together with Prof. Amartya Sen, entitled 'Mismeasuring our lives'. Sen discusses the role of social inclusion in discussions on climate change and building capacity. Stiglitz et al. (2010) stress the importance of building capability to value social and environmental goods as the basis for personal, social and planetary wellbeing. This is determined by investing in and building 'stocks for future generations of life'. They conclude that if all measures consider wellbeing in terms of *median* households, then consumption, capital and income could be compared across rich and poor households.

But the problem with the research approach of Stiglitz et al. (2010) is that measures of average cannot address the diverse emotions and cultural perceptions of 'quality of life', consumption and the capacity to live a full life (Nussbaum 2006). Instead, the measures detailed in this chapter are based on qualitative data on perceptions that are used to develop scenarios. The scenarios ranged from maintaining the status quo to making small changes towards living sustainably and achieving a perceived sense of wellbeing. These scenarios are used as a starting point for enabling participants to think about their own lives and the choices they are prepared to make.

Just as we cannot ignore externalities associated with profit, we cannot ignore the externalities of living life at the expense of others. So how can we address the issue of rights and responsibilities at a local level? Could this be the basis for scaling up management of our social, economic and environmental choices at a regional level?

The cost of greed is carried by the poor, the powerless and the planet. Helping the powerful to realize that complicity entraps the rich as much as the poor is perhaps one way out of the trap. Another way out of the trap is through putting in place a new architecture for democracy and governance that could balance individual and collective needs through a fairer distribution of social resources that value our relationship with others and the environment—thus leading to a reframing of economics.

Participatory design has a long history in the International Systems Sciences, International Sociological Association, the Action Learning and Action Research Association, for example. The rationale is that by testing out ideas with people who have lived experience as well as by people with professional expertise it is possible to enhance the quality of the decisions and to achieve a better policy response to people. It is based on the notion that the complexity of the decision needs to be matched by the complexity of the decision makers. This enhances the robustness of the decision and it is also more likely to be supported politically by those who are affected by the decisions. The process is vital to develop appropriate indicators of wellbeing that are linked to an interactive map of the perceived haves and needs of the population in the context of a post-carbon world in which the cost of resources is affected by the cost of oil. This is where the collaborative work on participatory democracy and governance is located.

The objective is to make a case for social change to address wellbeing not merely productivity for profit through transdisciplinarity and a reframed approach to wellbeing. The rationale for the book is that food, energy and water consumption need to be used sustainably and currently terms of reference applied by economics do not take these into account.

Reducing, reusing and recycling need to become the litmus test for households and local development as a means to redistribute resources to those in need and as a means to limit the misuse of scarce resources. Accounting and accountability at the local level need to be fostered by means of monitory democracy and governance.

The research applies this philosophy at the local level and advocates for its extension to post-national regional biospheres. How can neighbours think that they live in isolation from one another? How can we turn back those who seek assistance at our borders or worse 'turn back the boats' at sea in order to 'protect boundaries'?

Food and energy are the bases for human wellbeing and security. Current approaches to international relations and war (Etzioni 2004, 2011) are unsustainable. Post-nationalism needs to be buttressed by human rights, rights to protect biospheres and the law of the sea. As the experience of suffering becomes more widespread, the notion of class will become central once again, because 'the poorest people in the world will be the hardest hit' (Beck 2009, p 37).

Since the commission on wellbeing that was requested by Sarkozy and the book that resulted from it, called 'Mismeasuring our lives' (Stiglitz et al. 2010), the global financial crisis has escalated to a social and environmental crisis that continues to unfold.

The key policy message is that simple living is both elegant and ethical. This requires a new stoicism, based on a sense of responsibility for others.[29]

The challenge is that individualism has been taken too far as a result of the power associated with capital. It is possible that the low carbon footprint could be decreed from above as necessary for human survival, but that the elites will exempt themselves from the low carbon lifestyle. This could become increasingly likely if the media (print and digital) are owned by elites. This is why it is vital that cosmopolitan citizens hold elites to account.

How should we live and how can governance become more ethical through engaging people to think about their emotions and the consequences of their choices?

How can these choices be limited within the scope of what is fair to others and the next generation of life? How can whistle-blowing be achieved without lapsing into a distrusting society in which everyone lives in fear? How can we be the change when dollars and cents (not wellbeing) is the bottom line?

[29] How can engagement be enhanced so that the Orwellian future is avoided? How can designs reframe technology in ways that (a) reclaim designs from below and (b) drive policy so that they inform the final decisions? How can elected leaders be held to account on the basis of the lived experiences of the electorate as well as by those who are so-called discipline experts? How can the decision (or cut) be made by the elected representatives in ways that balance individual and collective interests—rather than the interests of elites? Creativity guided by humility and the willingness to care for others is needed to underpin the transformation from 'Wall Street' to 'wellbeing'.

2.8 Expanding Pragmatism: Praxis to Build Wellbeing Stocks for Future Generations of Life

This research is located in the domain of how to develop a new architecture in response to Dahl's pessimism about extending the scale of democracy and governance.[30]

The Intergovernmental Panel on Climate Change (IPCC) theorem (Charlton 2011) is as follows:

$$\mathrm{E}(\text{emissions}) = \text{Population} \times \text{consumption per person} \times \text{energy efficiency} \times \text{energy emissions}.$$

The options are as follows: business as usual and small adjustments for the long haul to achieve living in ways that do not risk our way of life (see McIntyre-Mills and De Vries 2011, 2012, for a detailed argument and the details of the software). The software provides a way to enable people to explore the question, how should we live? Participants are invited to consider what they have, they need, what their turning points are for better or worse and what the barriers are. Services that help them meet their needs are detailed as well. The software updates as it is used. The idea is that it will help people to make better decisions to address complex needs. Excel sheets are provided that give cross tabulations of socio-demographic details and the choices they make. The idea is that by thinking about their lives they will be able to consider the consequences of their choices on wellbeing. The entry to software is user name = test password = test.

The starting point is to listen to the three scenarios. The pathway address for local government is https://wellbeing.csem.flinders.edu.au/.

[30] Dahl's (1967) pessimism about choosing nested systems of governance—because democracy was designed for the city state—has long been overturned by the necessity to extend governance in the interests of sustainability. The signing of the United Nations Declaration of Human Rights has not lead to detailed covenants or the means to implement the noble ideas. The book makes the case for social change through exploring interdisciplinary frameworks to address environmental politics, ethics and legal frontiers as a necessity for human security. Social change frameworks to address greed and the commodification of the powerless and the environment will be informed by debates on ethics, human reasoning capability, environmental politics and the role of the market in achieving a sustainable future for the next generation. We face ongoing social, economic and environmental challenges that are unprecedented. The global economic meltdown needs to be used as an opportunity to change direction. Change requires necessity, desire and will in the sense used by Delueze and Guattari. We need to understand that 'we are the land'. Dualistic thinking needs to be recognized as part of a failed enlightenment project and we need to 'rescue the enlightenment from itself' (McIntyre-Mills et al. 2006a) through recognizing our codetermination of the environment of which we are a part. We need to understand that by identifying with others and with biodiversity (Lever-Tracey 2011) we extend the circle of those with whom we feel solidarity and compassion and redefine our identity with humility—then we may be able to transform the culture (Hulme 2010, 2011) which shapes the planet on which we depend. This requires some space for diversity and freedom and a sense of irony (Rorty 1989) which could ensure that corporatist responses do not sink the potential for balancing individual and collective needs in federalist regional biospheres.

2.9 Enabling Local Communities Through Fostering Cosmopolitan Values

Participatory design has a long history in the International Systems Sciences, International Sociological Association, the Action Learning and Action Research Association, for example. The rationale for this approach is that by testing out ideas with people who have lived experience as well as by people with professional expertise it is possible to enhance the quality of the decisions and to achieve a greater match. It is based on the notion that the complexity of the decision needs to be matched by the complexity of the decision makers. This enhances the robustness of the decision and it is also more likely to be supported politically by those who are affected by the decisions. The process is vital to develop appropriate indicators of wellbeing that are linked to an interactive map of the perceived haves and needs of the population in the context of a post-carbon world in which the cost of resources is affected by the cost of oil. This is where the collaborative work on participatory democracy and governance is located. The role of the good citizen is to: (a) enhance wellbeing of communities, (b) support the demographic transition and (c) enhance life chances for all through securing food, energy and water. The good global steward builds stocks for future generations and does not externalize the costs. Poverty, pollution and carbon emissions ought not to be shifted to future generations or other people. This requires post-national and post-disciplinary cooperation and new forms of governance. Could we start to see patterns in the statistics and in the stories that we cocreate as shared narratives that become increasingly harmonious song lines for a new society that is indeed post-materialist? The participants are residents of a local government area in South Australia, in the first instance.

The research explores whether using a computer-aided model could enhance data collection, analysis and ongoing engagement to address complex social, economic and environmental issues associated with climate change. The software is loaded onto the Flinders Website,[31] in the first instance, but has the potential for links with local governments elsewhere at a sub- and post-national level within the region. Part of the rationale for trialling the software was to establish to what extent computing per se is a useful way to engage different interest groups and whether it could be useful to enable managing large, diverse data sets spanning many diverse interrelated variables about which residents have strong values. A diverse range of values, emotions and opinions are associated with wellbeing, quality of life and

[31] Until broadband is made widely available, the software will run less effectively at peak hours. Participation is thus effected by the lack of broadband. This point was made strongly by the Thinker in Residence Genevieve Bell (2009) who was invited to review the potential for ICTs in South Australia in her report 'Getting Connected, Staying Connected, Exploring South Australia's digital futures'. Another challenge was the migration of data from one part of the server to another and the right to obtain access to log into the data systems by both users and administrators. The next hurdle will be to link the Flinders website to the Local Government Association (LGA) website. It is currently linked as a demonstration to the ISA wiki site and also to Abdushomad Muhammad's website. As a senior public servant in the Ministry of Religion in Indonesia and my PhD student at Flinders University, he is well placed to assist.

climate change. These can be regarded as a wicked problem, in the sense that it has many, diverse and interrelated variables that are viewed differently by people with different values (see the West Churchman Series 2006).

Our research (McIntyre-Mills and De Vries 2010, 2011) attempts to enable people to think through the 'if-then' scenarios, not merely to 'unfreeze' (to cite Lewin's concept) but also to work towards sustainable praxis, based on an understanding of our interrelatedness. This requires ongoing changes to learning (Schein 1996), 'habitus' (Bourdieu 1977) or ways of 'being in the world' (Haraway 1991, 1992, 2010). How can we extend our horizon of solidarity through enabling people to develop a greater ability to think about the bigger picture?[32] The design builds on research with Aboriginal service users and providers whose philosophy on wellbeing raised areas of concern which this research strives to address.

2.9.1 Typological Characteristics

'Business as usual' is characterized by the perception that: (a) physical space is segregated, whereas (b) conceptual spaces are individualistic and competitive. Typically, informants stress that 'time is money' and life is considered to be stressful and competitive. Adaptation is through increased expenditure and technological innovation, rather than a willingness to give up their standard of living.

Small steps towards sustainability are characterized by: (a) making more use of energy-efficient appliances and cars and a 'less is more approach' to living elegantly and ethically. At the time this paper was written, the responses from participants about what they perceived to be positive about their quality of life (Nussbaum and Sen 1993) are as shown in Table 2.1.

What engagement processes could be effective to address the policy and governance challenges of mitigation and accountability? This section addresses the program of research on representation, accountability and engagement to adapt to and mitigate the extent of risks. Thus, its emphasis is not merely to describe what the case is, but to discuss participatory action research that strives to design and prefigure alternative praxis as a seed for transformation. The research tests the principle of subsidiarity, namely that people ought to have the right to make decisions by drawing on their own experiences at the local level, but they have the responsibility to follow norms and laws that protect the interests of the public. In order to address convergent social, economic and environmental questions, it is necessary to address complexity, by making sense of issues through narrative and dialogue in order to understand the diverse, interrelated variables each of which is perceived differently

[32] De Grasse in conversation with Richard Dawkins explains that we need to see horizons as always changing, but we need to strive to think about larger assemblies and to make use of conceptual tools to enhance evolutionary consciousness. The limits are beyond us and always relative to where we are located physically and conceptually. http://www.youtube.com/watch?v=9RExQFZzHXQ&feature=related.

Table 2.1 Perceptions and emotional dimensions to quality of life. (Nussbaum and Sen 1993)

Sustainable future: growing seeds for transformation					
In basket	Out basket	Barrier factors	Have factors	Need factors	Turning points
A job that uses my education and challenges me More trees and shrubs	Greed and wasteful habits	Reducing dependence on supermarkets Greed and wasteful habits	Social inclusion	Economic means of transport	Join clubs (B) Lack of conscience, because individualistic (W)
Access to farmer's markets More walking	Mining gas seams and contamination of food systems	Saving money, stop spending, apathy	Stone house	Environmental community activities	Physical wellbeing undermined by greed and consumerism (W)
Bus service is declining More walking in the hills	Access to computer	Stuff/consumer goods Buses not running regularly	Rain water tank	Housing library	Buying a house that is not energy efficient(W) Fear of change (W)
Celebrate friends and family with food Own home	Air conditioning to heat home	Time to read Caring for dementia sufferer	Good public transport near home Travel for an hour by car each day	Good public transport near home Time to reflect	Leaning more about energy efficient living More money for community centre and youth centre
Community education—reading and meeting needs Own my own home	Avoid being stuck in traffic	Too much (stuff) is a problem Closed minds	Community garden 7 rain tanks Use grey water on garden	Community garden near to where I live Community education—reading and meeting	More spare time Work at home 1 day a week
Conserving water, electricity and switching off gadgets People to help me do things around the house I cannot do	Big house = too much cleaning	Use ceiling fan Cost of solar panels	Stone and wood house own my own home Fresh air	I work part-time on the weekends Efficient and effective public transport	Able to spend on social activities Doing things because I want to—not out of obligation

Table 2.1 (continued)

Sustainable future: growing seeds for transformation					
In basket	Out basket	Barrier factors	Have factors	Need factors	Turning points
Eating meals at home or with friends—to minimise costs Public transport	Buy recycled clothes	Use stone basement flat when hot Difficult when family or friends do not want to come to community events	My house suits my needs Need vegetable market	More money to buy the things that I need to live Fresh air	Saving on petrol (B) Downpipes fixed—so collect rain water (B)
Education Public transport so less cars on the road	Car	Wasting water Doubt about ability to make a difference	My job is enjoyable and has meaning Garden with mostly trees	I need a job that pays the bills and is sustainable More meaningful relationships	Extra exercise Increasing social networks
Employment Public transport to access services	Community development based on brochures	Excessive packaging Greater understanding of environment	I am a full-time university student	I need trees and plenty of space Emotional and physical space	Isolation because of cost of petrol so cannot meet friends Isolation
Energy efficiency standards Purpose—a reason to live	Computer—time spent on it	I don't own a car so rely on public transport high cost of local produce	I don't own a car so rely on public transport Rental housing	Discard petrol car Mental stimulation	Post-materialist lifestyle More street trees
Energy-efficient appliances Recycling centres for electronics	Conserving water, electricity and switching off gadgets	I will get rid of my car Instability in employment	Am just making ends meet each week Small retirement unit	Friends More money so less stressed	Conferences with like-minded people More cars will destroy our environment
Experience of the world Recycling in separate not split bins	Dependence on car	Laziness, isolation	Car–family are interstate	Money Low rise housing	Doing new things Help
Extra exercise Recycling wherever possible	Dependence on large business corporations	Less holidaying (away from home)	Study on a full belly	A job Shade	Apathy Low rise and low density

Table 2.1 (continued)

Sustainable future: growing seeds for transformation

In basket	Out basket	Barrier factors	Have factors	Need factors	Turning points
Food networks Renewable energy	Dependence on technology	Lack of public transport	Volunteering Strong family relationships	Relaxation Keep air unpolluted by traffic	Lack of time Lack if native vegetation
Fresh air Riding my bike	Discard car	Less small talk more on what matters Lack of time Less stress	Volunteering Big garden or access to it	Extra exercise Public transport	Sleep Wellbeing promotion
Friends Safer bikeways Full-time job Shade	Discard chemicals for use in garden or house Discard dishwasher and clothes dryer	Less useless packaging Loss of sight Long shower Low income	Relaxation Kindness to one another Family—general A sense of mission	Family—general Services to help caring A house Help with shopping	Lack of public transport Community Garden More support of local businesses Share more resources in the community
Garden with mostly trees Social contract	Discard high-energy use—turn off at the switch	Money spent on unnecessary food Money	Meaningful life Energy efficiency	Fresh and tasty food Help with community transport	Time outdoors Values—selfishness
Geothermal energy Social relationships—love, friends	Discard plastic bags	Overuse of power in the home More spare time	Connection with environment Initiative and confidence	Water Housing design	Savings on petrol Recycling wherever possible
Help with shopping Solar energy	Discard travelling distances for shopping	Plastic bin liners Poor public transport at night Less time to pursue interests if cannot take car to work	Hobbies	Air conditioning, double glazing and better insulation	Savings on car maintenance Overuse of power in the home
Holistic life Solar panels	Do not make new plastic	Recycling centres for electronics poverty	Lack of time Positive community	Shelter Quality of life in higher density areas is possible	Isolation if no public transport Growing awareness of the issue

Table 2.1 (continued)

Sustainable future: growing seeds for transformation					
In basket	Out basket	Barrier factors	Have factors	Need factors	Turning points
Home-grown produce Subsidies of small unobtrusive wind turbines	Double glazing and better insulation	Reduce chattels Remembering to take shopping bags	Aspirations Bike riding	Love Subsidise green technology for those on pension	Inconvenience due to limited services Advertising pressure to use domestic appliances
I know my neighbours Time		Resistance to change	Education Low-consumption light bulbs	Purpose—a reason to live Food security	Reducing car use Deterioration of resources as a result of inappropriate agricultural production of rice, cotton and other crops
I need more balance time on the beach		Social commitments	Social and environmental conscience Recycling rubbish Insulation	Public transport to access services Share more resources in the community	Increase recycling and water restrictions Downgrading public transport
Independence Time to read		Time	Exercise Food	Education Everyone needs access to rain tanks and solar	Growing own food Library at 'Middleville' and Mitcham
Independence in own home Time to reflect		Time it takes to catch three buses to work	Healthy critical mind Garden	Sleep Values—kindness to all	Growing own food Comfortable house
Less garbage Time to spend in the garden		Time to grow own food	A sense of adventure Riding my bike	Social relationships Love, friends Holistic life	High cost of local produce Second hand charity shops

Table 2.1 (continued)

Sustainable future: growing seeds for transformation					
In basket	Out basket	Barrier factors	Have factors	Need factors	Turning points
Less work and more community involvement		Greed	Spiritual respect for others	Validation	Less garbage
				Recycling wherever possible	Poverty
To help others			Community activities		
Low-rise housing		Unwillingness to change way of life	Use solar panels for water	More community involvement	Less landfill
Transport hubs near places of work					Living in one country and not commuting
				Full time job	
More community involvement		Way we perceive time	Not working—retired	Time	Remembering to take shopping bags
				Solar electricity	
Vegetarianism					Energy efficiency
More efficient ducted systems		Weather		Intellectual stimulation	Remembering to take shopping bags
				Mental wellbeing	
Volunteering					Waste and recycling
More meaningful relationships		Work commitments		Home grown produce	Healthy critical mind
				Positive community	More time to go bushwalking
Worm farms					
More money				More support of local businesses	Less work and more community involvement
Yoga					
				Water tanks	
					Use modern light globes and save
More social interaction				Experience of the world	Time to spend in the Garden
More sustainable housing				Healthy critical mind	
					Use ceiling fan
More spare time				Exercise	Conscious or mindful
More time to be creative				Good fun	more walking
More support of local businesses				Permanent job	Less cleaning products
				Books that inspire and challenge	Buy recycled clothes

Table 2.1 (continued)

Sustainable future: growing seeds for transformation					
In basket	Out basket	Barrier factors	Have factors	Need factors	Turning points
More time without obligations				Own home Indeed more balance More time to be creative More social interaction Riding my bike	Riding my bike Resistance to change Giving up, being overwhelmed Community activities
Small changes					
Water mManagement	Education	Native vVegetation	Solar panels and rain tanks	Eating less lollies and rubbish More street trees	Big business as usual High living costs
Social inclusion	Discard second car	Motivation	Energy eEfficiency Recycling wherever possible	Family Drive electric car	Efficient and effective public transport Scientific results on impact
I don't have anything to do with my neighbours	Reduce use of air conditioning	Resistance	Recycle as much as possible Solar energy	Health services accessible Solar street lights	Energy efficiency and water efficiency
Exercise	Lack of understanding of the long-term impacts of climate change	Wellbeing has nothing to do with climate change and vice versa	Air conditioned Drive energy-efficient car	Help with bush management Rain tanks	Environmental policy that supports sustainable future Lack of consistent action
Greater understanding of environment		Do not believe in climate change but do believe in protecting environment	Mental wellbeing Walking	Less energy use Insulation	More tolerance of other views Compost bin
Less energy use		Traffic affects safety when walking	A job Gardening using drought tolerant plants	Less resistance to change Solar energy	Solar hot water system Unscientific Information Undermines motivation to change behaviour

Table 2.1 (continued)

Sustainable future: growing seeds for transformation					
In basket	Out basket	Barrier factors	Have factors	Need factors	Turning points
Eating less lollies and rubbish		Un-scientific information under-mines motivation to change behaviour	A house	Less work	Solar panels
			Financial wellbeing	Support farmers with water allocations	Ignorant politicians
Less work			Good health	More community activities for elderly	Use solar panels for water
			Understand how climate change affects lives and livelihood	Government policy to subsidise renewables	Information and education on wellbeing
Environmental policy that supports sustainable future			Dependence on technology	More time to walk and cycle	
			Ability to adapt and change	More public transport	
Solar street lights			Satisfying work	More time with family	
			Building temperature control	Better—more accessible public transport	
More public transport			Loving family	More time with friends	
Compost bin				Safe pathways for crossing traffic	
Build more safe walking paths at the local level			Books	Reduce chattels	
			Energy efficient light bulbs	Double glazing affordable	
Access to information regarding changes—impact and time frame			Music	Social inclusion on–off switches for all appliances	
			Low-consumption shower heads		
Scientific results on impact			Videos	Solar panels	
			Vegetable garden	Information about likely changes	

Table 2.1 (continued)

Sustainable future: growing seeds for transformation

In basket	Out basket	Barrier factors	Have factors	Need factors	Turning points
Compost bin			Good mind Double glazing and better insulation	Time to read Information about what I can do	
Poultry for manure and local food			Efficient and effective public transport	Trees Less traffic	
Business as usual					
Community garden	Water management	Fire	Economic Physical wellbeing	Jobs that support environment Car	
Waste and recycling	Discard petrol car	Discard petrol car	Environmental Stress associated with lifestyle	Native vegetation More Aboriginal leaders	
Finances	Discard my couch	Cost of adaptation	Employment Need a job that pays bills and is sustainable	I would like to know my neighbours better Youth shelter for Aboriginals	
Drive diesel car		Loss of inspiration	Sport Access to computer	Access to fire manage resources Downpipes fixed	
Car		People bringing you down	Family Friends	Join clubs Mining gas seams and contamination of food systems	
Money			I don't have anything to do with my neighbours Have vocational opportunity as Tafe Student	More Spare Time No real community development [it is just] based on brochures	

Table 2.1 (continued)

Sustainable future: growing seeds for transformation					
In basket	Out basket	Barrier factors	Have factors	Need factors	Turning points
A job			Civil servants have energy awareness	More money Drive energy-efficient car	
More Aboriginal leaders			Dispute with neighbours	Drive diesel car Do not believe in climate change but do believe in protecting the environment Access to information regarding changes—impact and time frame	

by different stakeholders and then to work out socially and environmentally just decisions (Talpin and Wojcik 2010).

The idea is to use the scenarios as starting points to explore ways to enable people to live healthy, happy ethical lives that are not at the expense of others or the next generation of life. The scenarios are for Australia and we need scenarios from other parts of the world that reflect social, cultural, political, economic and environmental diversity.

It could help people to realize their dependency on their relationship with one another and the land and on one another for peace and security. The problem with current forms of governance is:

- Spatial: limited to the nation state but the resources to support quality of life are beyond the boundaries of the nation state.
- Temporal: limited to electoral cycle and this generation.
- Conceptual: Wellbeing not profit (economic) is the problem—addressed through education and transformation of ethics and law.

Perceptions and emotional dimensions to quality of life (Nussbaum and Sen 1993) could change not only as a result of laws to manage energy, water and food resources but also through engagement with a form of interactive software that helps to develop consciousness of our interconnectedness.[33]

It is likely that a greater balance will need to be achieved between individual and collective needs through emphasizing the determinants of wellbeing for this generation and the next. This requires a new approach to public education, democracy, governance and ethics that places food security at the centre of decisions. The role of local participation and governance thus becomes increasingly important (Schweber 2012). Our research strives to enable people to have a say about how scarce resources should be used, in order to inform elected representatives of their perceived social, economic and environmental needs. It is hoped that by thinking about what they have and what they need and what they are prepared to change (by being prompted to consider the consequences of our choices for others and for the environment), the notion of engagement in 'if-then scenarios' is helpful to

[33] It strives to enable a greater awareness of consciousness of our rights and responsibilities as global citizens. It is practical in that it attempts to acknowledge that localized, slow lives that are sustainable could lapse into the Orwellian nightmare of control from above—without surveillance from below to hold the elites to account. It is for this reason that the digital future needs to be shaped not only by the state military complex but also by those who wish to act as caretakers for the next generation. Members of the public need to be protected by a scaled-up version of the Aarhus Convention that gives residents within post-national regions the right to access information and to the right to be heard by the state (1998; see McIntyre-Mills 2011); thus, this report (a) discusses the theory of participatory democracy—based on the principles of subsidiarity and Ashby's rule of requisite variety—meaning that decisions need to reflect the complexity of the area of concern and (b) makes a case for new forms of accountability to support regional governance that is capable of extending the social contract beyond the nation state and thus to protect biospheres and the diversity within them. The governance decisions will need to be upheld by rule of law based on the axiom that we can be free and diverse to the extent that freedom and democracy is not undermined (McIntyre-Mills 2006 et al.).

enable people to develop sustainable social, economic and environmental decisions (McIntyre-Mills and De Vries 2011).

A sustainable local community is determined by a sustainable region in which food, energy and water supplies are considered as major determinants for wellbeing. No community can be expected to transform from a high-carbon lifestyle (or aspiring to this lifestyle) without being part of the design process and owning the decisions as to how resources should be used.[34] The exercise of 'thinking about their thinking' is an attempt to build new neural pathways in the mind—to rehearse a different way of 'being in the world', based on thinking about the consequences for themselves, others and the environment.

The research aims to establish if it is possible for cultural transformation to be scaled up to enable a shift towards sustainability.

The research is about cultural transformation. While enabling individual citizens to manage their pathways, the software enables analysis of the responses to inform and assist local government in matching service outcomes to the perceived needs of service users. It is conceived as an online process to work out where to 'draw the line' based on inclusive testing of ideas with those who are to be affected by the decisions.

It also enables comparisons across the different pathways taken from the three core scenarios to establish not only how the pathways differ but also how they overlap—and therefore to find common ground with regard to their views—their concerns, values, priorities and approaches to how they want to live their lives.

The objective is to make a case for social change to address wellbeing (not merely productivity for profit). By working in middle- to upper-income area, the aim was to establish to what extent this group of people (the majority of whom are employed and own their own homes) are able to think in terms of enhancing their wellbeing whilst lowering their carbon footprints. The central challenges for democracy, governance and ethics are as follows: (1) representation, (2) accountability, (3) sustainability and (4) engagement (McIntyre-Mills and de Vries 2011).

2.9.2 *Options for Engagement*

It is worth bearing in mind that even in this middle-class area only 66 % of the households had access to computers, according to the census in 2006. But the number could have increased by 2012, despite the tendency for cost saving on other household items. Thus, engagement relying solely on computer software access needs to be extended by means of mobile connections; however, those who cannot afford home computers or who do not have computing skills are unlikely to make more use of expensive mobile phones. The way forward will be tested through

[34] This research emphasizes the creation of multiple paths to form webs to wellbeing through critical, systemic engagement to ensure that local people get to know about local resources (that are listed in directories created by both service users and providers) and that their identity is protected. They are able to see the typical scenarios of what people have, need, are prepared to add or discard from their lives and what they think are turning points for better or worse.

linking with a range of sites and moving gradually towards social networking sites, once we are satisfied with the testing of the software through smaller pilots.

2.9.3 *Face-to-Face Engagement*

Participants were asked to consider the following scenarios as a starting point for answering the questions listed in the pro forma below. Each participant will have new ideas and they are just a starting point for asking you to share your own ideas about how we should live.

2.9.3.1 Business as Usual Scenario

We continue to believe in economic arguments that others believe ignore the social and environmental dimension. We continue to think that our way of life is sustainable and are not prepared to manage the perceived risks of climate change by changing our way of life. We attribute drought, bush fires and floods to one-off unrelated events or natural cycles, and deny that climate change can trigger rising temperatures in some areas and plummeting temperatures in others as melting ice affects the ocean currents.[35]

---

[35] The detailed scenario is as follows: We continue to believe in economic arguments that ignore the social and environmental dimension and we continue to think that our way of life is sustainable and are not prepared to manage the risks of climate change by changing our way of life. We blame the increasing risk of drought, bush fires and floods are on 'one-off' unrelated events or deny that climate change can mean rising temperatures in some areas and plummeting temperatures in others as melting ice effects the ocean currents. The sea is used as a dumping ground and it no longer helps to regulate our climate. More and more of us suffer from viruses and food poisoning. Animals are diseased. Most of our rivers are polluted and many have dried up. We fight over the last of energy and natural resources. We export our waste material to poorer nations who 'offer' to store it.

'The government' and 'the economy' are blamed for the problems, but we do not make any changes to our personal lives, because it is too hard, or not our problem. The corporate business sector continues to tell us that the market self-regulates. We compete with one another and are proud to wear designer labels or to carry designer packages. We engage in fundraising activities and give money to charity. These small gestures are to enable us to pretend that we are making a difference. We refused to an agreement in Copenhagen, because it is bad for the state of the economy. We continued to wrangle for after the inconclusive climate change talks in Copenhagen (18 Dec 2009). We cannot achieve agreement internationally as to how we will go about reducing our emissions and changing our way of life. We feel anxious, stressed or depressed and we use drugs, alcohol and shopping to provide temporary relief. We flop in front of television and watch mind-numbing programs or endless DVDs so that we ignore the problems in our neighbourhood. We withdraw and do not know the people in our street. We feel we cannot be bothered, because we are too busy making a living and worrying about our own problems. We base our decision on narrow pragmatism, because we think about the consequences only for ourselves and not others. We believe that our power and profit must be driven by self-interest and the bottom line, namely ensuring our powerful positions and our profits. We think that social and environmental considerations are 'externalities', rather than imbedded in the current system.

2.9.3.2 Small Changes for the Long-Haul Scenario

People make slow annual progress towards goals which they meet for the benefit of their children and grandchildren. People of all ages and from all walks of life who are able to join up the dots between the economic, social and environmental dimensions help to motivate movement towards a better future. We do not perceive these small changes as being too slow to sustain beyond our grandchildren, or we envisage that something else will happen by then to reverse the current trend. Governments and nongovernment organizations take the initiative. They hold workshops to demonstrate how people can make a difference. They listen to the people and help local groups to respond to local challenges. Together, they undertake model projects that demonstrate how it will be possible to live differently. They model different ways of thinking and through living the changes show that it is possible to balance individual and collective interests, because we are not selfish nor are we unable to create alternative ways of governing at a regional level.[36]

2.9.3.3 Sustainable Future Scenario

We live in an environment that can support this generation and the next. Housing is affordable and made of sustainable materials. We have faced up to the convergent social, economic and environmental challenges and we are resilient, because we live in clusters of homes, share rain tanks and solar grids that are subsidised by local governments. Our living and working areas are powered by alternative energy. The new status symbol is the environmentally friendly lifestyle. Public transport is green. The green economy supports a vibrant job market spurred by subsidies to enable packaging goods, housing people, transporting people and educating and entertaining the public. The carbon economy is replaced through innovative inventions. All members of the public are encouraged to share their experiences and ideas for living sustainably. The future's market has been reconstructed to take into account the air, water and earth we need to grow organic, safe food. We have thought carefully about the implications of treating people, animals and the land as commodities and we strive to care for ourselves, others (including the voiceless) and the land.

[36] The detailed scenario is as follows: People make annual progress towards goals which they meet for the benefit of their children and grandchildren. But they do not move quite fast enough. People of all ages and from all walks of life who are able to 'join up the dots' could help to motivate cultural transformation towards a better future. They are motivated by concerns for others and the environment and are becoming increasingly less selfish and more concerned about the common good. They empathize with others. Local governments and nongovernment organizations take the initiative. We hold workshops to demonstrate how people can make a difference. We listen to the people and help local groups to respond to local challenges. Together, we undertake model projects that demonstrate how it will be possible to live differently. We model different ways of thinking and through 'living the changes'. We show that it is possible to balance individual and collective interests, because we are unselfish nor are we unable to create alternative ways of governing at a regional level.

The idea is to use the scenarios as starting points to explore ways to enable people to live healthy, happy ethical lives that are not at the expense of others or the next generation of life. The scenarios are for Australia and we need scenarios from other parts of the world that reflect social, cultural, political, economic and environmental diversity.[37]

---

[37] The detailed scenario is as follows:

A best-case scenario: an inclusive, creative society that balances individual and collective interests

We live in an environment that can support this generation and the next. Women, children and men have a say in local public agoras. Some wish to attend the face-to-face meetings in the local town hall. Others log on to the website to follow the debates and to add their own ideas (using freely available software such as this software). The summaries of ideas update automatically and are shared horizontally with other local governments and with the state government who in turn shares the findings at joint meetings spanning all the states in Australia. These findings are shared by local government representatives at a regional forum every 3 months which is held to address quality-of-life concerns are being met in a timely, transparent manner. Quality of life is defined in terms of social, economic and environmental indicators by the people in terms of what works, why and how. Housing is affordable and made of sustainable materials. We have faced up to the convergent social, economic and environmental challenges and we are resilient, because we live in clusters of homes. We share rain tanks and solar grids that are subsidised by local governments. Poor local governments and rich local governments form twinning arrangements to support each other. No one in our community is homeless, because those who are ill or unable to work are assisted in community housing where they make a contribution in many different ways to public projects spanning home construction, food production, repairs, art projects and recycling materials. Our living and working areas are powered by alternative energy. The new status symbol is the environmentally friendly lifestyle. Public transport is green. Off-road vehicles are used only when appropriate. The green economy supports a vibrant job market spurred by subsidies to enable packaging goods, housing people, transporting people and educating and entertaining the public. The carbon economy is replaced through innovative inventions. All members of the public are encouraged to share their experiences and ideas for living sustainably. The future's market has been reconstructed to take into account stocks for the future, such as the air, water and earth we need to grow organic, safe food. People develop new economies and new trading systems that enable them to have time to enjoy many activities. The clothes and shoes we wear are made of renewable resources. The windmill and fabric shoes are the new chic! People understand that their carbon basket can be stretched further by growing their own veggies. Most waste is recycled locally and used for building or composting. Packaging is designed to ensure that waste is minimal. Animals live in a carefully monitored environment to ensure their quality of life and ours. We are better off because we respect ourselves, one another and a biologically diverse environment. Bird flu, swine flu and bovine disease are unheard of in this scenario, because governance standards for animal husbandry and farming are monitored and applied (Horvath and Odor 2010; the Union after and International Commission on the Future of Food and Agriculture 2007). We no longer take too many antibiotics, because we take time to recover from illnesses. We live in harmony with the people of our region and our economy prospers through being able to work in one another's countries. We learn many languages. We are enriched by the diversity of language and culture. We are free and diverse in our neighbourhood, subnational region and supranational region, to the extent that our freedom does not undermine the freedom of others. Each local area enables each resident to be heard. The concerns that they raise about living in the hills or on the plains or near the coast are given careful consideration when making complex policy and planning decisions. Community networks are formed to enable people to discuss their fears about bush fires, drought and the inundation of coastal properties. People who are worried or stressed are able to access specific services to address their mental health needs and their practical concerns about building regulations and

The software linked with this project is at https://socsci.flinders.edu.au/fippm/pathways_lg/.

Log in at wellbeing.csem.flinders.edu.au:

This is just one of the ways to enable participation—and we are studying the extent to which it is useful and relevant. It is free ware and can be used by anyone, anywhere in the world. It is in the pilot stage—so we value your ideas and criticisms—if using software appeals to you. Most importantly, if you are not keen to use software—then please just blog or email your responses to me at janet.mcintyre@flinders.edu.au.

Please remember this is a public space and any details that are lodged here are public. If you use the software or if you email me then the details will be confidential. The ethics form for this project is available on the project site or I will send to you the form by email on request.

For Those Who Like to Engage Online Please see the attached set of slides that explain how to use the software. The idea is to enable people to scale up participation at a local and regional level, in order to make careful use of resources and to ensure that we live healthy, happy lives that are not at the expense of others. The software is freeware and can be used by anyone. It is in the pilot stage—so we value your ideas and criticisms.

For Those Who Prefer Email Participants were invited to email their responses to us, if they did not feel confident using the software:

Pro Forma to Fill Out

- What is your age?
- Gender?
- Level of education (primary, secondary, tertiary)?
- Employment status (employed, unemployed, retired)?

---

the safety of their neighbourhood. The ideas of local people are scaled up through interactive democracy and governance software. People have a say in ensuring social and environmental justice. We are happy and creative, because we have time to sleep, make slow food, talk to our neighbours, work in communal gardens, irrigated by water harvested and saved in many ways. We have green parks where the trees look healthy because they thrive on grey water. We play sport and express ourselves in a range of art forms. We have hope for the future. We do not commute long distances to work. We teleport to virtual communal areas and congregate in streets. We have technology that is inexpensive. Our desire for recognition and status is supported through being rewarded for innovation that supports the next generation by living in ways that not only sustain, but regenerate resources. We live not only for ourselves but also for others and the environment. We understand and remember what the first nations have taught us that we are the land and we are the earth to which we return. We base our decisions on an expanded form of pragmatism based on thinking about the consequences for our own family and neighbours and also for the next generation of life. We understand that what we do to others and to the environment, we do to ourselves.

- How many people live in your household?
- What is your place of birth (Australia (post code), Africa, Asia, Europe, North America, South America, Pacific Islands, Other)?
- Are you Aboriginal/Torres Strait/non-Aboriginal?
- What is your religious affiliation (Aboriginality, Agnostic, Atheist, Baha'i, Buddhist, Christian, Hinduism, Islamic, Jewish, Jainism, Sikhism, Spiritualism, Taoism, Other)?

Please think about your own life in terms of the consequences of these choices, for example:

I have the following things in my life—understanding of human rights, respect for biodiversity, fear for the future/hope for the future, a confidence, or lack of confidence, loss of home due to natural or other disaster, no family/community support, responsibility to care for others and very high levels of stress.
My own story is:
I need in my life—a home, a sense of safety, a place near public transport and hope for the future.
My own story is:
I will add to my life—more community supports from a range of services and/or more community engagement to lobby for resources, more connection to nature.
My own story is:
I will discard from my life—a sense of hopelessness, a sense of entitlement, excessive consumption.
My own story is:
Self-reflection on *the turning points* for better or worse—hope that consumption can be replaced with greater sense of attachment to others and the environment.
My own story is:
Consideration of the barriers that currently exist and consideration of what could be done to transform society and our relationship to the environment.
My own story is.

The results can be displayed in excel sheets and by means of word queries to cross-tabulate concepts such as:

Independent variables:

- Age
- Gender
- Level of education (primary, secondary, tertiary)
- Employment status (employed, unemployed, retired)
- Number of dependent children
- Number of dependent elderly
- Place of birth (Australia (post code), Africa, Asia, Europe, North America, South America, Pacific Islands, Other)
- Aboriginal/Torres Strait/non-Aboriginal
- Religious affiliation (Aboriginality, Agnostic, Atheist, Baha'i, Buddhist, Christian, Hinduism, Islamic, Jewish, Jainism, Sikhism, Spiritualism, Taoism, Other)

X:

The following systemically linked variables:

- Scenario with which they identify: A (business as usual), B (small adjustments for the long haul) and C (sustainable futures)
- Social, economic and environmental factors drawn from what participants consider that they have in their lives (material and non-material resources that make them resilient)
- Social, economic and environmental factors drawn from what participants consider they need (resources to enhance their lives):
- What they wish to add
- What they wish to discard
- Turning points for better or worse
- Barriers
- Services and actions

The extent to which demographic variables (age, gender, level of education, place of birth, home language, Aboriginal/non-Aboriginal, religious affiliation, type of occupation or employment status) make a difference to:

- With which scenario they identify
- What they perceive they need to *add to* their lives to make a difference to mitigating or adapting to climate change
- What they perceive they need to *discard* from their lives to make a difference to mitigating or adapting to climate change
- What they perceive are the *turning points* for better or worse, what the barriers are and what services make a difference

Telling a story and thinking about what we have and what we need and what we are prepared to add or discard from life is part of stepping into another conceptual space.[38] The evaluation of the level of importance of multiple and a simultaneously important issue is important by reflecting on one's life in terms of different scenarios and the consequences of these choices, for example:

I have the following things in my life—understanding of human rights, respect for biodiversity, fear for the future/hope for the future, a confidence, or lack of confidence, loss of home due to natural or other disaster, no family/community support, responsibility to care for others and very high levels of stress.

I need in my life—a home, a sense of safety, a place near public transport and hope for the future.

I will add to my life—more community supports from a range of services and/or more community engagement to lobby for resources, more connection to nature.

I will discard from my life—a sense of hopelessness, a sense of entitlement and excessive consumption.

Self-reflection on *the turning points* for better or worse—hope that consumption can be replaced with greater sense of attachment to others and the environment.

Consideration of the barriers that currently exist and consideration of what could be done to transform society and our relationship to the environment.

[38] This needs to be a therapeutic process and cannot be rushed. The time taken is part of the emotional connection with a different *way of being*. It involves thinking about being a different person. It is the same kind of process as taking an oath or making a vow (Collins 2004), or entering into a contract to undertake certain actions.

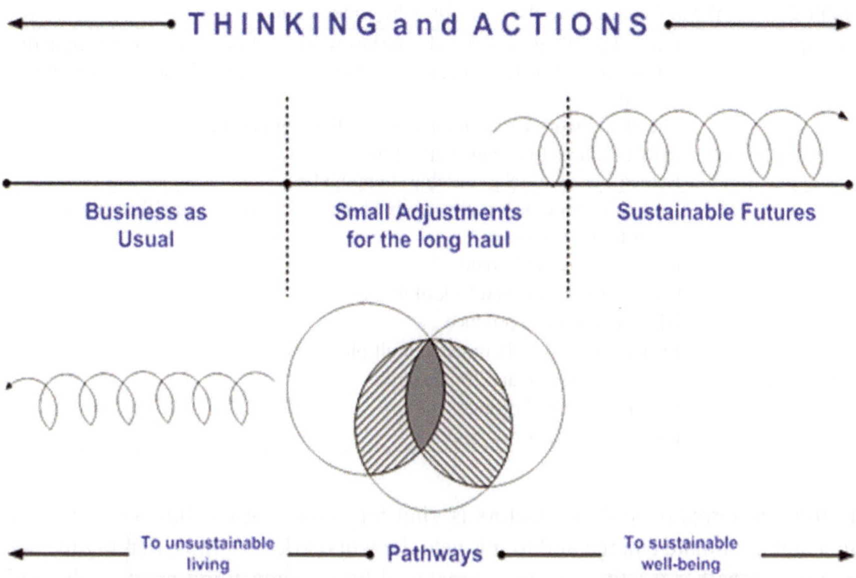

Fig. 2.1 Conceptualisation of the continuum of praxis from business as usual to sustainable futures

Typological characteristics

'Business as usual' is characterized by the perception that: (a) physical space is segregated, whereas (b) conceptual spaces are individualistic and competitive. Typically, informants stress that 'time is money' and life is considered to be stressful and competitive. Adaptation is through increased expenditure and technological innovation, rather than a willingness to give up their standard of living (Fig. 2.1).

Small steps towards sustainability are characterized by: (a) making more use of energy-efficient appliances and cars and a 'less is more' approach to living elegantly and ethically. At the time this report was written, the responses from participants about what they perceived to be positive about their quality of life (Nussbaum and Sen 1993) are shown in Table 2.2.

Sustainable living extends *the less is more* approach to supporting wellbeing for this generation and the next by *being the change*. Those without the means to install new technology stressed the need to provide subsidies and for building codes to ensure the quality of accommodation for all. Those who rent and are unable to afford to purchase their own homes are at a disadvantage. Few fit into the ideal of sustainable living. But the overlaps across all three include a willingness to save energy and water—driven by price, fines and user standards that are determined by the public sector. Installing energy-saving devices and expenditure on new technology is the main way in which the groups who favour business as usual adapt to rising temperatures and the rise in energy prices. Small adjustments are characterized by being prepared to make material changes if they can afford to do so. Capability

Table 2.2 Highlighted concerns as the basis for policy intervention

Social	Lack of public transport and poor bus service—buses not running regularly
	Cannot discard petrol car, less time to pursue interests if cannot take car to work
	Social and work commitments make slow living difficult
	Unwillingness to change way of life
	Remembering to take reusable shopping bags
	Loss of inspiration, apathy, doubt about ability to make a difference, People 'bringing you down'
Economic	Unwillingness and greed
	Cost of adaptation and lack of money
	High cost of local produce
	Lack of time to walk or catch multiple buses
Environmental	Native vegetation and fire hazards
	Extreme heat and drought
	Lack of time to grow food

to think in terms of multiple factors is vital for enhancing our human capabilities to adapt to climate change and to mitigate the worst effects—thus, making us more resilient, whether we live in areas threatened by drought, flood or other dramatic climate change events.

2.10 Findings: Cultural Ambivalence

In the first instance, the data are analysed according to how each informant wishes to live. The majority think that they are living sustainably or are prepared to 'make small adjustments for the long haul.' The factors include the material and non-material conditions that each informant perceives that they have *or need,* in order to experience a sense of wellbeing and so-called quality of life and that they are willing to *add or discard* from their lives, in order to enhance their quality of life in the future and the conditions that they consider to be *turning points for better and worse.*

The challenge is that most participants seem to combine a range of thinking and actions, some of which lead them towards sustainable living and some of which are unsustainable. Only a minority of respondents have chosen 'business as usual' as their preferred way of life. But a running list of those who have refused to participate indicates that a willingness to engage is also indicative of openness to change. Furthermore, once the actual choices are analysed in terms of what they are prepared to do to make a difference, it is clear that the majority are clustered closer to the midpoint in the continuum. This is because so many of the small actions such as recycling, etc. are counterbalanced by the other choices made. Nevertheless, with the increasing direct and associated costs associated with the use of energy and water will mean that local living will have increased benefits.

The savings associated with living locally, engaging in local food production, sharing the resources and developing local recreation and volunteering opportunities

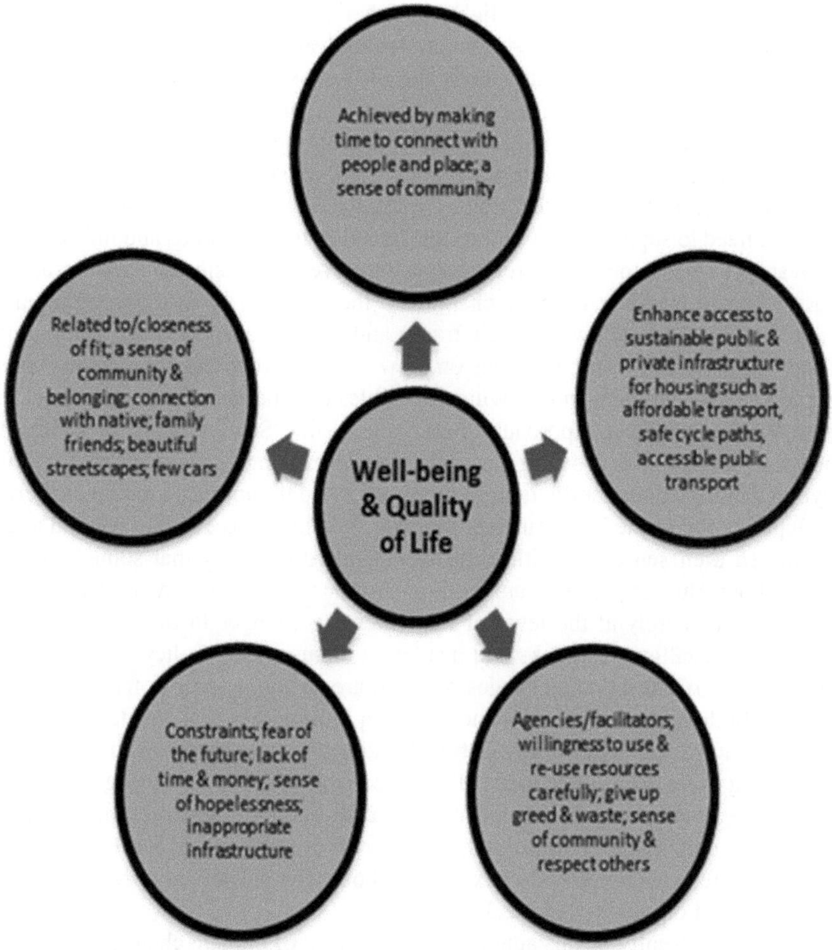
Achieved by making time to connect with people and place; a sense of community
Related to/closeness of fit; a sense of community & belonging; connection with native; family friends; beautiful streetscapes; few cars
Well-being & Quality of Life
Enhance access to sustainable public & private infrastructure for housing such as affordable transport, safe cycle paths, accessible public transport
Constraints; fear of the future; lack of time & money; sense of hopelessness; inappropriate infrastructure
Agencies/facilitators; willingness to use & re-use resources carefully; give up greed & waste; sense of community & respect others

Fig. 2.2 Interrelationships that support wellbeing and quality life

will make investment of time in the community more attractive. For more wide-ranging changes to occur, there will need to be transformations that are driven from below and above (Fig. 2.2).

To date, a preliminary analysis of the factors shows that the following are the most frequently mentioned non-material responses to change: water conservation through introduction of rain tanks, installing solar panels and using air conditioning more responsibly. But the cost of making these changes are a barrier for some. Only those who are in full-time employment or with access to capital are able to make these changes. The more affordable options are using public transport more frequently and walking or cycling. The barriers are lack of time to spend waiting for public transport and concerns about safety—due to inadequate pathways for cycling or walking and inadequate public lighting. Other non-material changes are community-based gardening and home-based gardening leading to the sharing of produce. For some, this is about growing seeds and also transforming people's attitudes to one another and the earth. In the process of engaging in community gardening, they learn to share and to grow more connections with the land and one another. The keeping of livestock on a small scale was raised, in Middleville, a suburban area, but bylaws will need reconsideration in Middleville. The state needs to be persuaded of the need to support changes through subsidies to households and incentives to innovators in all sectors. More regulations that give market signals need to support those who are prepared to make changes to their homes, or who are prepared to make use of public walkways, cycle tracks and public transport. Their community gardening philosophy and emphasis on slow transport (cycling and walking), getting to know neighbours and growing vegetables together has made a tangible step towards a 'less is more' approach to community life. Some emphasize wellbeing changes—a lifestyle of growing local food and developing greater concern for those beyond the immediate family to include the wider community and global concerns. An appreciation of the importance of kindness to others was emphasized and a few questioned their sense of entitlement to a standard of living that some can only dream about. But the predominant cultural shift or 'habitus' or way of being (Bourdieu 1977) is merely at the level of implementing changes to the housing stock, in terms of installing rain tanks and insulation or suggesting policy changes to infrastructure. To sum up, the changes required are social in order to free up time to spend on building the community and fostering links with others, the desire to build a creative, active and renewable lifestyle through growing vegetables, living locally and relying more on local produce. The processing of rubbish, reusing, recycling, growing vegetables, making compost and sharing community harvest are the basis for growing community in Middleville. A future is possible where local, sustainable living is a lifestyle choice will coexist with those who are forced to remain in one area as a result of poverty (Fig. 2.3).

Adaptation usually means adapting to *the effects* of climate change at the local level, which requires awareness, whereas mitigation usually means responding *to the causes* through changing policy on emissions. But the latter requires adaptive responses to new policy and governance requirements. Adaptation is through reducing the effects of emissions through spending money or living differently, whereas responding to heat, for example, involves installing air conditioning. Adaptation to fires requires changing designs for living and our expectations about consumption and the commodification of life. For example, in the words of an informant: 'Even taking out the rubbish is a spiritual matter.' He explained that sorting out the rubbish carefully is a matter of respecting others and the environment. A strong sense of community is also displayed by the organizers of the community garden and the Opportunity Shop linked to St Middleville's Church. The notion of reusing and recycling is demonstrated in the way in which all waste is recycled from the community op show. All items that are not sold are sent to Statewide Cleaning Cloths, Australia. Surplus is also sent to the 'Anglicare NGO or to Korea and Africa'. This contrasts with the exasperation expressed by some informants who said that

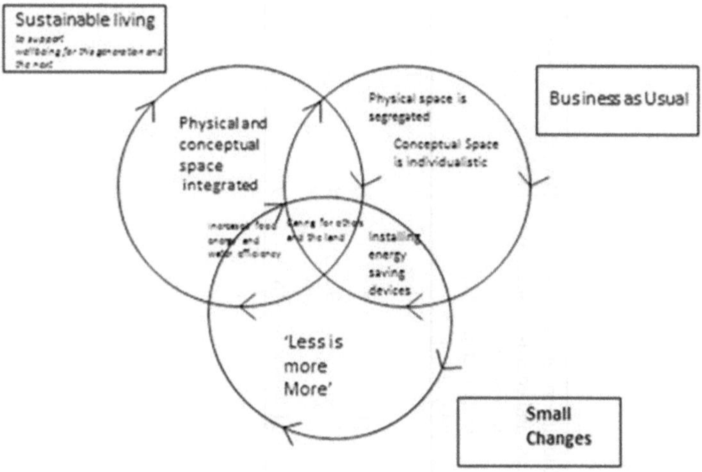

Fig. 2.3 Overlaps and turning points for better or worse

'Climate change is natural' but 'we do care about the environment.' Clearly, the politicization of the carbon tax that became official on 1 July 2012 played out in the federal election. This research strives to make a contribution to gathering data on perceptions that can be summarized without losing the fine-grained detail and the emotions of what people are saying. It is vital to be able to gather large data sets on perceptions if policy engagement and community education is to be achieved. Clearly, the desire to engage more in the community and to have more spare time is shared by the majority of participants. Energy awareness does not however translate into a willingness to change greed and wasteful habits. Poverty was considered a barrier by those without financial security or facing poverty. The weightings given to perceptions were obtained by analysing data from a matrix spanning the following snapshot of factors downloaded from the publicly accessible software in June: For example, these are the findings on 1/07/2012, but the research is ongoing and the data set continues to grow as it is extended (Table 2.3).

Sustainable living extends *the less is more* approach to supporting wellbeing for this generation and the next by *being the change*. Physical and conceptual space is considered to be integrated. Time is perceived to be constructed as 'we are the land'. Those without the means to install new technology stressed the need to provide subsidies and for building codes to ensure the quality of accommodation for all. Those who rent and are unable to afford to purchase their own homes are at a disadvantage. Few fit into the ideal of sustainable living. But the overlaps across all three include a willingness to save energy and water—driven by price, fines and user standards that are determined by the public sector. Installing energy-saving devices and expenditure on new technology is the main way in which the groups who favour business as usual adapt to rising temperatures and the rise in energy prices. Small adjustments are characterized by being prepared to make material changes if they can afford to

Table 2.3 Weightings of perceived areas of concern based on the number of responses per category

	Social inclusion needs + turning point	Less waste and more recycling needs and turning point	Energy awareness as a need or turning point	Financial and job security as a basis for change	Greed and Waste habits as a barrier	Spare time	Sustainable transport as a need	Information and education on climate change adaptation	Food security	Poverty as barrier	Housing quality
Business as usual	9	2	7	8	1	2	0	3	0	1	1
Small changes	9	6	28	4	3	7	5	11	7	0	1
Sustainable future	63	23	52	17	16	35	20	7	9	8	11
Total	81	31	87	29	20	44	25	21	16	9	13

do so. Capability to think in terms of multiple factors is vital for enhancing our human capabilities to adapt to climate change and to mitigate the worst effects—thus, making us more resilient, whether we live in areas threatened by drought, flood or other dramatic climate change events.

2.11 Future Policy and Research Direction to Address Representation, Accountability and Sustainability

The majority of suburban participants in this local study made partial changes, rather than embracing a post-materialist lifestyle and the costs associated with implementing it. The local prefiguring project will have little potential unless it is scaled up through other organizations in Adelaide and through other participating local governments. Simultaneously, the testing and engagement is being extended through working with a network of colleagues, current and past PhD graduates. The findings will be shared iteratively with the other groups, using the Delphi technique to build a sense of overlaps and differences. Organizations such as 350.org[39] could be used to share the free software and by linking, for example, the work of PhD students and graduates on the relevance of critical systemic thinking. Cultural narratives that foster sustainability are a starting point for democratic transition. But narratives that remain untranslated into equitable governance destroy trust and lead to cynicism. We welcome the opportunity to work with you to continue the research.

The research attempts to develop the case for monitory democracy and participatory governance people to develop a wider sense of responsibility for the environment within and beyond their neighbourhood.

The software is in the process of being piloted to make it more intuitive for those who are not so computer literate. It needs to be used in ways to complement other forms of engagement for planning and to respond to user's needs and not only those engaged in governance or policymaking. In a discussion on the research at a workshop on the 10th of August, 2012, the following points were made by a diverse group of participants spanning diverse beliefs and cultural experiences in Australia, Indonesia Africa and Europe.

B.W., an Aboriginal mentor for the research, made the central point that dependency on the land needs to be recognized as a key determinant of policy decisions. Human beings are not dependent on city infrastructure in the final instance. This

[39] 'In the end, everyone needs to remember that the goal at Copenhagen was not to get a "victory," not to sign an agreement. It's to actually take steps commensurate with the problem. And those steps are dictated, in the end, by science. This negotiation, on the surface, is between America and China and the EU and India and the developing world; between industry and environmentalists; between old and new technology. But at root the real negotiation is between human beings on the one hand, and physics and chemistry on the other. Physics and chemistry have laid their cards on the table: above 350 the world doesn't work. They are not going to negotiate further. It's up to us to figure out, this year and in the years ahead, how to meet their bottom line.' http://www.350.org/en/understanding-350#4, accessed 10/04/2012.

dependent relationship has been understood by Aboriginal Australians prior to colonisation.

B.D. But denial is a problem, how do we address denial? How do we enhance engagement? People who deny there is a problem—such as the effects of climate change—generally do not wish to be engaged, but they are the people with whom we most wish to engage. It is a case of anticipating what interests them, in order to draw them into the conversation and to make it relevant. That raises the question of whether incentives are needed, what forms those may take and how acceptable they may be to what we are doing.

J.M. I agree, but we also need to acknowledge that we are 'consuming the land to excess'. We need to address the risks urgently and the problem is that people do not necessarily change unless they realize that they have no other choice. Research on complex needs with "long term" alcoholics (recovering from addiction) highlighted that people only stopped being addicted when they faced up to the fact that if they continued their way of life that they would not survive. The tipping point has been reached. Long-term addicts talk of "hitting the wall" or hitting rock bottom and realising that the only way to address their approach to consumption is to change their lives. Similarly, the risks associated with change in temperatures and weather patterns are such that it will affect our food, energy and water supplies.

We also need to remember that we are dependent on our neighbours in Australia and within the Asia Pacific region to secure food, energy, water and safety.'

A.M.S. stressed that people need to engage in dialogue to understand one another better and to cocreate shared meanings of how we should live together within the region by getting to know one another. He discussed (after the meeting) the difficulties faced by those with different views on the Muslim faith and said that moderate viewpoints need to be fostered through engagement and the development of integrated curricula.

J. highlighted that we need to be thinking about ways to address the risks—energy, water, food and how we will work together to achieve shared goals.

P. D. stressed that the core point is 'a change of heart'. This is necessary to foster sustainable wellbeing. We forget that we are dependent on the land and that without bees our food security is under threat. Decisions need to ensure that ecological land value is placed foremost in decisions when undertaking urban planning. Our relationships with the resources that sustain us are critical to the long-term viability of our cities if we are going to learn from the past demise of great civilizations. Cities can only exist in harmony with the land on which they are dependent. A shared understanding of value, outside our current economic financial status symbols, that redefines our economic systems, will drive a different paradigm of engagement with our neighbours and our environment. When the value of shares is based on TBL (Elkington 1992, 1997) outcomes rather than straight financial return, we will know that our fundamental economics of our system have changed.

B.W.: In the Southern Region (of Adelaide), partnerships have been created with Aboriginal people to achieve better wellbeing outcomes. The challenge is to match services to complex needs, but to realize that the final determinant of decisions is 'how sustainable is this for the land?'

J.M: Nation states are becoming increasingly diverse and it is important to meet diverse needs of people irrespective of age, culture, gender, level of income or where they live. People in some geographical areas face particular risks, as the droughts and bushfires and floods have demonstrated in recent times.

B.D. stressed that people were making passionate comments and that emotions play a central role in decisions. The project allows for people to express their own perceptions (which may be diametrically opposed to others' perceptions) so that their ideas are not lost in the engagement process.

D.H.: Some of the decisions to address challenges such as water shortages such as the de-salination plant are not sustainable. We could have made better use of storm water and given more support for rain tanks and rain catchment for example.

N.F. made the point that some of the infrastructural changes made in Middleville such as installing solar panels have been undertaken, because it is a way to cut living costs and perhaps to earn money by returning power to the grid. It is not necessarily a change of heart towards the environment.

V.L. added that alternative power supplies like wind farms can be subject to community choices—for example, in the Goyder council area wind farms that were supported initially but are not going to go ahead because of community concerns that the noise will be bad for health. Communities and individuals sometimes have the dilemma of philosophically agreeing with sustainable practices, but there is a limit if concerns about health impacts are involved. This issue is clouded by legislation which has set separation distance limits (in this case, 1 km but which the people living in the area think is not far enough away).[40]

J. M: Legislation will need to balance the needs of local people with the overall need to reduce the size of our carbon footprint. So perhaps people will need to live within a safe distance from the turbines. If the distance is supported by credible research, then this will need to be applied as a national law to protect and balance the individual rights and the collective good.

D. H.: Laws should teach people the right choices to make. For example, parking fines teach people to make responsible choices. Smoking legislation or wearing seat belts has led to changed behaviour and then changes in values follow.

J.M.: Yes, the 'big brother' threat is one to worry about, but we need laws in a democracy to ensure that people do the right thing. The trouble is that in democracies some people are now more interested in their own rights than their responsibilities.

J.M.B. stressed that social justice needs to be supported by the law—we do not have democracies without the rule of law. He based his comments on the basis of his doctoral research in the DRC and his work in a social justice in Australia.

[40] The politics associated with the approval of wind farms may be driven less by concerns for the wellbeing of the residents and have more to do with the politics of the so-called coal base load, as suggested by Tim Flannery (2012, p 29). The argument is that wind farms cannot provide adequate amounts of base load energy for a functional economy and household usage. The planning permission for wind farms is also required in Victoria. http://www.dpcd.vic.gov.au/planning/planningapplications/moreinformation/windenergy. According to Friends of the Earth, the planning permits undermine the renewable energy industry (see http://melbourne.foe.org.au/?q=node/1007 Accessed 20/01/2014).

Many of the social, economic and environmental policy choices that have been made in Middleville achieve only small overall steps towards wellbeing. This is an upper middle class community, but the approach to sustainability is still middle of the road. The major shifts are in terms of material infrastructural changes by those who can afford them. But steps towards sustainable living is demonstrated by those who foster community organic gardening, share the community harvest, recycle resources, volunteer time to help and include others and use public transport or bikes. Some understand the importance of living sustainably but they stressed that time was one of the most important determinants in living slow, community-oriented lives. If 'time is money', people tend to become more selfish and concerned with personal, rather than community, needs.

The 'small is beautiful' philosophy of Schumacher resonates with the notion of caretaking stressed by Aboriginal Australians. As populations increase in size, compete for scarce resources and emphasize 'time is money' in a fast carbon-based economy, we are at risk of forgetting our dependency on the land.

Existential risk is ignored by politicians, but also by the majority of research projects that do not 'join up the dots'. The loss of species to pollinate plants and the degradation of soil could lead to a grim future. The prospect of a Dubai-type urban landscape where the elites live in digitally controlled, secure-gated communities and the rest live outside in the wastelands is already on the horizon—unless we reconsider how we ought to live. This project is not merely about looking at current risks to wellbeing—it is about exploring a way to do things differently. Cosmopolitan rights and responsibilities have been stressed by David Held and Ulrich Beck who stress the boomerang effect of poverty, pollution and a carbon-based economy on this generation of life and the next. Sir Nicholas Stern has stressed that we need to make changes now to reframing economics.

Strengths The software works as a prototype. It enables people to think about whether they identify with:

- Business as usual.
- Small changes.
- Sustainable living that support wellbeing now and in the future.

It also enables people to rank what they have in their lives to support wellbeing and what they need to make their lives better in terms of quality of life and wellbeing. Each of the items needs to be thought in sequential terms so people get a sense of the consequences of having, for example, a large status-symbol car that guzzles fuel or a large, badly insulated home and to give each item a weighting.

Then people are asked to consider what they need to help them improve their lives. These items also need to be thought through in sequential terms so people get a sense of the consequences of using a more energy-efficient vehicle or using public transport.

People are prompted to think through what they are prepared to add or to discard. Linked with this process are services to help them achieve their perceived needs.

Then they are asked to think through turning points for better or worse, the barriers and they are able to print out their own report.

The benefit is that people are able to add concepts to an ever-growing list of social, economic and environmental indicators of wellbeing.

The administrators are able to summarize the data on excel sheets.

Weaknesses Whilst the software is robust, it is not sufficiently intuitive as yet. The identified weaknesses are iteratively tested by members of the team with volunteers with varying levels of skills.

Some participants will never engage online, but the software needs to be as easy to use as possible on as many forms of computers, iPads and iPhones as possible. Or to enable people to engage face to face in groups and then to share ideas with the facilitator who loads the data, or to merely fill in the email online. Current forms of democracy and governance need to enable more engagement with diverse people and to enable people to think not only about rights but also about their responsibilities to enhance their own resilience and to adapt to risks within their neighbourhood and the wider national and post-national region in which they live.

Opportunities The long-term policy aim is to extend the testing of the research in post-national regional biospheres. The open democracy forum was the starting point for research. The local and regional scorecards could be developed by scaling up the process to respond to social, economic and environmental needs.

Dialogue helps to explore one argument and an opposing argument and to try to achieve a synthesis or weaving together of ideas. By telling and listening to stories, we are capable of unfolding values and emotions whilst 'sweeping in' the social, cultural, political and environmental context. As West Churchman reminds us, decisions are based on what we include or exclude, whether to say yes or no. But openness to change needs to be based on constant reviewing, rather than merely unfreezing and refreezing as Lewin suggested (Schein 1996).

Threats People tend to deal with information or fear through denial. McLuhan and Powers (1989) expressed reservations about the ability of people to override the sense of overload as a result of exposure to images and information by cutting off from the world. But with increasing exposure to a sense of global issues through a range of media not only the elite global knowledge workers have a sense of being global citizens.

2.12 Systemic Praxis to Protect Regional Biospheres

Planetary wellbeing: Meeting challenges begins with monitory democracy and governance at the local level to ensure greater equity across households. One way to implement this is to develop traditional strategic plan based on indicators. Policy contradictions result from an inability to think critically and systemically. They are evident in the following seven primary areas of focus for action. But the problem with undertaking research based on linear approaches is that it can lead to the following sorts of lists, that contain within them contradictions that are not acknowledged in the report entitled: 'Strategic New Directions for South Australia' which stresses the need for the following:

> Clean, green food industry, the mining boom and its benefits, Advanced manufacturing, A vibrant city, Safe and active neighbourhoods, Affordable living, and Early childhood.

In South Australia, the use of uranium to bolster the state economy contradicts with the idea of a sustainable clean green food industry. How will water supplies remain uncontaminated? Where will nuclear waste be stored? Does the idea that new forms of nuclear power generation will reduce waste provide little long-term security?[41] It also does not take into account the implications of the 'two-speed' economy in which those who are employed in this sector contrast with those who are in agriculture or manufacturing.[42] The social contract (limited to voters within the nation state) is now in jeopardy as a result of trying to sustain the unsustainable. Space, time and our relationships to one another, the land and future generations are in need of reconceptualisation. It does not require learning new lessons—merely remembering the lessons from people who live more closely with the land.

Meeting the needs of a burgeoning region will become increasingly challenging. Wellbeing requires seeing ourselves as one of many species in biospheres. This has implications for identity, ethics and governance. Local identities are increasingly global in their connections but remain somewhat ambivalent to the extent to which they have cosmopolitan loyalties and affinities.

Australia is part of a broader region. Nation states face social, economic and environmental challenges. Indonesia has 17,000 islands and a population of over 250 million of which 43.7% are under the age of 25 years.[43]

2.12.1 Recognition of Vulnerability and Interconnectedness

The need for new forms of good governance that address regional biospheres and that involve multilevel and multi-agency approaches to governance is becoming

[41] The recent revelations about the Fukushima disaster highlight the importance of monitory democracy and the need to think systemically. The Fukushima reactor could have been abandoned by the company and this could have released a chain of nuclear reactions. The governance directive for the company to take control and for workers to be sent in to maintain the reactor has resulted in containment. But the margin for error was so close that the lesson is not that the nuclear power option is safe. Alternative measures are preferable—even if the nuclear power option is used very cautiously to buy time for green economies and green technology to be implemented widely.

[42] Meeting the needs of a burgeoning region will become increasingly challenging. Wellbeing requires seeing ourselves as one of many species in biospheres. This has implications for identity, ethics and governance. Local identities are increasingly global in their connections but remain somewhat ambivalent to the extent to which they have cosmopolitan loyalties and affinities.

[43] http://www.indexmundi.com/indonesia/age_structure.html. Accessed 25 February 2014.

increasingly important. The UNDP 2013 report stresses the need for new forms of governance that span nation states and that enable greater transparency and cooperation.

The creation of the new Development Bank by the BRICS[44] nations is interesting in a context of the shift in the axis of power away from the west. The forum was set up in 2009 in response to the global financial crisis.[45]

Just as the axis of power and development in the West led to the founding of the World Bank after the Second World War to balance the influence of communist countries offering development, now the developing countries are in a position to offer aid as they move ahead of the old centrist powers. Smugness and complacency ought to be challenged by the window dressing of the flawed process of the top-down Millennium Goals.

Complicity denies the role of the privileged in creating and enabling the wicked problem of growth to the extent that it poses an 'existential risk' (Bostrom 2011) through undermining the social and natural fabric of life. Complicity—in the sense it is used in this book—means not appreciating the rights of future generations and the need for new configurations of identity.

The research detailed in 'Identity, Democracy and Sustainability' (McIntyre-Mills and De Vries 2011) and in this book explores the potential for participation supported by decision-making software to match services to need, mitigate the causes of risk and adapt to the consequences of climate change. It makes the case that the following are amongst the greatest challenges facing humanity and that they potentially pose an 'existential risk':

- Representation of the increasingly diverse populations within nation states,
- Accountability to ensure that resources are used fairly, equitably and sustainably and
- Engagement to enhance the capability of people to understand that attitudes towards consumption have profound implications for social and environmental justice issues.

We need to ensure that we remain open to the ideas of others in order to test out the consequences of our choices. Nation states will need to work together to address a common threat. If we hope to achieve conscious evolution and we do not wish to rely on chance, then we need to find ways to engage local people in thinking through the implications of their choices.

In democracies when the truth gets out, governments can be voted out and criminal sentences can be applied. In totalitarian states, threat and fear prevent the story

[44] BRICS countries set up new development banks. Brazil, Russia, India, China and South Africa met last week in Durban and discussed a 'new paradigm' for development. Guardian Weekly 5/04/2013

[45] It represents '43 % of the world's population and 17 % of trade.... Most analysts expect the bank to be dominated by China, whose economy is about 20 times the size of South Africa and 4 times as big as Russia's or India's...Brazil's president Dilma Rousseff, said the BRICS alliance has proved the doubters wrong...calling on the IMF and World Bank to become more democratic to reflect the growing influence of developing countries....'

from reaching the media or the courts. The question must be asked to what extent Western democracies have remained true to this mission? Unless governments are held to account by a monitory democracy, 'lying in politics' becomes a norm, not an exception.[46] The links between politics and research are also strong in democratic societies. Arendt stresses in her chapter 'Lying in Politics in Crises of the Republic' (Arendt 1969, pp 11–13) that democracies rely on manipulating the truth. Long before 'spin' became a topical term, Arendt links the role of researchers in propping up political agendas. According to Arendt (1969, p 12):

> Reasons aversion to contingency is strong: it was Hegel, the father of grandiose history schemes that philosophical contemplation has no other intention than to eliminate the accidental. Indeed much of the arsenal of political theory—game theory and systems analyses, the scenarios written for imagined 'audiences', and the careful enumeration of usually three options…whereby A and C represent the opposite extremes and B the logical middle of the road solution of the problem—has its source in this deep-seated aversion…. The kind of thinking that presents both A and C as undesirable, therefore settles on B, hardly serves any other purpose that to divert the mind and blunt the judgment for the multitude of real possibilities. What these problem solvers have in common with down to earth liars is the attempt to get rid of the facts and the confidence that this should be possible because of the inherent contingency of facts….

In response to the Vietnam War (1969, pp 17–19), Arendt writes about the way in which America tried to establish a reputation of power and leadership by examining the Pentagon papers; she stressed that the lengths they were willing to go should be a cause for alarm, rather than a cause for celebration from friends who could rely on USA. This is why the forthcoming book for the Contemporary Systems Series stresses a critical systemic approach, based on the concerns raised by West Churchman, but flows across a range of knowledge domains. The critical heuristics approach can be used to address the concerns about contingencies and the way in which different stakeholders see the world very differently and present different accounts of the truth.

Butler (2006), who holds the Hannah Arendt Professorship, stresses the continuum of ethical behaviour from those who chose to be sadistic and those who were coerced and prisoners to help maintain the functioning of the camps. The blurring of boundaries may be acceptable when giving an account or self-reflection, but drawing the line is necessary in law and being able to draw the line in one's own moral choices. Being open to critical self-reflection is always important. Maintaining this praxis is at the heart of being ethical.[47] The danger is that when giving an account

[46] 'Representative government is in crisis today, partly because it has lost, in the course of time, all institutions that permitted the citizens' actual participation, and partly because it is now gravely affected by the disease from which the party system suffers: bureaucratization and the two parties' tendency to represent nobody except the party machines' (Arendt 1972, p 89). We have forgotten the importance of cooperation and compassion as we engage in the feeding frenzy of eating our future.

[47] 'What is to give an Account of Oneself?' Public open lecture for the students of the European Graduate School EGS, Media and Communication Studies department program, Saas-Fee, Switzerland, Europe, 2006, Judith Butler. Uploaded on May 5, 2007. Political action and discourse are, in this respect, essential to the constitution of collective identities. http://www.egs.edu/ .

the truth can be distorted. Responsibility can be denied. This is where evidence needs to be brought to bear on a topic. The design of inquiring system allows this to occur through sweeping in a range of insights—empirical, historical and perceptive—in order to be accountable. This approach strives to enrich the testing of ideas through 'sweeping in' variables and unfolding values of diverse stakeholders guided by a 'design of inquiry' that is open to the knowledge and experience of others. The problem with operations research is that it sought to control humans and nature as human and natural resources for development. The mechanistic and systems-oriented approach however was not necessarily intended by West Churchman who understood the importance of human values when considering an area of concern. Thus, he called his approach an open systems approach and was open to criticism. For this reason, the starting point for this book is that design interventions need to become part of a way of life.

But in a cosmopolitan context, these need to be married together—whilst still providing space for diversity.

The ironical argument developed by Donna Haraway on the danger of essentialist identity categories in 'A Cyborg Manifesto' makes this point. In accepting our nonessentialism, it does not undermine Margaret Somerville's point on a sense of the sacred.[48] We can choose or ignore the sacred, depending on our will to power. Human beings can choose to rise above difficulties as did Victor Frankl (1955) who survived the atrocities of a prison of war camp by his capability of thinking about the future and by making sense or meaning out of what was going on around him. It was his choice to believe and not to be crushed. He discusses the importance of making meaning and on the ability of human beings to choose, because of their human spirit. This ability to show compassion and humanity is not however an entirely human capability nor should it be used as a terrible justification of being cruel to other species, just as being a member of a particular race was used as an excuse for racism or slavery. Frans de Waal, a primatologist, argues in *The Age of Empathy* that survival is based not only on competition but also on the ability to cooperate. Thus, emotions and not rationality also play a significant role in evolution and emergence. It thus provides a challenge for Dawkins who I argue confuses genes and dualism/digital either/or thinking as the basis for enlightenment and rationality. Knowledge is based on many ways of making sense, informed by all our senses—feeling, emotions and intuition are as important as sight, sound, touch, taste.

Human beings are not merely digital genes that switch on or off. They are able to respond to complexity in ways that are unique and based on their ability to think and feel. This perspective does not need to be essentialist in the sense used by Somerville and Frankl who consider this the essential difference between human beings and animals and that this gives human beings more rights than other sentient creatures.

---

[48] The competitive logic that plays out between human beings in competition for jobs and resources is unsustainable. We can evolve through cooperation. Competition is not the only basis for survival or the only basis for evolution as stressed by De Waal (2009) and discussed in: 'Identity, Democracy and Sustainability' (McIntyre-Mills and De Vries 2011).

Instead, I argue that appreciation of our connections with others can help us to emerge from our fixed identities and help us to recognize our interconnected rhizomatic connections.[49]

How can you blow the whistle if you do not have the right to a voice? This applies to asylum seekers. It also applies to those who are unprotected by the social contract, namely prisoners, young people, those who are disabled sentient beings who do not have a voice. We also need to be careful of philosophies that protect human beings without considering the continuum across all sentient creatures.

The local prefiguring project described in the first two chapters will have little potential unless the free software is scaled up through other organizations in Adelaide and through other participating local governments.

Cultural narratives that foster sustainability are a starting point for democratic transition. But narratives that remain untranslated into equitable governance destroy trust and lead to cynicism.

It is for this reason that the digital future needs to be shaped not only by the state military complex but also by those who wish to act as whistle-blowers. Members of the public need to be protected by a scaled-up version of the Aarhus Convention that gives residents within post-national regions the right to access information and the right to be heard by the state (1998; see McIntyre-Mills 2011); thus, this book (a) discusses the theory of participatory democracy—based on the principles of subsidiarity and Ashby's rule of requisite variety—and (b) makes a case for new forms of accountability to support regional governance that is capable of extending the social contract beyond the nation state and thus to protect biospheres and the diversity within them. The governance decisions will need to be upheld by rule of law based on the axiom that we can be free and diverse to the extent that freedom and democracy is not undermined (McIntyre-Mills et al. 2006).

We cannot wait for a cultural transformation—behavioural change needs to precede cultural values transformation. Laws and rules can lead to values transformation as people learn to conform to laws that will uphold rights and responsibilities. Regional scorecards can be developed that respond to social, economic and environmental needs and to the rankings people achieve along a continuum from 'business as usual' to small changes to living in ways that support wellbeing now and in the future.

---

[49] When human beings understood that the world is not flat, it is spherical; it had profound implications for explorers. When human beings understand that the universe is not finite or infinite, but instead, it is a continuum—perhaps a Mobius band that results in flux and flow. I am wading out of my depth, as I am not a physicist. The challenge of course is that political decisions must be decisive. So where do we draw the line and how? The answer is perhaps to ensure that the decisions are as inclusive as possible. Thus, diversity of thought is as important as biodiversity for human survival. See also the argument developed by Freeman Dyson, who anticipates the limitations of the digital and this explains why Dawkins (1976, 2006) is incorrect to argue that human beings are shaped by their genes. Dyson, F http://www.edge.org/3rd_culture/dyson_ad/dyson_ad_index.html, downloaded 11/3/2013. Dyson is professor of physics at the Institute for Advanced Study, in Princeton. His professional interests are in mathematics and astronomy. Among his many books are *Disturbing The Universe, Infinite in All Directions Origins of Life, From Eros To Gaia, Imagined Worlds, and The Sun, The Genome, And The Internet.*

Sustainability cannot be allowed to fall under the limitations of competitive nation states. The sovereign nation state has treated the planet as zero sum—when in fact the notion of externalities is quite wrong. Kantian personal ethics, public ethics (interstate) and cosmopolitan ethics need to be applied in overlapping regions that override zero-sum approaches. In order to achieve better forms of distributive governance, the mechanism is as follows—adapted form of Tuvalu test building on TBL accounting and accountability.[50]

People need to rank what they have in their lives to support wellbeing and what they need to make their lives better in terms of quality of life and wellbeing. This requires building 'stocks for the future'. This requires reframing not only economics but also our relationships to one another and the land. Stiglitz et al. (2011, p 15) use a multidimensional measure of wellbeing spanning:

> 1. Material living standards (income, consumption and wealth), 2. Health, 3. Education, 4. Personal activities including work, 5. Political voice and governance, 6. Social connections and relationships, 7. Environment (present and future conditions), 8. Insecurity, of an economy as well as a physical nature.

Each of the items people think about as relevant to their own wellbeing needs to be thought in sequential terms so people get a sense of the consequences of having, for example, a large status-symbol car that guzzles fuel or a large, badly insulated home and to give each item a weighting. Then people are asked to consider what they need to help them improve their lives. These items also need to be thought through in sequential terms so people get a sense of the consequences of using a more energy-efficient vehicle or using public transport. People are prompted to think through what they are prepared to add or to discard and how closely related the listed items of haves and needs are to achieving wellbeing. Linked with this process are services to help them achieve their perceived needs. Then they are asked to think through turning points for better or worse, the barriers and they are able to print out their own report. The benefit is that people are able to add concepts to an ever-growing list of social, economic and environmental indicators of wellbeing. The administrators are able to summarize the data on excel sheets.

[50] Please consider: what material and non-material things you have in life—positive and negative—such as rented accommodation, a mortgage, a supportive family, a job? What you need—a well-insulated home, a bicycle, access to public transport? What you could add/discard—exercise/costly vehicle? What are the positive and negative turning points—adding solar panels, learning more about sustainable gardening? What are the barriers—lack of motivation, lack of subsidies for green technology? What local government services can be used and in what combination? Each personal pathway to wellbeing can be printed out and kept for personal review and revised online. The aggregated data on the pathways could help service providers provide better responses to social, economic and environmental challenges. The data could build a statistical picture of socio-demographic perceived needs by diverse geographical areas spanning hills, plains and coastal areas. See https://socsci.flinders.edu.au/fippm/pathways_demo/ excel sheets by domain.

2.12.2 Outcomes of the Research

The research made use of many forms of engagement to help participants to consider the potential consequences of their choices. These approaches span narrative (to explore complexity and to enable a creative flow of ideas), dialogue and questioning to reformulate boundaries. Scenarios were also explored spanning 'business as usual', 'small steps towards a sustainable future' and achieving a sustainable future through building up 'wellbeing stocks' (Stiglitz et al. 2010).

Just as we cannot ignore externalities associated with profit, we cannot ignore the externalities of living life at the expense of others.[51] The challenge to move beyond the rhetoric of cosmopolitan citizenship and to address both justice and sovereignty. The nation state needs to be held to account by an Earth Charter that is supported by overlapping regional institutions (supported by inclusive regional research institutions, policies, the rule of law including parliaments and courts). The book discusses participatory action research to prefigure a means to hold the market to account—to ensure that the use of resources that are necessary for the common good are accessible and equitable. It explores the implications of developing localized living in regions that support appropriate technology and use solar or biofuels to run digital systems that monitor from below and enable alternative forms of democracy and governance based on the principles of subsidiarity (Schumacher 1973).

Some emphasize wellbeing changes—a lifestyle of growing local food and developing greater concern for those beyond the immediate family to include the wider community and global concerns. An appreciation of the importance of kindness to others was emphasized and a few questioned their sense of entitlement to a standard of living that some can only dream about. But the predominant cultural shift or 'habitus' or way of being (Bourdieu 1977) is merely at the level of implementing changes to the housing stock, in terms of installing rain tanks and insulation or suggesting policy changes.

Existential risk is ignored by politicians, but also by the majority of research projects that do not 'join up the dots'. Denial of the toxic effect of the way we live needs to be addressed. The addictive culture consumption is unsustainable and so enabling people to understand that decisions to support the mitigation and adaptation to climate change are rooted in enhancing wellbeing. Joseph Stiglitz, past president of the World Bank, has stressed (at the invitation of the Australian Productivity Commission) that the bottom line is wellbeing—this requires building *stocks for the future.* Wellbeing is crucial to redesigning economics. Encouraging

[51] These public interests include environmental considerations. Today, the decision to, for example, to use energy selfishly and excessively has implications for other communities who may be more affected by extreme weather events as a result of our choices. For example, we may choose to drive an SUV when it is unnecessary or when it is possible to walk to meet our friends. We may use water excessively for forms of agriculture that will have a downstream risk to other communities needs to be governed by laws that protect the common good. Furthermore, complex decisions need to be informed by those who will be affected by the decisions Ashby's rule of requisite variety (1956) to establish ways to enhance representation, accountability and engagement.

people to enjoy walking, making friends in their local community through community gardening and local sport helps to support slower more locally based lives. This requires wellbeing and sustainability decisions and reconsidering our democratic rights and responsibilities by using participatory engagement aimed to match services to needs—within limits—so that local communities make the best decisions that minimise social, economic and environmental risks and that shape 'policy from below' by enabling people to engage in a process of thinking about what *material and non-material* resources they have to support wellbeing, what they still need, what they are prepared to do to enhance their social, economic and environmental wellbeing, what they are prepared to discard and then to consider what they personally consider to be the social, economic and environmental turning points for better or worse.

They are also asked to consider the barriers that are experienced in achieving wellbeing. All their decisions are based on their own perceptions about material and non-material facets of their life.

The software updates as they add their new ideas and these help to inform others who see only the list of de-identified social, economic and environmental factors and the particular local resources that are available to assist them to move from (a) business as usual to (b) making small changes and (c) sustainable wellbeing.

The scenarios are for Australia and we need scenarios from other parts of the world that reflect social, cultural, political, economic and environmental diversity.

The research makes the case for systemic matching of governance options in context through a range of engagement processes; social change to address wellbeing is not merely about productivity for profit and transdisciplinarity and a reframed approach to wellbeing. It also makes the case that through the process of monitory democracy and participatory governance people will develop the capability to engage and thus increase their awareness. But current forms of democracy and governance are not engaging people actively. It merely enables a passive vote for their rights, whilst forgetting their responsibilities to other classes, other cultures or other nation states. A different kind of democracy and a different kind of identity is required. We need to develop a wider sense of responsibility—accountability and representation are quite inadequate today.

Wellbeing rests on mindfulness of our relationships with others and with the environment, not on status or ability to live 'high-carbon lifestyles' of our own choosing that are epitomized by mobility for pleasure, maintaining family connections or for work purposes (Elliot 2012). Mobility that is enforced could become greater as a result of increased regional conflict as a result of resource scarcity, disaster or climate change. Whilst there is resistance to this scenario at the moment whilst many live according to the principles of conspicuous consumption,[52] because

[52] Originally, conspicuous consumption was possible only for the leisure class and now they are more widely emulated, in order to keep up appearances in capitalist society. 'Conspicuous consumption of valuable goods is a means of reputability to the gentleman of leisure. As wealth accumulates on his hands, his own unaided effort will not avail to sufficiently put his opulence in evidence by this method. The aid of friends and competitors is therefore brought in by resorting to the giving of valuable presents and expensive feasts and entertainments. Presents and feasts had

carbon-based lives are still within the reach of the middle classes—it is likely that this will be increasingly the preserve of the super-rich elites. The monitoring of scarce resources will become increasingly important for the democracy project, in order to ensure that cynicism and distrust do not alienate electorates.

This requires many kinds of engagement—ranging from face-to-face focus groups to community agoras with an 'online' link to regional parliaments. This could enable all those who live within a region to voice their opinions. Giving 'a voice to the mob' is regarded as being fraught by liberals and neo-liberals—not only because majorities do not always uphold social and environmental justice but also because the current status quo could be overturned! But in a post-consumerist world, wealth would need to be re-evaluated and reconceptualised[53]. But the problem is that the nation state has not acted in the interests of freedom and democracy as Keane (2009a, b) points out which is why cosmopolitan politics is so important.

Emotions run high as resources run out, but it is pointless to polarize emotional and rationalist responses to climate change. Our capability as human beings to think about our thinking requires reflexivity. The more we are able to think about our emotions and the emotions of others, the more likely we are to make decisions that are rational. At times of high risk, this becomes increasingly important for policymakers. The subjective, objective and intersubjective domains of knowledge are vital, and as Habermas has stressed it is the latter that require the most work in policymaking. Reflexivity is both emotional and rational (see Holmes 2010). The recognition of the symbolic meanings people attribute to ideas needs to be given attention (Collins 2008, 2010). Human agency to respond to rising temperatures cannot be avoided and will require rational responses that take into account diverse emotions—particularly the outrage of the disenfranchised.

probably another origin than that of naïve ostentation, but they acquired their utility for this purpose very early, and they have retained that character to the present; so that their utility in this respect has now long been the substantial ground on which these usages rest. Costly entertainments, such as the potlatch or the ball, are peculiarly adapted to serve this end. The competitor with whom the entertainer wishes to institute a comparison is, by this method, made to serve as a means to the end. He consumes vicariously for his host at the same time that he is a witness to the consumption of that excess of good things.' Project Gutenberg's *The Theory of the Leisure Class,* by Thorstein Veblen's eBook or online at www.gutenberg.orgTitle. Accessed 25/06/2012.

[53] To draw on, adapt and apply Einstein's well-known aphorism: We cannot solve the economic and environmental problems of today with the same ideas of *property and consumption* that created the problem of an *unsustainable* way of life. But to enable freedom of thought in science and democratic testing out of ideas requires a democratic state.

Chapter 3
Facing Up to Fin De Siècle culture

3.1 The Pervasive Banality of Evil: Implications for the Notion of Whistle-Blowing, Complicity and Transformation

We live in interesting times. The outgoing chief scientist Sir John Beddington warned that the rising demand for energy, food and water will create a perfect storm by 2030.[1] Systemic monitory democracy and governance need to ensure that some users do not profit at the expense of current and future generations of life (Murray 2006). This requires a different approach to praxis and a different architecture for governance and democracy. The chapter introduces the following questions: What is cosmopolitanism? What are the arguments and what is the evidence as to why sovereign states or global citizens should strive towards a more cosmopolitan approach towards democracy and governance? What organisations would be appropriate or viable to address social and environmental justice? What are the pitfalls? Volume 2 is devoted to addressing the ethical implications raised by these questions in more detail. But this chapter will sketch out a line of argument. Thus, each of these questions will be addressed, in order to make a case for systemic praxis that balances individual and collective needs within and beyond nation states (in federalist overlapping regions).

Arguments by idealists, pragmatists and realists differ. A way to bridge the divides is discussed through considering the consequences of our decisions for current and future generations by addressing wellbeing and developing governance systems to ensure that stocks for the future are developed through limiting the way in which production processes and distribution practices benefit the minority at the expense of the majority. Young people (Osler and Starkeyb 2005), the disabled, asylum seekers and sentient beings (Nussbaum 2006) along with future generations live 'precarious lives' (Butler 2005). Those perceived as different are not protected (Young 1990). The ability to show compassion underpins cosmopolitanism

[1] 'Ashes to Ashes', the Guardian Weekly, pg. 22 5/04/2013 and http://www.bbc.co.uk/news/science-environment-21357520

http://www.theguardian.com/public-leaders-network/blog/2013/feb/15/government-scientific-skills (accessed 7/4/2013).

J. McIntyre-Mills, *Transformation from Wall Street to Wellbeing*,
Contemporary Systems Thinking, DOI 10.1007/978-1-4899-7466-2_3,

(Butler 2011). Her work stresses 'the need to rethink the human as a site of interdependency'. Butler stresses that humanity needs to be able to ask for assistance and we need to be able to anticipate that we will be heard and that people will respond with compassion. Unless this is possible, it leads to a life that can be unbearable. Should we challenge the notion of rights and responsibilities as Butler (2006) asked in a videoed conversation with Sunaura 'because in this world we need each other, in order to meet our basic and needs?'[2]

The threefold aims are:

Firstly, to give the reader a sense of the arguments for and against a weak versus a strong cosmopolitanism. It develops an ethical argument based on considering rights, responsibilities and empirical evidence, in order to address the realist arguments about why strong cosmopolitanism is not merely a discourse of the weak. It considers the inadequacy of the nation-based social contract to address the wide-ranging consequences of consumption on the quality of life of future generations.

Secondly, it sums up the literature on systemic approaches to the vexed challenge of how to bridge the false dualism of pitting the environment versus profit. Approaches that polarize the planet and profit miss the point that it is possible to reframe designs to address wellbeing as the bottom line for all development decisions.

Thirdly, it makes a case for developing cosmopolitan approaches that scale up local engagement and that enable monitoring from below. The process of monitoring needs to be supported by means of the principle of subsidiarity and buttressed by international law.

3.2 Statement of the Problem

The greatest challenges are the *consequences of inaction* that will potentially pose an existential risk to humanity. These challenges include *representation* of the increasingly diverse populations within nation states along with a*ccountability* to ensure that resources (e.g. water, food and energy) are used fairly, equitably and sustainably in local and regional biospheres. Better forms of e*ngagement* are needed to enhance the capability of people to understand that attitudes towards consumption have profound implications for social and environmental justice. Governance and democracy approaches that polarize the planet and profit miss the point that it is possible to reframe development designs to address risk and resilience.

[2] Butler explores the violence towards 'the other' and other species…in NominalistWay·6 videos. She discusses telling stories or 'giving an account of oneself'. In a conversation with a young woman (Examined Life: Judith Butler and Sunaura Taylor 720p.avi), she discusses the right to move in space and to use parts of the body that are not usually used. In conversation, Sunaura explains that disability is socially constructed through the disabling way people respond to you…. Just organising myself ordering a coffee and demand help is a political protest…we all need help…. We are all interdependent…. Impairment is the medical fusion of bones and the way it affects movement. Being able to move through space and to feel the right to express themselves…being able to move through space. 'When I did walk…told I walked like a monkey… where do our boundaries lie as a human…? Monkeys have always been my favourite animal…in a way I was flattered….'

The research made use of many forms of engagement to help participants to consider the potential consequences of their choices. These approaches span narrative (to explore complexity and to enable a creative flow of ideas), dialogue and questioning to reformulate boundaries. Scenarios were also explored spanning 'business as usual', 'small steps towards a sustainable future' and achieving a sustainable future through building up 'wellbeing stocks' (Stiglitz et al. 2010).

3.2.1 Representation

Protecting the environment is a cosmopolitan concern that ought to be above factional politics. The idealism of the Left and the idealism of the Right can lapse into Nazism or environmental destruction in the name of job opportunities. The fragmenting of politics is an indicator of the problems facing democracy and governance.

The problem is that the nation states are too small to respond to the big issues of the day, namely widespread poverty linked with environmental degradation and climate change. But paradoxically they are *too big* to enable diverse citizens to express their diverse needs. The challenge is the social and civil need to listen to the voices of diversity within and beyond nation states in overlapping regional biospheres that support diversity and freedom within sovereign states, to the extent that policies do not undermine the rights of others.

The state is too big to address some challenges. It needs to represent the many voices of people with diverse views to build a sense of the needs of all. Currently, parliamentary representatives at the Australian Federal level do not represent the diversity:

> Just more than one in four Australians is born overseas (26.1 % of all those who stated a birthplace on last year's census). Less than half that figure is reflected in the parliament, where 11.0 % of all members and senators came here from somewhere else.... The explanation for their inability to appreciate the diplomatic harm being done by the standoff in parliament is their life experience. They see politics in narrow terms, as a fortnightly contest for the favour of a polling firm. They can't calculate the damage to social cohesion at home, or our reputation abroad, because it's just politics to them. Immigration is one part of the national memory where hardship is understood. Another part of Australia where prosperity is not taken for granted is in Indigenous communities. Yet the NT, which has the largest proportion of Indigenous people in the nation, has no local born in Canberra....[3]

On the other hand, the nation state is *too small* to address the diverse energy, food and water needs at the regional level.

This requires post-national intervention if we are to avert the development of ever-increasing urban slums managed by Orwellian top-down intervention to prevent chaos. Services could breakdown as the overloaded cities and the shrinking arable land become unable to support their needs. The elderly rich could be unable to maintain ever-increasing services by means of excluding others without the use force so that those who are outside the net are abandoned. This is already happening

[3] Megalogenis, G (2012) Reform blues stem from parliament's monochrome demography Inquirer Weekend Australian July 21–22, p. 22.

as the turning back of boats justifies the limit to compassion is likely to be protected by networks that serve their needs and control those outside the net.

As stressed elsewhere (McIntyre-Mills 2012a, b), this approach could be mediated by a form of bottom-up monitory democracy that ensures the accountable use of resources in post-national biospheres that are supported by international laws, covenants and policies. The mobile carbon-based economy is currently centred on urban development that outstrips the land. The aging population in the developed world will need ever-increasing services. But technology is not reified—it is a product of design that could be liberative and could reflect a different approach.

Technocratic ideas about risk and responses to risk need to be guided by ethics. Of course, ethical views are shaped by culture and we are likely to see the world differently if we are no longer fully human. Speciation and evolution can happen or we can consciously guide the direction that we wish to develop. This is why democracy, governance, research and ethics need to be guided by an ability to test out ideas and to think about our thinking. Our emotions and fears need to be acknowledged and thought about carefully, in terms of the consequences for ourselves, others and the environment. This takes idealism to new expanded territories that respect not only human rights but also the rights of future generations of life. Emotions can shape thought just as thought shapes emotions—we can be conscious and lack self-consciousness or compassion, because we are in a passionate rage—this is why being capable of reflecting on our ideas is important. If consciousness is a continuum—what is human consciousness? How is it different from machine and animal consciousness? This is the wrong question—we are human animals and we are in some ways organic machines. We also have a human spirit that enables us to think about ourselves and enables us to design ourselves and our environment. The fact that animals are also capable to a certain extent to achieve some self-awareness—does not lower our sense of worth—it merely makes us responsible for respecting the diverse abilities of others. Once we abandon the notion that we are better off at the expense of others—then we are able to build solidarity, based on ensuring quality of life for all sentient creatures (Nussbaum 2006).

Social movements are required to develop rights and responsibilities across the state, market and civil society to hold the market and the state to account. But they will need to be supported by post-national regional systems.

To sum up, because the nation state is too small to address the convergent challenges and too big to represent diversity, we need to find ways to balance individual and collective needs.

We need to foster a new approach that ensures that communication for science, democracy, governance and ethics is based on appreciating many forms of human and animal knowing including quantitative numbers, qualitative experience of taste, smell, intuition, the ability to respond to the environment,[4] imagination, emotions as

[4] Not only primates but also a wide range of creatures have been shown to have an ability to think conceptually and to apply their sense of self to solving complex challenges. Octopi are able to work out how to escape from confined spaces and to teach and learn from one another. They have the ability to adapt and respond to their environment is ways that exceed human intelligence. http://www.sbs.com.au/documentary/program/804.

well as perceived, sounds and images. Thus, we need to re-evaluate our values. We need to factor in emotions. The approach used in the research is to enable people to reflect on their lives and to share their reflections with others. Their ideas provide conceptual pathways that are the basis for others to think about and extend. Thus, the approach is iterative and inclusive, not exclusive as the ideas grow through engagement—with the view of finding areas of overlap, whilst respecting diversity to the extent that it does not undermine the rights of others.

So the problem with current forms of democracy and governance are that they do not cultivate inclusion and they continue to work along the old dualistic lines of compartmentalized silos. In Australia, for example, one has to choose parties that are associated with capitalism (business as usual and some support for entrepreneurship), Labour (working conditions and social contract as usual) or Greens (environmental and social justice that extends the social and environmental contract).

The problem is that people need to think in terms of what is sustainable. The inconvenient facts are that the total world population is growing and moving to cities that are reliant on a carbon economy. The mobility of people, goods and most importantly food depends on water, energy, arable land and sustainable seeds. In developed economies, such as Australia, the population is aging (1946–1965), and after retirement will continue to expect a standard of living that will need to be supported by the Generation Xs (1966–1982) and Generation Ys (after 1982).

3.2.2 Accountability

The social contract is too narrow to address the food, water and energy challenges and it is not accountable to those who fall outside the mantle of the nation state or who are under the voting age of 18 years.

The policy and governance decisions taken within the boundaries of the nation state have an impact on the wider region and on the next generation.[5] Contained responses are inadequate to address challenges that span national boundaries.[6]

3.3 Rationale for the Research

The rationale is to explore the dominant cultural narratives on the relationship across humans, other animals and the environment. Language reveals the false assumption of humanity's right to hold dominion over others and the environment!

[5] This has been discussed by Joy Murray (2007) as the Tuvalu test, which suggests that we need to consider how our choices make a difference to others. She suggests that carbon choices made in developed nations impact on rising sea levels, for example. The social contract also excludes non-citizens and those too young to vote, including sentient beings that are voiceless.

[6] The challenge for governance, democracy and ethics will be to achieve a much broader sense of solidarity with others. This has implications for the way in which we engage with others. Complex problems can be addressed by human beings if they make use of many ways of knowing and if they are open to reading the landscape.

The examination of discourses is revealing, for example, the bottom line is 'protection of borders', 'tacking climate change', 'destruction of a business model' or 'developing a brand name', in order to 'tackle or tame' so called 'wicked problems'.

According to Gamble (2000), the basis for sound economic governance is stability through full employment and a stable currency that holds its value. This needs to be supported by development that invests in human and physical capital. But Gamble neglects to factor in what Stiglitz has called 'stocks for future generations', or diminishing returns and the opportunity costs of destroying the means of our common survival. Most importantly, he does not factor in the dimension of care and the time to build respectful relationships with one another and the environment or the tensions that exist between regional neighbours within and beyond the nation state

A case in point is the ongoing tension within the region over fishing and resources in contested territories within the region. These are points of tension that test the nerve and power of USA, China, Vietnam, Japan and Korea. http://www.bbc.co.uk/news/world-europe-22744728

Just as the Mekong River causes tensions between neighbouring nation states who resent the development of hydroelectric power in the upper reaches of the Mekong, because it impacts on fishing in Laos and Cambodia, the residents of South Australia understand the tensions around water usage in the river Murray and the implications for the sale of Cubby Station, because the property dams water that could flow downstream, according to some participants in the debate. The question remains how to balance individual and collective rights at a regional and post-national regional level. Recently, Australia passed legislation to limit fishing off our shores by a super trawler. The standoff between the Australia and the Norwegian trawler echoes the tensions within our region in the East and South China Sea *over access to fishing and mineral rights.*

China and India have economies that are growing faster than the USA and they too need to protect 'stocks for the future' (Stiglitz et al. 2010).[7] Decisions need to be informed by connecting many kinds of knowledge.[8]

[7] It is undeniable that the approach to development needs to respect the environment. It is pointless for Held to say that the philosophy underpinning the consensus cannot be blamed on John Williamson (Held 2005, p. 8) who developed the neoliberal theory about the free market, because the way it has been applied no longer applies to his original ideas. The market failures Held (2005, p. 15) anticipates fall short of what has actually occurred. The problem is not only concerning externalities that are not factored into calculations of the degradation to the environment, it is a way of thinking and 'being in the world' that shifts the extraction of profit to where labour is cheaper and where governments and citizens are less likely to complain about degradation of environment. Short-term profits are made at the expense of future generations. This undermines the conditions of employment so that full-time employment becomes less available. The globalised market needs post-national controls to ensure control of the movement funds (see McIntyre-Mills 2011). Enabling a transformation of identity through consciousness raising and governance is the challenge for governance which has become increasingly difficult in the wake of the convergent crises.

[8] But the problem with media control in any nation state—is that they could lead to an erosion of democracy per se. It is better to be able to develop critical systemic thinking skills so that one can read through newspapers and are able to locate the different arguments in commentary and editorials that are pro the zero-sum or containerist approaches, pro-market and unaware of or denying the interconnections or the impact on wellbeing. The *Mail and Guardian* newspaper editor stressed

One of the central policy challenges is the way in which the market is seen as sacred and requiring a stability or conformist culture to respond to the needs of the market (Tognato 2004, 2012). In some ways, the reified symbol becomes sacred and conformity[9] perpetuates the religion of the market and selfishness. Related to this perceived sanctity is lack of time. Instead of investing time in transformation, time is invested in supporting the current culture of disposability and waste. Gamble stresses that nation states can no longer control markets, because they are subject to large corporations. But in fact they are also subject to a rampant banking system and inhumane organisations that are disrespectful of staff members who are seen as disposable. The concern is that those who see themselves as 'lucky enough to have jobs' barely have the time or energy for leisure activities, let alone volunteering or social action for the poor and voiceless. But those who are unemployed have led to masses of protests by those who have time and who have nothing to lose. This may (eventually) lead to wide-ranging changes towards more socialist governments in Europe.[10] Many socialist movements focus on human rights and do not see their integral relationship with the other and the environment.

Held proposed that the core challenges of the day are to address the vast differences in the standard of living between the rich and the poor through reforming world trade and through using the market to address global warming by means of a global covenant that prevents unilateral interventions.

Held responds to his critics by arguing that he accepts post sovereignty and networks and those tools such as the Internet and co-operations of NGOs such as Civicus will need to develop future governance. Desai's arguments rest on accepting that people will move to find jobs and that multinational companies will eventually have more power than nation states and they will 'demand a uniform standard of environmental or accounting practices, in order to operate across the world'(Desai 2005, p. 69).

People will need to change the world from below, but the question remains how to balance individual and collective rights? The debate that began earlier in 2004 reveals how many of the points of criticism are correct. Thompson (2005) stressed that the US economy is fragile and that assuming that the Washington Consensus

---

that self-regulation is vital for democracy. McDermott, S.K. 2012 'Clash of paradigms' as editors defend self-regulation, Feb 01 2012.

[9] A sense of the sacred and the need to protect the common good is discussed in identity, democracy and sustainability (McIntyre-Mills and De Vries 2011) in which I draw links across the need to understand that the zero-sum approach does not apply and that evolution requires developing a sense of the sacred (inspired by open religions) rather than a closed religious mindset (2006), a renewed respect for the law of the land and an understanding that human beings are caretakers of the land (see McIntyre-Mills 2012) for a discussion of religion and a sense of the sacred, evolution and the way that De Waal has critiqued Dawkins (1976).

[10] This may or may not support the green movement in Europe. In Australia, a backlash against the Greens has been launched by the right faction of the Labour Party (July, 8th, ABS), in a bid to distance itself from the Greens in preparation for the next election.

and security agenda should be the starting point for discussion is problematic.[11] In some ways, it is hubris. China and India have economies that are growing faster than the USA and they lack planning to protect 'stocks for the future' (Stiglitz et al. 2010). It is undeniable that the approach to development needs to respect the environment.

3.4 Policy Context and Distributive Governance

Specifically the research responds to the policy context, in order to achieve better forms of distributive governance adapted from Murray et al. (2007) Tuvalu test and Local Agenda, triple bottom line accounting (Elkington 1992, 1997), Hayden (2010):

- The 'United Nations Local Agenda 21 and variants that strive to scale up triple bottom line accountability not only at a local-level, but whether networks of local organizations internationally could effectively implement the approach. 2a Accept that with the right to own manage and use natural resources comes the duty to prevent environmental harm and to protect the rights of people. 9a) Guarantee the right to potable water, clean air, food security, uncontaminated soil, shelter, and safe sanitation, allocating the national and international resources required.10a) Promote the equitable distribution of wealth within nations and among nations. The Aarhus convention as a means to implement 13a uphold the right of everyone to receive clear and timely information on environmental matters and all development plans and activities which are likely to affect them or in which they have an interest.
- 13b Support local, regional and global civil society, and promote the meaningful participation of all interested individuals and organizations in decision making' (cited by Hayden in Brown and Held 2010, p. 369).
- Common Future and UN Declaration of Human Rights and Earth Charter in particular—4a Recognize that the freedom and rights of each generation is qualified

[11] It is pointless for Held to say that the philosophy underpinning the consensus cannot be blamed on John Williamson (Held 2005, p. 8) who developed the neoliberal theory about the free market, because the way it has been applied no longer applies to his original ideas. The market failures Held (2005, p. 15) anticipates fall short of what has actually occurred. The problem is not only concerning externalities that are not factored into calculations of the degradation to the environment, it is a way of thinking and 'being in the world' that shifts the extraction of profit to where labour is cheaper and where governments and citizens are less likely to complain about degradation of environment. Short-term profits are made at the expense of future generations. This undermines the conditions of employment so that full-time employment becomes less available. The globalised market needs post-national controls to ensure control of the movement funds (see McIntyre-Mills 2011). Enabling a transformation of identity through consciousness raising, humility and governance is the challenge for ethical systemic governance which has become increasingly difficult in the wake of the convergent crises. Morality becomes politically disposable, because of a lack of understanding of our interconnected existence.

by the needs of future generations. 6c. Ensure that decision-making addresses the cumulative, long term, indirect, long distance, and global consequences of human activities. The Millennium Goals cannot be met unless these are addressed.

The architecture of governance (Archibugi 2008) needs to respond to environmental needs that protect the wellbeing of global citizens (Haydon 2005).

Sovereign nation states need to consider regional rights and responsibilities in a series of overlapping organisations that apply the rule of law to ensure equitable and fair distribution of rights and responsibilities for food, energy and water.

The research is about developing post-national organisations to ensure human rights. Disaster management, movement of people fleeing disaster or injustice, securing food, energy and water are concerns that span boundaries (spatial, conceptual and temporal). We need to appreciate that stewardship to address convergent social, economic and environmental challenges span generations, disciplines and nation states. Stewardship requires trust and better communication so that we understand one another better.

The purpose is not to rehearse the same arguments about rights and responsibilities—these are taken as a given.[12] The research is also not about 'what is the case' or 'what ought to be the case' in terms of stating that social injustice and inequality exist and that the disappearance of biodiversity will make a difference, because the ecosystem is a web. The loss of insects, the unbridled greed and hubris will indeed impact on food security—just as it will jeopardize seed security.

Instead this research is located in the domain of reframing, developing and prefiguring a new architecture in response to Dahl's (1967) pessimism about extending the scale of democracy and governance.

[12] The Brundtland Report (1987) on our Common Future stressed our interconnectedness and the rights of future generations. Clarke (2000) stressed that the planet is a system, but all the policy documents and conferences to date have been limited by the containerist philosophy echoed by the rights of sovereign states (UN 1992, COP and Cancun) to make decisions on the use of resources—most particularly in connection with the carbon-based economy. If we are to balance the interests of the planet as well as ensure the rights of less developed nations to re-dress poverty—then we must find a way not only to innovate—but also to limit the misuse of resources and to enable the fair (Rawls 2009) distribution of rights and responsibilities to ensure food, energy, water supplies that underpin quality of life and wellbeing. The United Nations declaration of human rights will remain rhetoric unless new forms of governance that respect diversity and freedom to the extent that the diversity and freedom of the next generation of life is not undermined. Democratic governance requires listening to perceived needs and responding within the architecture of rights and responsibilities that are in line with cosmopolitan law to protect human rights and the human environment, as outlined in Our Common Future and the Earth Charter of 1997 that outlines world environmental citizenship, namely to: Build rapport, and trust—counter the realist approach to international relations through:

Deciding how best to use scarce resources
Drawing on local wisdom
Drawing on creative ideas of local people
Enabling participation to match responses to perceived need but also through
Enabling people to blow the whistle on mis-use.

We could develop surveillance systems *from below* to monitor Big Brother and blow the whistle on corruption—in order to avert control *from above* and to ensure that local areas do not lapse into the so-called ungovernable zones of 'warlordism' (Elliot and Urry 2010). But the paradox is that in the resource-rich cities of the world mobile people spend their time rushing from one appointment to another. They use mobile technology in ways that can make life frenetic. But digital technology can be used in different ways—not to constantly reschedule meetings but to enable life to be lived at a slower pace. It could be used to enable people to think about alternative ways of living and to 'join up the dots'.

It is likely that a greater balance will need to be achieved between individual and collective needs through emphasising the determinants of wellbeing for this generation and the next. This requires a new approach to public education, democracy, governance and ethics that places food security at the centre of decisions. The role of local participation and governance thus becomes increasingly important.

A sustainable local community is determined by a sustainable region in which food, energy and water supplies are considered as major determinants for wellbeing. No community can be expected to transform from a high carbon lifestyle (or aspiring to this lifestyle) without feeling part of the design process and owning the decisions as to how resources should be used.[13]

The United Nations declaration of human rights will remain rhetoric unless new forms of governance that respect diversity and freedom to the extent that the diversity and freedom of the next generation of life is not undermined (Table 3.1).

We need to face up to our own complicity.[14] Global citizenship ought to become a concept supported by international law and social justice movements

[13] Our research strives to enable people to have a say about how scarce resources should be used, in order to inform elected representatives of their perceived social, economic and environmental needs. It is also hoped that by thinking about what they have and what they need and what they are prepared to change (by being prompted to consider the consequences of our choices for others and for the environment). The notion of engagement in 'if then scenarios', is helpful to enable people to develop sustainable praxis decisions (McIntyre-Mills and De Vries, 2011).This research emphasizes the creation of multiple paths to form wellbeing webs through critical, systemic engagement to ensure that local people get to know about local resources (that are listed in directories created by both service users and providers) and that their identity is protected. They are able to see the typical scenarios of what people have, need, are prepared to add or discard from their lives and what they think are turning points for the better and worse. The aim is to enable people to think about their attitudes to consumption of resources and the implications of these attitudes for their relationships with others and the environment.

[14] Systemic monitory democracy and governance need to ensure that some users do not profit at the expense of others and future generations of life (Murray 2006). This requires a different approach to praxis and a different architecture for governance and democracy. Overlapping federations of nation states need to consider biospheres without jeopardizing the ability of states to uphold social and environmental justice.

'Representative government is in crisis today, partly because it has lost, in the course of time, all institutions that permitted the citizens' actual participation, and partly because it is now gravely affected by the disease from which the party system suffers: bureaucratization and the two parties 'tendency to represent nobody except the party machines'. (Arendt 1972, p. 89). Law, stewardship, culture and behaviour and the way that architectures for democracy and governance are designed

Table 3.1 Capacity building for ethical governance requires structures based on norms, facilitated by processes and implemented as thinking and practice (praxis)

Structures	A priori norms concerning the principal/agent relationships that protect regions
	A posteriori checks and balances that are supported by cosmopolitan democracy and governance that enables government representatives and individuals living and or working within a state to have a say
	Tax base should be developed by means of global taxes to address the high, medium and low incomes of individuals and corporations. A super tax on the top 1 % would be transparent
Processes	Whistle-blowing by individuals, states and organisations
	Monitoring informed by critical systemic toolkit (McIntyre-Mills 2006)
Actions/tasks	Social, economic and environmental actions to enhance representation, accountability and sustainability, in terms of what we have, what we value and what we are prepared to change through our actions and relationships

(McIntyre-Mills 2000). The four themes of citizenship discourses are: 'inclusion, erosion, withdrawal and expansion', these 'reflect the foci of contemporary discourses on citizenship' (Kivisto and Faist 2007, p. 13).

The ongoing work in progress (McIntyre-Mills and De Vries 2011, 2012) addresses a means to operationalize environmental protection through engaging members of the public in the process of developing appropriate measures of wellbeing.

This is a vital step in cultural transformation as it raises awareness. Participants are also asked to create a contract concerning their consumption choices and the tradeoffs they are prepared to make in the public, private or volunteer sectors, such as being prepared to do more re-cycling and re-using resources in a responsible manner.

The burden of responsibility ought not to be shifted to locals without the private sector, welfare sectors and all levels of government playing an equal role.[15]

This governance research explores a way to reframe architectures for representation, accountability and sustainability. It builds on and applies the concept of fostering wellbeing stocks (Stiglitz et al. 2010) through valuing social and environmental

need to balance individual and collective needs. Law can be characterized as monist, dualist or based on harmonization to draw on international law. I argue for the latter *as a means* to strive towards justice based on quality of life for all. One truth (monist) responses defended by grand narratives; no truth (postmodernist) approached defended by relativism or conflict; mediated (harmonized) responses are based on co-created meaning (McIntyre-Mills 2000; Crowder 2003, 2004) based on the principle of subsidiarity that can be summed up by the axiom that freedom and diversity at the local level needs to be encouraged to the extent that it does not undermine the common good. The notion of stewardship is thus also entailed by the axiom.

[15] According to Heycox et al. (1997, p. 4): 'Data published by the ABS on the environmental protection expenditures by the public sector, including local government, is derived from the public sector finance collection which is based on an international Classification of the Functions of Government (COFOG). The problem arises due to the structure of COFOG that was designed long before collecting data on public sector transactions. It does not enable the environmental component of transactions…to be separately identified.' But separation or disaggregation is quite the wrong way to approach the problem. This is why a systemic approach is vital and why the research supports the promotion of wellbeing as an integrated measure for a sustainable future.

dimensions in our accounting systems so that we are more accountable to both current and future generations. It attempts to reframe economics through participatory governance and democracy to enable a transformation in what, why and how we value social and environmental factors.

To sum up, the research develops a process by which a suite of measures can be developed with local stakeholders within a region.[16]

According to Barbara Dickens from the Urban Renewal Department:

> Pathways to Wellbeing software offer a unique avenue for ongoing, long-term engagement between local residents and local government. It facilitates considering the consequences of our choices for ourselves, others and the environment. These considerations are used to shape evidenced-based policy to inform decision-making at the local level. By asking residents to make choices from Pathways to Wellbeing scenarios, participants are invited to make changes in their lives. It aims to help them think through the implications and consequences of their choices for themselves and future generations. The choices relate to sustainable living and the extent to which people are prepared to adapt their lives to mitigate the effects of climate change. It is hoped that this will help people to adapt to the convergent challenges and that they will be able to change their socio-economic choices through adapting their culture. Thus, the research is about cultural transformation.

Whilst enabling individual citizens to manage their pathways, the software enables analysis of the responses to inform and assist the local government in matching service outcomes to the perceived needs of service users. It provides a means to work out where to 'draw the line' based on inclusive testing of ideas with those who are to be affected by the decisions. It also enables comparisons across the different pathways to establish not only how the pathways differ but also how they overlap—and therefore to find common ground with regard to their views—their concerns, values, priorities and approaches to how they want to live their lives. The book considers the potential for a digital scorecard to address social, economic and environmental factors that support or undermine adaptation to the challenges and mitigation of the effects of climate change. It evaluates the extent to which the

[16] An alternative form of governance architecture is developed by considering the challenge posed by Stiglitz (2010) to the Australian Productivity Commission, namely to foster an understanding that the wellbeing of humanity is dependent on the global commons (McIntyre-Mills and Binchai 2013). The focus of the research is on addressing social, economic and environmental factors that help to mitigate and adapt to climate change. Joseph Stiglitz, past president of the World Bank, has stressed (at the invitation of the Australian Productivity Commission) that the bottom line is wellbeing—this requires building stocks for the future (Stiglitz et al. 2010). Wellbeing is crucial to redesigning economics, but it depends on the recognition of flows of resources.

It explores the potential for participatory democracy and governance to (a) monitor, (b) match services to need and (c) mitigate risk and adapt to climate change. This is vital for ethics and stewardship on behalf of future generations. It discusses an alternative form of governance and democracy and grapples with ways to address wellbeing. The right to equal opportunities versus equal outcomes is a core policy and political consideration. The responsibility to ensure that some do not prosper at the expense of others is a core challenge. It considers the potential of human beings to address social, economic and environmental factors that support or undermine adaptation to the challenges and mitigation of the effects of climate change. It evaluates the extent to which interactive engagement approaches enable the community to consider their perceived assets and risks and the implications of their consumption choices for developing wellbeing stocks.

approach enables the community to consider their perceived assets and risks and the implications of their consumption choices for developing *wellbeing.*

Resilience is defined as the adaptive capacity of the physical environment, of an individual or of a group. It concerns factors such as the capacity of members of a community to act together and to be able to modify or even transform existing ways of life (Rose 2004, 2005, Hulme 2009) and thus personal, community or regional resilience, measured by a human sustainability footprint.

3.5 Culture, Identity and Post-national Solidarity

Unlike O' Connor and Lines (2010) who argue that border controls are vital to limit the size of the Australian population, this approach stresses the importance of post-national controls that provide an institutional framework to support mindfulness of our place in the world—not a limited approach to national boundaries that attempts to 'shift the burden' of climate change elsewhere.

The issue of national identity versus global identity has never been more important. The problem is that as people compete for scarce resources they fracture the shared identity that is so important for a sustainable world. The scaling up of digital technology can either enable us to achieve our potential which could, in the words used by John Man, turn us into 'cells in a planet sized brain' (Florini 2003, p. 195) or it could lead to our becoming increasingly disconnected with people in face to face situations, because we spend so much time connected without digital technology, that we forget how to be connected and engaged with people and our surroundings in real time (Greenfield 2008).

Engaging with one another in real time requires being able to connect emotionally with one another. The capability to communicate in many ways and to respond effectively and quickly to increased risks is the topic of this book.

Telling and listening to narratives does not necessarily enable people to see things differently, unless they are asked to consider the implications of different scenarios. Ways forward out of this contrived way of life pose a challenge.

The process of enabling people to think about their thinking and to consider the emotional dimensions of their choices is vital (McIntyre-Mills and de Vries 2011).

Educational processes to address this gap need to enable people to:

- Work with complexity.
- Rebuild the connections with one another and with the environment. These connections have been forgotten in the hype of hyper reality. Participatory democracy will achieve little without specific laws to prevent excessive consumption. The bricolage of existing laws, covenants and conventions provide the first step towards liberating design from the lobster pot, in order to establish post-national federations within regional biospheres.

The Aarhus Convention requires engaging people at the local level in local decision-making in line with the principle of subsidiarity. An expanded form of Aarhus

Convention (see Florini 2003; McIntyre-Mills 2010a, b, c) could enable the United Nations Local Agenda 21—that provides guidelines for local engagement—to address systemic transformation. Globally within each nation state, the diversity of citizens is becoming greater. Even more importantly, rights are only accorded to citizens, not to residents who by virtue of age, place of birth, level of ability may fall outside the mantle of protection. The diverse legal heritage of multiple cultures needs to be reflected in a responsive legal system that is designed to protect social and environmental justice. Public conversations are needed to make a case for enabling people to think about their mental maps and the consequences of their praxis.

We need both *centralized* controls to protect the sacred global commons that sustains life and *decentralized* engagement to test out ideas and to co-create a sense of ownership of the ideas.

Where and *how* we draw the lines of inclusion and exclusion will be relevant for our survival.[17] This could be achieved by acknowledging that we are part of the biosphere and as human beings our narratives need to support systemic stewardship praxis. Flannery (2010, pp. 241–242) suggests that biodiversity needs to be protected through 'satellite monitoring from above'. This needs to be supplemented by a range of social participation sites 'from below'.[18]

The process for monitoring and local contextual details needs to be monitored by local people with local knowledge. This requires decentring the humanist approach to entitlement fostered by the enlightenment without lapsing into an elevation of nature that leads to totalitarianism (in the process of protecting the biosphere on which we depend). This will in turn elevate planetary wellbeing not as kitsch, but to the level of a sense of 'the sacred', collective good.

An example of nested governance process that is worthy of consideration and development is the process developed by the Tuvalu test (Murray et al. 2007). A resilient biosphere supports a sustainable carbon footprint within and across overlapping regions and as such needs to be protected and supported by systemic governance. This is a sine qua non of social and environmental justice. It is arguably appropriate to combine cycles of open discursive democracy with cycles of rational, structured dialogue. The role of Internet-supported e-governance and e-democracy software is partly able to address this concern. The former enables the generation of ideas and relationships in respectful conversation. The latter enables better matches of service responses and greater attachment to rational, sustainable decisions through engagement with values, ideas, feelings and their implications for decisions on the length and quality of life of people—living within overlapping regions.

[17] Darwin argued that evolution was driven by both competition and co-operation (De Waal 2006, 2009). The 'twice wise', or *Homo Sapiens Sapiens* (Banathy 1996) need to think about their thinking and their practice if they are to evolve beyond the addictive consumption of the planet.

[18] The conceptual basis for the research is discussed in 'Wellbeing, mindfulness and the global commons' (McIntyre-Mills 2010). It is developed in more detail in 'Identity, Democracy and Sustainability' (McIntyre-Mills and de Vries 2011). The pilot stage of the ongoing research is described in 'Transformation from Wall Street to Wellbeing' (McIntyre-Mills and de Vries 2012).

The aim of the research detailed in Chap. 1 is to enable participants to monitor their footprints based on the Max Neef (1991) Human Sustainability Scale. The approach is also inspired by the work of Joy Murray et al.'s (2006, 2007) Tuvalu test. This test asks to what extent our personal choices impact on the rights of others. She suggests that our personal lifestyle choices shape the life chances of others in our region. This research strives to apply West Churchman's (1971, 1982) approach to testing ideas through 'sweeping in for example: social, cultural, political, economic and environmental variables' and 'unfolding the values' of diverse stakeholders.

This approach could be scaled up by means of the policy suggested in the Aarhus Convention (1998). According to the European Commission website[19]:

> The Aarhus Convention establishes a number of rights of the public (individuals and their associations) with regard to the environment. The Parties to the Convention are required to make the necessary provisions so that public authorities (at national, regional or local level) will contribute to these rights to become effective. The Convention provides for:

1. The right of everyone to receive environmental information that is held by public authorities ("access to environmental information"). This can include information on the state of the environment, but also on policies or measures taken, or on the state of human health and safety where this can be affected by the state of the environment. Applicants are entitled to obtain this information within one month of the request and without having to say why they require it. In addition, public authorities are obliged, under the Convention, to actively disseminate environmental information in their possession;
2. The right to participate in environmental decision-making. Arrangements are to be made by public authorities to enable the public affected and environmental non-governmental organisations to comment on, for example, proposals for projects affecting the environment, or plans and programmes relating to the environment, these comments to be taken into due account in decision-making, and information to be provided on the final decisions and the reasons for it ("public participation in environmental decision-making");
3. The right to review procedures to challenge public decisions that have been made without respecting the two aforementioned rights or environmental law in general ("access to justice").

Florini (2003) suggests the potential of the Aarhus Convention could be scaled up to enhance accountability. This book argues that social, economic and environmental accounting could be assisted by means of participation to make this so-called triple bottom line accountability viable. Thus, the participatory action research grasps the nettle to address the challenge posed by the Earth Charter: 'Everyone shares responsibility for the present and future wellbeing of the human family and the larger living world' (cited by Hayden, 368).The challenge is to move beyond the rhetoric of cosmopolitan citizenship and to address both justice and sovereignty. The nation state needs to be held to account by an Earth Charter that is supported by

[19] http://ec.europa.eu/environment/aarhus/.

Table 3.2 Architecture for governance in overlapping domains to maximize changes towards a more sustainable future

	Structure	Process	Action
Micro-level individuals	Aarhus Convention (1998)	Questions raised and posed to local government by individuals	Local government, NGOs and individuals
Meso-states and regions	Aarhus Convention linked to Global Covenant	Online monitory democracy and governance to address state/market/civil society concern	Networking NGOs and INGOs to address representation and accountability
Macro-cosmopolitan governance	Legal structures to support the Global Covenant, Aarhus Convention and Biospheres Convention	International Criminal Court United Nations	Global action to pass laws to protect social and environmental justice in overlapping biospheres

overlapping regional institutions (supported by inclusive regional research institutions, policies, the rule of law including parliaments and courts).

The GFC and the environmental melt down seem to be seen as two problems—not one. Human beings cannot achieve new growth through increased extraction of profit. Instead we need to live elegantly and well through re-distribution of resources and living a simpler lifestyle (supported by green economies, reciprocal sharing of resources and skills in green communities, and energy efficient systems (see Table 3.2 and 3.3)).

Ideally, a universal respect for social and environmental justice could enable subsidiarity as a means to support freedom to the extent that it does not undermine the quality of life of this generation or the next.

Dualist thinking pervades our consciousness and is reflected in socially unjust and environmentally unsustainable designs for society.

Designs need to be supported by constitutions, based on a priori *norms,* and consequentialist or a posteriori *approaches,* based on testing out ideas within context and with future generations in mind.

Global axioms to protect future generations and the poor of this generation need to guide legal constructs and legal decisions at the local level.

The principle of subsidiarity could rest comfortably with global axioms—provided that the caveat is made that—*people at the local level can be free and diverse to the extent that their freedom and diversity does not undermine the rights of others or future generations of life.*

This challenge of balancing individual and collective social, cultural, political and economic concerns needs to be buttressed by regional parliaments and courts that focus on social and environmental justice at a post-national level.

The desire of the rich to consume and the desire of the majority of the poor to leave the ghetto are expressed through emulating the rich.

Table 3.3 Cosmopolitan democracy: design implications for protecting human security. (Source: Adapted from Archibugi (in Wallace Brown and Held 2010, p. 322))

Distinctive features	Cosmopolitan democracy model by Archibugi	Cosmopolitan architecture for democratic governance McIntyre-Mills adaptations
Components	Both individuals and governments have their own representatives in the global sphere	Representatives of all states will sit on a Global Covenant protectorate to ensure that member states comply with the axiom that people have the right to be free and diverse to the extent that they do not undermine the freedom and rights of current or future generations of life
Citizenship	Together with their citizenship of the state, individuals also acquire cosmopolitan citizenship. This envisages a minimal list of rights and duties vis a vis constituting cosmopolitan institutions	Rights and responsibilities are enshrined in a set of guidelines monitored locally through an adapted and extended form of UN local Agenda 21 and Aarhus Convention
Membership criteria	Admission to intergovernmental organisations is regulated by the principle of effective control over a given territory, excluding only governments that violate fundamental human rights (e.g., genocide and apartheid). Cosmopolitan institutions accept only delegates deemed to be legitimate representatives of their respective peoples	Genocide will be interpreted as individuals who act in ways that undermine the fabric of life Human security will be managed in terms of social, economic and environmental indicators spanning household, community, regional and post-national levels
Decision-making	Intergovernmental institutions are based on equality among the states, as guaranteed by the principle of 'one state, one vote' Cosmopolitan institutions are based on equality among citizens, as guaranteed by the principle 'one individual, one vote'	Decision-making will be guided by means of software to enable complex decision-making to be made in ways that enhance comparisons across social, economic and environmental indicators The process and dynamics could support local choices and diversity in line with the principle of subsidiarity. Those who undermine social and environmental justice would be responsible to regional courts that protect biodiversity. These courts would in turn be responsible to the International Criminal court linked with the Global Covenant Protectorate. The representatives would span all member states and the chair would rotate every 6 months and be subject to the scrutiny of the international criminal court at all times. The judges of this court will be selected from nominations spanning all the member states and their appointment will be subject to an open voting system

Table 3.3 (continued)

Distinctive features	Cosmopolitan democracy model by Archibugi	Cosmopolitan architecture for democratic governance McIntyre-Mills adaptations
Internal sovereignty	The internal sovereignty of the states is limited by global constitutional rules and is aimed at ensuring effective self-determination	The internal sovereignty could prevail to the extent that the freedom and diversity of actions of the state did not undermine the global covenant
External sovereignty	The external sovereignty of the states is replaced by a global constitutionalism. The union has the task of solving conflicts by negotiation	The conflicts could be resolved by ensuring that the fine-grained detail of managing water, seeds, air are governed by rules to protect the global covenant and rules that ban the patenting of life
Powers of coercion	The states retain their own armed forces. Humanitarian interventions to prevent acts of genocide are managed by cosmopolitan institutions	Perpetrators will be policed by global commons protectors who comply with the rules of the International Criminal court
Jurisdiction of states	The member states accept the compulsory jurisdiction of the international courts. Although the union has no means to enforce the decisions, it can use sanctions	The Aarhus Convention could be used to enable monitoring from below to ensure the fair distribution of resources. It could be a constitutional requirement that all member states agree to comply with the social, economic and environmental indicators that are developed in the proposed architecture outlined in *Wall Street to Wellbeing*
Criminal jurisdiction	A criminal court is envisaged which has compulsory jurisdiction and can intervene in the case of crimes not punished or pursued by national legislations	A biosphere court is envisaged to govern the distribution of resources to ensure social and environmental justice, based on the Helsinki principle and operationalized by means of monitoring from below the resources that are equitably shared in terms of federalist, overlapping regions
Participation	Participation is voluntary and revocable. It nevertheless requires consulting the citizens in addition to their governments. In cosmopolitan institutions, the union can resolve to accept citizens also representing states that do not intend to participate	Democracy could be enabled through monitoring the resources that are allocated by biosphere courts. The judges on the panel could be required to work with transdisciplinary jurist panels to practice stewardship of wellbeing stocks
Territorial delimitation	In the case of disputes among or within the state, the territorial modifications are indicated by the union with a view to enforcing individual rights and self-government	Rights are permitted to the extent that they do not undermine the rights of others or lead to exploitation or pollution of 'downstream states' This is a synecdoche of water management applied to demonstrate the concept of flows

On the one hand, socio-demographic research shows that debt and bankruptcy in developed nations—such as the USA and nations within the EU—are driven by advertising, easy credit and the desire to 'keep up appearances' by emulating the standards of the very rich (Frank 2007; Wilkinson and Pickett 2009).

On the other hand, the designer 'rip off' label may be an attempt to emulate conspicuous consumption—or it may be a 'cast off' worn—simply because it is all that is available, as in the case of an 'I love Paris' shirt worn by an Aboriginal woman at a camp site in Alice Springs. Making and invoking treaties and conventions that control commodification needs to be a priority and needs to be ongoing if justice is to be maintained. The approach could be buttressed through federations supported by, for example, the Lisbon Treaty (Horvath and Odor 2010) which requires that social, economic and environmental legal considerations be met. Unfortunately, the structural and process mechanisms of the EU are not able to manage the distribution of power or funding (Rhodes 1997). Clearly, if the EU is to survive it needs to be supported by a means to balance individual and national interests with the collective good of the union. More and more members of the union are disenchanted for a number of reasons.

3.6 Capacity Building for Better Governance Through Ongoing Monitory Democracy

Hannah Arendt (1963, 1969) stresses that evil is comprehensible. It results from the way in which policy is made and practiced through the architecture of governance.

Complicity denies the role of the privileged in creating and enabling the wicked problem of growth to the extent that it poses an existential risk through undermining the social and natural fabric of life.

But it is easier to blame the 1 % for everything. The other problem is that everyone else strives to emulate them! Cultural transformation requires respect for simplicity and dignity. Complicity—in the sense it is used in this book—means not appreciating the rights of future generations and the need for new configurations of identity. Arendt has criticized the systems approach for imposing change through 'ABC-type scenarios' that pose a false dichotomy or an oversimplification of options and then encourages a compromise through option C.[20]

[20] The sociologist Hannah Arendt (1969) criticised the systems approach used to plan the Vietnam War in her book *Crises of the Republic.* Hannah Arendt (1969) criticized closed systems and the Operations Research Approach for imposing change through simplistic scenarios that pose a false dichotomy or an oversimplification of options that encourage a compromise without exploring wide-ranging systemic complicity (Arendt 1963). The critical tradition of the Frankfurt School, critical heuristics and open systemic intervention (Midgley 2000) underpin this research. Arendt has criticized the systems approach for imposing change through ABC-type scenarios that pose a false dichotomy or an oversimplification of options and then encourage a compromise through option C. Whilst the criticism is fair for closed systems and operations research, it does not apply to the work of critical heuristics or open systems that cut through the governance game and the minutiae of bureaucracy that is pervasive, banal and part of the complicit, wicked problems.

Whilst the criticism is fair for closed systems and operations research, it does not necessarily apply to the work of critical heuristics (CH)[21] or open systems. Hannah Arendt's legacy is demonstrating that the crimes against humanity were not the preserve of a single monster; they were the result of the banal complicity of many people in society.

Arendt stresses that lying in politics occurs in democracies and in totalitarian states. The comments she makes about America post the Vietnam War are relevant today[22] to other developed nations that are equally complicit.

I listened to the inauguration speech by Obama.[23] The fine speech was listened to by hundreds of thousands of supporters. The statements about the need for peace after a decade of war, the need for rallying to support appropriate sustainable energy supplies and the rights of all American people. He stressed that those with skills who wish to enter the USA should be given a place. He stressed that gay unions should be given equal rights. The issue of marriage was not raised in his speech, nor was the issue of immigrants (without skills) and asylum seekers remain outside the concerns of the state, which only represents citizens' interests, but not the interests of those outside the mantle of the state who for example are fleeing war, poverty or natural disaster. So the problem of extending the social contract, in order to enhance human capabilities remains a challenge for human rights.

Arendt stressed the need to revive democracy and to continue the efforts to improve the life chances of all.[24] This requires a social movement beyond the boundaries of any one state.

> Representative government is in crisis today, partly because it has lost, in the course of time, all institutions that permitted the citizens' actual participation, and partly because it

[21] CH 'unfolds values' and 'sweeps in' the social, cultural, historical, economic and environmental dimensions.

[22] Arendt stresses in her chapter 'Lying in Politics in Crises of the Republic' (Arendt 1969, pp. 11–13) that democracies rely on manipulating the truth. Long before 'spin' became a topical term, Arendt links the role of researchers in propping up political agendas. According to Arendt (1969, p. 12): 'Reasons aversion to contingency is strong: it was Hegel, the father of grandiose history schemes that philosophical contemplation has no other intention than to eliminate the accidental.' Indeed much of the arsenal of political theory—game theory and systems analyses, the scenarios written for imagined 'audiences', and the careful enumeration of usually three options…whereby A and C represent the opposite extremes and B the logical middle of the road solution of the problem—has its source in this deep-seated aversion…. The kind of thinking that presents both A and C as undesirable, therefore settles on B, hardly serves any other purpose that to divert the mind and blunt the judgment for the multitude of real possibilities. What these problem solvers have in common with down to earth liars is the attempt to get rid of the facts and the confidence that this should be possible because of the inherent contingency of facts….' In response to the Vietnam War, Arendt writes about the way in which America tried to establish a reputation of power and leadership by examining the Pentagon papers (17–19): She stressed that the lengths they were willing to go should be a cause for alarm, rather than a cause for celebration from friends who could rely on the USA. The mainstream media and elected governments in Western democracies such as the USA focus on the banal.

[23] http://www.bbc.co.uk/news/world-us-canada-21122015.

[24] This argument is in line with the approach advocated by Crocker, 1995 in the chapter entitled 'Functioning and Capability' in Nussbaum and Sen (Ed) 'Women, culture and development'.

> is now gravely affected by the disease from which the party system suffers: bureaucratization and the two parties 'tendency to represent nobody except the party machines'. (Arendt 1972, p. 89)

In democracies when the truth gets out, governments can be voted out and criminal sentences can be applied. In totalitarian states, threat and fear prevent the story from reaching the media or the courts. Unless governments are held to account by a monitory democracy, 'lying in politics' becomes a norm, not an exception.

The links between politics and research are also strong in democratic societies. The *will* to change and the ability to understand the pervasive nature of the problem are the dual challenges.

This book is filled with suggestions—drawn from experience and research. It amounts to an attempt to respond to the emotional despair of 'doing nothing' and a hope that it is possible to redesign, remake and transform our relationships with one another.

> All over the world, people believe that they are being lied to, that the figures are false, that they are being manipulated…. And there are good reasons for their feeling this way. For years, people whose lives were becoming more and more difficult were told that their living standards were rising. How could they not feel deceived? For years, people were told that finance is a powerful engine of growth, only to discover one day that the risk it had accumulated was so great that it had plunged the world into chaos. Who could fail to understand why those who had lost their home, their job, their pension, would not feel deceived. For years the statistics portrayed increasingly strong economic growth as a victory over scarcity, until it came to light that this growth was endangering the future of the planet and was destroying more than it was creating. Is it any wonder that those whom we are now asking to make efforts and sacrifices and change their way of life before it too late feel deceived? (Sarkozy cited in Stiglitz et al. 2010, p. viii)

The problem is that even if the statistical measures that have been created and collected are accurate, they are not measuring the right concepts. The gross domestic product or the gross national product are economic market measures within the boundaries of the nation state.

Productivity measures do not take into account the costs to the environment, society and the individual human beings who do not have leisure to enjoy time with their families or friends or their communal environment.

The exhaustion felt by workers is a reflection of the exhaustion of stocks of energy—social, cultural and environmental—that will impact on future generations of life. This is why we need to develop new ways to live with one another and the environment.

The surveillance 'from above' by governments needs to be countered by surveillance of governments 'from below' by members of social and environmental justice groups.

Given the accusations cyber espionage of state versus state and state surveillance of citizens the containerist approach to democracy and governance is passé.[25] The role of engaged monitoring by cosmopolitan citizen whistle-blowers needs to

[25] Cyber spying dominates US–China talks http://www.afr.com/Page/Uuid/59df94f0-d186-11e2-b5de-529bd24c91c8 Accessed 17 June 2013.

be shared more widely.[26] The nation state is no longer relevant to a world where food, energy and water security are dependent upon a resilient global commons that spans nation states. The cosmopolitan citizen understands her or his responsibilities to others, sentient beings and the environment. The axiom on which cosmopolitan citizenship rests is that we can be free and diverse to the extent that freedom and diversity does not undermine the rights of others, the environment and the next generation of life.[27] Stoicism needs to receive more attention.

But unlike classical stoicism, this approach places humanity within ecosystems, rather than above the environment and other animals. It also does not assume that controlling emotions today means something similar to controlling emotions in the time of the early Stoics!

Times have changed; human beings have evolved (for better or worse) in response to their environment and to the ever-growing list of perceived rights that are met only if you are part of the privileged 1 % of humanity (who live their lives at the expense of others). Similarly, the old institutions of marriage and child rearing as a normative right needs to be discussed in terms of the consequences for the next generation of life, without the 1 % blaming those with large families and few rights.

The Kantian doctrine that the social contract ought to be extended needs to be translated into active politics supported by a new architecture of governance to protect the planet. The philosophy of the stoical freed slave Epictetus invoked human beings to make the best of things and live in ways that respect the harmony of nature. He distinguished humanity from animals because they could observe their own behaviour. But human animals have the right to develop their full capability as do other animals (Nussbaum 2006).

New Stoicism is about applying rational thinking to control our emotions and desires for more and more.[28] Unlike traditional stoicism, it emphasizes the stewardship of nature for the benefit of this generation and the next. Stoicism underpins stewardship and caring for the voiceless, including other species and those with disabilities. By showing compassion to the voiceless we attain self-respect which ought to be the goal of humanity and it ought to be buttressed by laws that protect the quality of life for all. Epictetus[29] (tr. by Carter 1910, p. 16) stressed that rational thought needs to raise our choices through thinking through the implications of our

[26] http://www.guardian.co.uk/world/2013/jun/11/edward-snowden-nsa-whistleblower-profile Accessed 17 June 2013.

[27] This axiom guides stewardship decisions that consider the consequences for this generation of live and the next.

[28] New Stoicism is about applying rational thinking to control our emotions and desires for more and more. Unlike traditional stoicism, it emphasizes the stewardship of nature and caring for the voiceless, including other species and those with disabilities. Compassion for others stems from our understanding of our relationship with other animals. The pain of other sentient beings cannot be dismissed as irrelevant. What we do to others we do to ourselves. The stoicism of hope translated into courageous action needs to be more than a role for women carrying a triple work load of mother, carer of children and worker within the paid labour market or unpaid worker who volunteers time to keep a business viable and then volunteer hours to keep a community viable.

[29] Rhys, E. (Ed) 1910. *The moral discourses of Epictetus: Mrs. Carter's Translation* Everyman's Library. Published by J M Dent, New York.

choices and the careful examination of discourses to avoid 'being taken in by appearances'—thus critical thinking is of primary importance.

Unlike Nussbaum, who develops a case for strong cosmopolitanism, weak cosmopolitans argue that the problem of what constitutes justice needs to be protected by the social contract and that this contract entails obligations to citizens who are given priority. The argument is that morally we feel more obligations to those closer to us.

At this point, it is useful to introduce the realist criticism of cosmopolitanism, namely that states will only serve the interests of their own citizens and will follow up on human rights when it is in their interests to do so.

As Goldsmith and Posner (2005, pp. 27–35 cited by Beardsworth) stress:

> Consistency of much state action with international human rights law simply means, regarding liberal democratic governments, coherence between domestic and international law. (Goldsmith and Posner 2005, pp. 86–90 cited by Beardsworth 2010, p. 58)

But normative law holds 'no *explanatory* purchase on international legal reality: they are prescriptive only…' (Beardsworth 2010, p. 57).

Criticisms from the Right and from realists rest on the impossibility for post-national institutions to be democratic. But although in the past this was less likely, the argument made by strong cosmopolitans is that architectures for strong cosmopolitan governance do exist. And that for social, economic and environmental well-being to be achieved—responsible global governance protected by international law needs to be implemented (Archibugi 2009).

In this respect, strong cosmopolitans differ from so-called weak cosmopolitans. The latter stress moral principles without providing any means to implement them.[30]

---

[30] Weak cosmopolitanism supports the principle of universal human rights enshrined in the Universal Declaration for Human Rights, but it argues that democracy per se is best served within the boundaries of the nation state. Citizens of nation states (albeit diverse) need to debate issues of common interest and to elect representatives to act as their agents within national governments, who in turn negotiate on their behalf on the international stage. Miller (1999) argues that we feel more responsibility towards those who are closest to us, family members, relevant others who are more connected to us. Linklater (1999, p. 473) strongly links cosmopolitanism with social justice, in order to address the rights of those who are not protected by states: 'The strong do what they can and the weak suffer what they must, boldly expresses the realist theme….' Miller along with Rawls, Nagel, and Pogge can be broadly characterized as weak cosmopolitans, albeit for very different reasons, ranging from their concern about the local participation of local people—who are best served within sovereign states—that are in turn responsible for sustaining human rights and environmental protection to the idea raised by Nagel that because all powerful states can do harm that a global state could be more trouble than it is worth. He also argues that states are more likely to do harm before being prepared to assist others. But Cosmopolitan justice is served through identifying the need for global rights and responsibilities to protect a sustainable and 'common future', in the words of the Brundtland (1987) Report. The challenge will be to enable people to extend their national identity and concerns to regional biospheres (of which we are part) and thus to include responsibility for others. This has spatial and temporal requirements, namely extending political responsibility to a wider region and to future generations. Miller's, Rawl's and Nagel's approach to justice is more minimalist than Nussbaum's approach (2006) which stresses that the moral boundaries of species and nationality need to be reconsidered, because the social contract is too narrow to protect those that fall outside the mantle of the nation state. The strong argument

Critiques of cosmopolitanism stress that normative wish lists are insufficient to address the real challenges posed by poverty and the will to power. Strong cosmopolitans stress that practical engagement and the capacity for understanding the point of view of other people is vital to bridge differences.[31]

Dialogue on a small scale (to create meaningful relationships at a face-to-face level) is important for building trust and for respecting why people see the world in particular ways.

Capacity building for the so-called good governance requires structures that represent the people and future generations of life. This in turn requires norms, facilitated by processes and implemented as praxis.

The problem is that state sovereignty is an outdated notion, because the problems of social and environmental poverty and injustice are the result of intermeshed problems that span national boundaries. A further challenge is that the convergent social, economic and environmental problems are perceived very differently by diverse stakeholders who are no longer isolated from one another. They jostle on the same global stage simultaneously. How can people become more capable of extending their horizons?

Noam Chomsky argued that language structures are shared by all humanity and that common meanings are linked by a common grammar which could support public education for the common good.

---

for cosmopolitanism is not necessarily undermined by postmodernists, such as Derrida or Foucault who argue that the normative approach needs to be informed by diverse voices, because the powerful frame or decide what constitutes knowledge. The strong cosmopolitans believe that rational reason ought to guide international law to protect the individual subject. But rational decisions need to also be guided by compassion for the powerless. 'Postmodernists stress that law per se does not protect the human or for that matter non-human life, it is complicit in supporting domination and control, but it can be used in a liberative manner. Foucault's work has been interpreted to address the way in which the state is complicit in allowing the patenting of some forms of life and the selective protection of those who fall within the social contract, thus removing rights from others….' (Beardsworth 2010, p. 181). But the post-modernists caution that what constitutes morality may shift according to the context and thus a bridge across the argument for universality, national sovereign approaches and the local is an approach based on the notion that the complexity of a decision needs to be matched by the complexity of the decision-makers and that the scaled up approach to decision making in overlapping regions may provide a way forward, along the lines suggested below. This will be a vital consideration in addressing the challenge of climate change.

[31] The difficulty of whether understanding and forgiveness need to be translated into legal forgiveness and leniency for those who are guilty of war crimes is another issue. The extent to which the perpetrators of widespread atrocities can be punished is a concern that cannot be swept aside. But the complicity of entire societies cannot be denied either. The widespread acceptance of the right to label others and to treat them differently provided the conditions for atrocities to be committed in Germany, Cambodia, Palestine and South Africa. Truth and reconciliation are perhaps the only ways in which transformation can occur. The corrupt treatment of people, the environment and animals in the name of profit is so widespread that laying the blame on the privileged 1 % without also accepting the everyday complicity of every middle-class person is very problematic. This is why the research is about middle-class people. I am part of this research project and complicit in that live a mobile lifestyle.

Diversity in terms of this argument could be underpinned by shared structures to communicate with one another in ways that respect diversity—to the extent that diverse ideas and values do not undermine the common good.

Creativity is needed to underpin the transformation from 'Wall Street' to 'wellbeing'. Wellbeing ought not to be conceptualised in narrow economic terms as an economic stock. Instead, wellbeing needs to be seen as a relationship or a flow of many factors resulting from our choices pertaining to '*being, having, doing and interacting*'.[32]

As the experience of suffering becomes more widespread, the notion of class will become central once again, because 'the poorest people in the world will be the hardest hit' (Beck 2009, p. 37). But the suffering and survival of other species whose fate is entangled with ours—should also be uppermost in our minds. Mitigation and adaptation to climate change through sustainable living needs to be explored. In particular our use of food, energy and water needs to be carefully managed locally, regionally and internationally. The strong cosmopolitan approach stresses the need for praxis, not only fine ethical rhetoric. It is based on the idea that what we do to others we do to ourselves and future generations of life.[33]

---

[32] It needs a wider movement to ensure that age and gender roles are acknowledged in ensuring viable communities within viable regions. The megacities are not sustainable. The grid lock in Jakarta and the haze of pollution in Beijing are recognized as unsustainable at conferences held in 2012 at both the University of Indonesia in Depok, J and at the Chinese Academy of Social Sciences Conference in Beijing. Protecting the global commons at the local and regional level is the focus of this ongoing research program in public policy and public administration, which has implications for education and the transformation of organizations spanning the state, market and non-government. For example, the Jakarta Post (March 3rd, 2012) highlighted the case of 33 law makers sent to jail who were involved in the election of Miranda S. Goelton for bribery, involving travelers checks to enable buying oil plantations in North Sumatra. The article was entitled: 'Nunan attends first trial session for bribery'. Corruption by the powerful at the expense of the environment also has implications for the way in which economics is framed and the way in which we govern. Specifically, it has implications for productivity for wellbeing and not for profit. Negative externalities are fiction, because the costs borne by the voiceless, marginalized, future generations and the environment. The theme of corruption and stealing from the next generation in developed and developing nations needs to be addressed. Cross-generational piracy could be a theme for research.

[33] The strong cosmopolitan argument is that the basis for containerist thinking is fallacious. According to realists, the problem with cosmopolitan politics is where do governments of nation states draw the line as to how they support those who seek refuge and asylum? The norms of hospitality are unrealistic they say. But, our fates are interlinked. The onus is upon all nations to rethink the notion of democracy and governance. The economy cannot continue to extract profit at the expense of the wellbeing of current and future generations. Wellbeing—not the economic bottom line needs to be the focus of our attention for cultural transformation, according to Stiglitz et al. (2010). But this requires re-conceptualizing culture. The strong cosmopolitan stresses the importance of recognizing the value of the environment on which we depend and thus recognizes that we are either part of the change—or complicit in contributing to the problem of 'consuming the planet'. Thus, Elliot and Urry (2010) stress the implications of developing a non-carbon economy for cultural transformation. Transformation will require changing the way in which we care for others (Mukta 2010, 2005). This will imply re-conceptualizing how we engage with one another and our attitude towards commodifying people, animals and the environment. The neo-conservative market uses people and the planet without care of the consequences. It extends the argument by

Developing nations such as Indonesia will be the leading global economies (along with China India and Southern Africa). These nation states will have more and more citizens not only aspiring to unsustainable middle-class lifestyles but also achieving them in the short term. But the middle-class lifestyles (as they are currently designed and lived) are based on heavy consumption and exploitation of human and natural resources.

Sustainability and resource management are central to the mitigating and adaptation process. The central ways to address the size of our carbon footprint is through minimizing our use of non-renewable energy. The challenge is to make a difference sooner, rather than later. The drive to succeed at the expense of others is based on false dualism. We cannot profit at the expense of others (human or animal) without some sort of systemic fallout. Furthermore, in order to be capable of distributing more resources to others, developed nations need to use *less resources* through *less wasteful living and more emphasis on fostering creative policy to support sustainable living.*[34] These aspects impact not only on our responsibilities to others, but also on rethinking what our rights ought to entail.[35]

Kant on hospitality to strangers by stressing the importance of the recognition of transnational agreements and law on environmental concerns and human rights (Nussbaum 2006). The strong cosmopolitan will define human security (Kaldor 2003, 2004) in terms of meeting human rights for all and avoiding a Eurocentric approach when addressing human rights. Cosmopolitanism as a concept has developed through responding to the critics such as Babar and Derrida who emphasized the difficulties associated with universalism and the colonial and imperialist overtones.

[34] Vidal, J. 2013 'Toxic e-waste dumped in poor nations', warns UN, *The Guardian Weekly*, 20.12.13.

[35] The toxic life of excess will lead to an unsustainable footprint. As human animals, we have the responsibility to look after current and future generations of life through considering the size of our footprint. This requires a change of culture. The inequality between the 1 % and the rest of the population is the key problem. According to Vidal (2013), illegal e-waste is shipped to developing countries: 'Few countries understand the scale of the problem, because no track is kept of all e-waste, says the European Environment Agency, which estimates between 250,000 t and 1.3 m t of used electrical produces are shipped out of the EU every year, mostly to West Africa and Asia.'

Chapter 4
New Regionalist Monitory Democracy and Governance: A Reply to the So-Called Problem of Cosmopolitan Politics

4.1 Introduction: How Can Democracy Avoid Being a So-Called 'Neo-Liberal Fantasy'?

Is democracy a 'neo-liberal fantasy', as suggested by Jodi Dean? Firstly, democracy or representative approaches involving degrees of participation are not the preserves of western capitalist societies. According to the historical research by Keane (2009), democratic engagement originated within an agrarian community in the Middle East in an area now known as Syria.

Dean (2005, p. 82) has stressed that the problem with democracy is that the discourse of the university stresses what democracy ought to be, in other words what it ought to look like and what it ought to do according to procedures. These normative accounts of the ideal may or may not be translated into practice. That depends on the vigilance of citizens who are prepared to defend the interests of the marginalized and voiceless within and beyond the boundaries of the nation state.

The Rawlsian approach has been extended by Nussbaum and Singer albeit from different ethical premises. But even if this expanded form of rights and responsibilities is accepted, the issue remains, how can praxis be achieved at the local and international level? This is my area of concern.

Dean has stressed in a videoed lecture on her book *Communist Horizon* (2012) that it is vital to ensure that working class rights are not eroded.

Dean was asked to comment on some practical ideas she had developed for making a difference. She listed talking and listening to people and then developing a transportation network to redistribute resources so that they could be shared with those who were in need. These ideas are compatible with an ideal form of social and environmental democracy and *ought to underpin* working towards the common good.

For this to occur social and environmental resources need to be valued appropriately through new forms of accounting to ensure that 'mismeasurement' (Stiglitz et al. 2010) no longer occurs.

Ideally, the fabric of life comprising the global commons ought not to be measured, because this could lead to commodification. This would be the ethical high

J. McIntyre-Mills, *Transformation from Wall Street to Wellbeing*, Contemporary Systems Thinking, DOI 10.1007/978-1-4899-7466-2_4,

road. But the low road to a more ethical and sustainable future developed in this book is that in the short term—by placing a value on water, biodiversity, freedom of expression, time to connect with others and the land and compassion for sentient creatures—then more ethical and sustainable governance measures could be put into practice.

The rule of law in overlapping Republican states would need to be a part of cultural transformation to protect the rights of the voiceless and future generations of life on the planet.

What is meant by accountability for the environmental protection? Who should be held responsible? The argument is that it ought to begin with local government, in order to ensure that the elitist or oligarchical tendencies of socialism (see Michel's 1915) and capitalism are averted.

Dean (2009) dismisses Butler's work (2005) but by 2012 she stressed the need for openness to the ideas of others, but within the limits of working towards the common good. Why does working towards the common good have to start with the label communism?

It is better to work without the baggage of any solution. It is useful to look to history for empirical lessons and for ideological inspiration (or cautionary tales), but the future can be written afresh with the wisdom of hindsight.

Dean characterizes all non-communists as mainstream, but her use of reflexivity resonates in many ways with the critical approach used by Butler—who stresses that appreciation of another's point of view is vital, in order to enhance reflexivity and in order to be responsive.

Totalitarian approaches are part of communism, so how can we continue to move towards the horizon? What empirical examples of communism work? The corrupt elitism evident in communist societies is as problematic as the corrupt elitism in capitalist societies. This is why the horizon needs to be always extended through monitory democracy and governance. Governance needs to be accountable to the people. The technology can enable an expansive principle 'from each according to his ability to each according to his need.'

According to Jodi Dean, digital communication makes some things possible, such as increased *exploitation of workers,* but it also makes it possible to share information and to expose corruption by sharing experiences with many groups of people.

Three options exist for transformation: centralist interventions, anarchist and negotiated discursive dialogues with a focus on expanded pragmatism. Reducing waste, reusing resources, saving resilient seeds and recycling wherever possible need to become the litmus test for households and local development, in order to redistribute resources to those in need and as a means to limit the misuse of scarce resources. Accounting and accountability at the local level need to be fostered by means of monitory democracy and governance.

Our research applies this philosophy at the local level and advocates for its extension to post national regional biospheres. The notion espoused by policy thinkers that representation needs to be carefully controlled (to support democracy) is fallacious.

If people are required to participate and to engage in 'if-then scenarios' they are likely to be able to understand one another's viewpoints better and more likely to make connections, provided that the axiom is maintained that we can be free and diverse—to the extent that our freedom and diversity does not undermine the rights and freedoms of others. This is the point raised by researchers such as Murray et al. (2007) in the Tuvalu Test to address the use of resources equitably within the region.

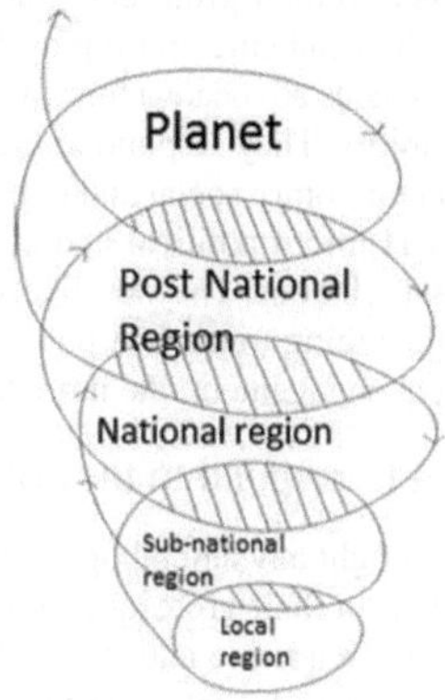

Transformation to a sustainable future through social movements such as 350.org could make a difference to the way in which we live, work and engage in leisure. It could be used as a means to ensure that those who fall outside the mantle of the nation state are given a voice.

The role of personal self-reflection and community engagement to consider 'if-then scenarios' could provide a means to achieve an alternative economic structure that values wellbeing as the bottom line through day-to-day choices and changes to thinking and practice.

Firstly, democracy or representative approaches involving degrees of participation are not the preserves of Western capitalist societies. According to the historical research by Keane (2009, p. xxv), democratic engagement occurred in an area of the Middle East, now known as Syria and it was born in an agrarian society. It has existed in many contexts and whether it is wise to label all these different approaches to representation democracy per se or forms of representative participation and governance is a moot point. What is important is that a balance is kept between rights and responsibilities locally, nationally and internationally.

The Rawlsian approach has been extended by Nussbaum and Singer albeit from different ethical premises. But even if this expanded form of rights and responsibilities is accepted, the issue remains, how can praxis be achieved at the local and international level? This is my area of concern. As stressed previously, governance and democracy have to deal with three options pertaining to truth (Crowder 2003; McIntyre-Mills 2000): (a) one truth response defended by grand narratives or conflict, (b) no truth (postmodernist) approached defended by relativism and (c) mediated (harmonized) responses based on stewardship. This book makes the case for social change through exploring interdisciplinary frameworks to address greed, the commodification of the powerless and the environment. It will be informed by debates on ethics, human reasoning capability, emotions and environmental politics and the practical implications for social democracy (Judt 2010).

Although I sympathise with Dean (2005, p. 123), I disagree with her authoritarian argument:

> …conservatives have resolved to fight any and all opponents to the death and neo-liberals have been every more emboldened in their grotesque grabs for greater and greater shares of the world's wealth, many of the academic and typing left have urged peace, love and understanding. These influential voices advocate a turn to ethics, a generosity to difference and awareness or mutual vulnerability. They respond to the religious, nationalist or market fundamentalisms dominating contemporary social and political life by rejecting dogmatism and conviction, advocating instead micro political and ethical practices that work on the self in its immediate reactions and relations. They are likely right that engaging others with affirmation and generosity is a nice thing to do. But politically it is suicidal. The more the left refrains from divisive political engagement, the more the right advances…[1]

Dean (2005, p. 123) argues that to respond to the crises as follows:

> As conservatives have resolved to fight any and all opponents to the death and neo-liberals have been every more emboldened in their grotesque grabs for greater and greater shares of the world's wealth, many of the academic and typing left have urged peace, love and understanding. These influential voices advocate a turn to ethics, a generosity to difference and awareness or mutual vulnerability. They respond to the religious, nationalist or market fundamentalisms dominating contemporary social and political life by rejecting dogmatism and conviction, advocating instead micro political and ethical practices that work on the self in its immediate reactions and relations. They are likely right that engaging others with affirmation and generosity is a nice thing to do. But politically it is suicidal. The more the left refrains from divisive political engagement, the more the right advances…

The extensive criticism of Butler by Dean for emphasizing agency at a personal level, based on striving to suspend judgement and to understand the other as a precursor to connecting with them, seems unjustified, in her bid to stress the important role of political action to draw the line against what ought to be condemned. But Dean falls into a trap of her own making.

> But for all our hatred of Bush and his wars, for all the protests and petitions, for all the energy our anger provided, we remained unable or unwilling to take the next steps of imagining, organizing, and creating another world… (Dean 2005, p. 174).[2]

---

[1] See Jodi Dean (http://www.guernicamag.com/features/the-limits-of-communication/) in Oct 2012. Extending hours has a limit, even when workers are accessible via their technology. The exhaustion and overload is one reason for these limits, but nevertheless the potential to organize social movements and to use digital media with discretion has changed the nature of democracy and governance. Although Dean criticizes the way in which digital technology has been used to exploit workers and to extend the market, it could also be used to enable the distribution and sharing of resources. Perhaps digital cooperatives could be part of the transition—to a new phase in human history?

[2] Jodi Dean on *The Communist Horizon* at the Utube site 'Not an alternative'. Democracy is problematic…'mounts a response to the economic and social crisis 'Democracy is no panacea: Politics are not dead. Communism didn't end in 1989.' Drawing on *The Communist Horizon,* she asks: 'How can we organize against the current gridlock?' Dean stresses the limits to communication (http://www.guernicamag.com/features/the-limits-of-communication/ in Oct 2012). 'Extending

Condemnation, drawing the line and using law to support justice require working out with others what ought to be condemned. To create a cosmopolitan politics, we will need to establish conversations with diverse interest groups.

Class pleasures such as excessive consumption may be nauseating to those who understand the reason why excess is toxic to oneself, others and the environment.

But rights and responsibilities can only be upheld within a framework of law and governance. Butler is right to criticize the way in which USA has acted outside the Geneva Convention. But Dean has a point that compassionate connection is insufficient to uphold justice. Nevertheless, communication is the basis for democracy and for ethical practice. A society that does not support compassion and communication with others (whether or not we agree with them) is a society that is on the wrong track, a track towards authoritarianism. This applies to any society—be it consumer capitalist, socialist or communist.

Dean was asked to comment on her book *The Communist Horizon* about practical ideas she has for making a difference. Talking and listening were listed first and then developing a transportation network to redistribute resources so that they can be shared.

These ideas are compatible with an ideal form of social and environmental democracy and ought to underpin working towards the common good. She makes a fair point that no real choices are provided within current liberal democracies. But the point that needs to be stressed is that wellbeing needs to be supported by means to ensure justice and the appropriate distribution of resources. Social and environmental resources need to be valued appropriately as a precursor to new governance processes being implemented.

How can this be achieved without new forms of accounting to ensure that 'mismeasurement' (Stiglitz et al. 2010) no longer occurs? A response could be that the fabric of life comprising the global commons ought not to be measured, because that could lead to commodification.

The argument developed in this book is that, on the contrary, by placing a value on water, biodiversity, freedom of expression, time to connect with others and the land and compassion for sentient creatures, appropriate governance measures could be put into practice.

The rule of law in overlapping Republican states will need to be a part of cultural transformation to protect the rights of the voiceless and future generations of life on the planet.

What is meant by accountability for the environmental protection? Who should be responsible? The argument developed in Chap. 1 is that it ought to begin with local governance,[3] in order to ensure that the elitist tendencies of both socialism (see

hours has a limit, even when workers are accessible via their technology. The exhaustion and overload is one reason for these limits, but nevertheless the potential to organize social movements and to use digital media with discretion has changed the nature of democracy and governance. We need to look at the relationships of exploitation and the way in which people, animals and labour are commodified.'

[3] Heycox, J., Meadows, P. and Vernon, B. 1997. 'Environment and Energy Statistics Section Australian Bureau of Statistics. Measuring environmental expenditures and revenues in Local Govern-

Michel's 1915) and capitalism are averted through ensuring monitory democracy and governance checks from below:

> In 1993 the United Nations published a handbook describing the conceptual basis for implementing an Integrated System of Environmental and Economic Accounting (SEEA) SEEA is a comprehensive framework which outlines a range of potential and monetary measures of the environment/economy relationship which could be used to support integrated social, economic and environmental policy and planning. SEEA outlines a number of possible accounts and sub-accounts which relate to different aspects of the interactions that occur between the environment and the economy. The ABS has based its environmental accounting program on the accounts outlined in SEEA…. (Heycox et al. 1997 cite UN 1993, p. 3)

The research outlined in Chaps. 1 and 2 addresses a means to operationalize environmental protection through engaging members of the public in the process of developing appropriate measures of wellbeing. This is a vital step in cultural transformation as it raises awareness. It also requests contracting at a household level as to the trade-offs they are prepared to make. Nevertheless, detailed accounting and accountability ought not to create a legalistic environment where attempts are made to find ways around the letter of the law. Sanctions can never replace ethical responsibility. Values, not law, are the most vital consideration for cultural transformation. Furthermore, the funding of environmental protection activities needs to be supported by all levels of government[4] and by the private sector. The users of services, the providers of services and the beneficiaries all need to make contributions. The

ment: report on a pilot project with 21 local governments in Australia.' The Australian Centre for Regional and Local Government Studies. Working Paper No 2. University of Canberra: 'Based on adaptation from international frameworks for environmental accounting, the survey sought information from councils about their outlays and income related to environmental protection, natural resource use and management, and addressing the repercussions of damage from environmental events…Most councils….found it difficult to provide the information sought since their accounting systems are not usually structured to separately identify environmentally related transactions. Nonetheless, the estimates provided suggest that the 12 responding councils spent a collective total of $ 232 million in 1994–1995 or 1995–1996 on environmentally related activities and received around $ 259 million in revenue related to those activities. By far the largest category of these expenditures and revenues was related to environmental protection activities, particularly waste waters (sewerage and storm water) and waste management services. Natural resource use and management was the other substantial activity in budgetary terms for many types of council. Expenditures on activities such as protecting biodiversity and landscape were found to be a very small proportion of environmental transactions by these councils.' According to this report, local government is responsible for approximately one third of public sector expenditure of sanitation and protection of the environment each year according to ABS (Osborn 1997b cited in Heycox et al. 1997). But according to this source (op cit.) the classifications 'do not provide details on the types of environmental protection activities being undertaken.'

[4] According to Heycox et al. (1997, p. 4): 'Data published by the ABS on the environmental protection expenditures by the public sector, including local government, is derived from the public sector finance collection which is based on an international Classification of the Functions of Government (COFOG). The problem arises due to the structure of COFOG was designed long before collecting data on public sector transactions does not enable the environmental component of transactions…to be separately identified.' But separation or disaggregation is quite the wrong way to approach the problem. This is why a systemic approach is vital and why the research supports the promotion of wellbeing as an integrated measure for a sustainable future.

problem with neo-conservative versions of communitarian arguments is that the burden of responsibility ought not to be shifted to locals without the private sector, welfare sectors and all levels of government playing an equal role.

Dean was asked the following question: 'Who are the Left? How do they relate to class…?' It is worth considering the question carefully. The representatives of the Left are part of the elite. The class dimension is blurred, because the representatives do not have to be responsive to those they represent on the shop floor. As stewards, they are paid large salaries. But the casual labourers who make up the working class poor in USA, for example, have no representation and no awards to protect them.

Who are the people who comprise the 1 % who make up the elite? A Wall Street trader may be a member of the 1 % in terms of salary, but he may lose his job tomorrow and if he does not have capital of his own or assets, he too could become a casual labourer as depicted in 'Down in Jungleland', an Australian Broadcasting documentary about the non-recovery of the US economy, post 2008.[5] The trader reflected (perhaps defiantly) that he was 'still not a liberal' but that he was more concerned about how difficult it was to work until 2 am as a bartender and then to get up to work a second job the following morning.

Although it may be better to earn US $ 2.13 an hour than to exist on US $ 2 a day, we cannot say that because people in USA or Europe[6] are relatively better off than in the Democratic Republic of Congo, as a way to sell the extreme capitalism to the working poor and unemployed. We need to look at the relationships of exploitation and the way in which labour and the land is commodified. The unemployed and the working poor in South Africa have seen some changes. According to Calland (2013, p. 13):

> Adult literacy under five mortality, access to water, levels of sanitation and rates of poverty have improved. Notably, the proportion of people living on less than two dollars a day, an internationally accepted measure of poverty, has declined either from 16.2 per cent in 1996 to 2.7 per cent in 2011 (if one considers South African sources) or from 39.9 per cent in 1995 to 31.3 % in 2009 (if one considers World Bank data).

But the gap between the incomes of the rich and poor has widened. According to Calland (op cit.):

> [the] Gini coefficient, which measures the extent of such inequality (0 indicating perfect equality and 100 indicating that one person owns all the wealth), has worsened by 6.6 points. Meanwhile, the income share of the top 10 per cent of earners has risen by 6.6 percentage points, and the share of the bottom 20 % has declined by 0.9 percentage points. Indeed, South Africa now enjoys the dark accolade of being the most unequal society in the world. While we have slightly improved our Human Development index score (a composite of life expectancy, education and income per capita), our ranking among our emerging market peers has slipped. Finally and most worryingly, the unemployment rate, which considers both the formal and informal employment, has worsened by approximately 5 %.

[5] Down in Jungleland, http://www.abc.net.au/foreign/content/2013/s3874510.htm details the working conditions of Americas working poor.

[6] http://jdeanicite.typepad.com/i_cite/2012/11/europe-faces-a-multi-national-general-strike-against-austerity-timecom.html

4.1.1 *Old-Style Democracy Does Not Represent the Will of the People*

Fragmentation of policy ideas and non-participation by voters within a nation state can lead to the election of leaders who are not widely representative of the people. The costs of old-style democratic elections means that only those who are able to muster large amounts of funding have a hope of being elected.

At a post-national level, democracy does not protect human rights. The right to water security and the implications for food security are raised by Shiva in *Water Wars* (2002). This builds on her other work in the area of global corporations who patent seeds and who destroy crop diversity.

4.1.2 *Food Security Through Overlapping Regional Domains*

The bottom line is that food security is essential and agricultural land must be protected. Agrarian approaches need to be delinked from any one specific known political option. Humanity has the capacity to be a competitive mobile hunter-gatherer and a cooperative, parochial agriculturalist who engages in reciprocal exchanges. The challenge is to find cultural balance along with alternative forms of energy. New regional approaches to food security will require transnational approaches that place security and protection of the global commons at a post-national level. This does not mean that the state ought not to play a role in federalist regions. But the local, national and international domains will need to be seen as integral or part of a systemic whole.

According to Morton (1998, p. 6):

> The concept of think globally and act locally 'underlines the importance of local government involvement in environmental management. Local government operates at the local level not only as a service provider but also as a planning, regulatory and coordinating agency. This multi-functional role provides a capacity to combine both economic instruments and regulatory provisions to achieve specific environmental management objectives in an efficient and effective manner. The principles of Ecologically Sustainable Development (ESD) are also an important element of local environmental management, typically underpinning the land use planning and control functions delegated to local authorities. The location, intensity and form of human settlement within an area tend to pose threats to the environment which need to be addressed....

Morton (1998, p. 6) does not address the additional and systemic issue which is the security of human settlements from disaster. Instead, he focuses on the threats to the environment as:

> Wasteful use of scarce natural resources; loss and/or pollution of natural habitats and associated water and reduced biodiversity; production of greenhouse gases and associated global warming; air and noise pollution through factors such as excessive use of private vehicles and poor settlement planning and location.

We need to learn from all these options. Dean (2005) stresses the limitations of politics in America as a debate between pseudo-opposition. The Right and the Left are complicit in supporting neo-liberalism. Transformation requires openness to change plus a reconceptualization of what it means to sustain the wellbeing of the planet. Rights and responsibilities must be reframed, but it is unlikely to occur within establishment politics, because the choices are limited. Using digital technology more responsibly could help to enable communication to support agriculture, but it is debatable whether mobility per se will be reduced by digital technology. It is used to augment communication with those who maintain some face-to-face connectivity (Elliot 2012).

4.2 Designing Multilevel, Multi-Agency Governance for Social and Environmental Justice

The current system is failing the majority, as the following data reveal:

> The rates of temporary work in Australia are staggering with around a quarter of employees having no paid leave entitlements Spain is the only country in the OECD with a higher rate of temporary employment than Australia. (Evans 2013, p. 21)

Evans discusses the bill to amend the Fair Work Act that was introduced by the Greens MP Adam Bandt. Lack of job security removes the ability to plan ahead and it has implications for the ability of part-time workers to own a home.

From the days of the Eureka Stockade in Australia, socialist movements have stressed that workers' rights are not given without assertive action. The taxes were levied at a time when miners (diggers) could ill afford to pay them.

According to Evatt (1984, p. xx):

> It may fairly be said that the Eureka Stockade put an end not only to an unjust tax upon labour, but to a brutal and tyrannical method of enforcing the tax. It procured for the miner's equality in political status, a franchise both in the general government of the colony and in the local administration of the mining laws…In the end public opinion and popular agitation prevailed over mere legalism.

According to Evatt (1984, p. xxiii):

> When the people of Melbourne were informed of the truth—that the miners had been attacked while sleeping within their stockade….they were aflame with indignation. The Age insisted that the resistance of the miners was not against the Crown, but against the pollutions and abominations covered by its sanction…. A great public meeting of Melbourne citizens attributed the tragedy to the 'coercion of military force' and to the 'harsh and imprudent recommencement of digger hunting….

The testimony and historical account by Raffaeollo Carboni underlines the point that careful testimony based on empirical evidence as well as solidarity with the public and the press can help to transform society. The skills of translator and political awareness obtained in Italy as a member of the Italian Risorgimento (Evett 1984, p. viii) provided the groundwork for local action that helped to establish worker's rights in Australia.

Raffaeollo Carboni's contribution to worker's rights was informed by experience working for justice in Europe.

Can cosmopolitan politics address the criticism raised by the Left, namely that politics needs to strive for debate that ensures the pseudo-politics of the Right and Left in capitalist society leads to a transformation of the neo-liberal market? The Islamic movements in Africa, Asia and America and Asia Pacific argue that this is the case. The victory by the French troops in Mali announced from Timbuktu was highlighted by Hollande as just that, a small victory in an ongoing battle that will need to face up to the unsustainability of current ways of life and the danger of allowing a narrow determinism that could undermine critical thought and all that this would entail for democracy, science and ethics.

In 'White-papering the cracks', Hugh White (2013) argues that the policy direction of both Australia and the USA fails to recognize the shift in the power dynamics to Asia and that Australia should recognize that geographically it is Asian and that policies should not strain Asian relationships. White does not follow through with any alternative policy suggestions.

Emotions need to be acknowledged when striving to think and act ethically, but they need to be tempered with empirical evidence. This was the strength of the first-hand account by Carboni, who wrote the following at the outset of his narrative:

> I undertake to do what an honest man should do, let it thunder or rain. He who buys this book to lull himself to sleep had better spend his money on grog. He who reads this book to smoke a pipe over it, let him provide himself with plenty of tobacco—he will have to blow hard.

Designs could harmonize our desires, wants and needs, so that we develop new forms of solidarity based on an understanding that what we do to others, we do to ourselves and the next generation of life.[7] This is the crux of the argument. Thus, it provides an answer to the realists who are concerned about self-interest or national interests and those who think it is impractical, or a sign of weakness to have compassion for others. Life depends on relationships with others and sustaining the interconnections of life.

Has 'seeing like a state' (Scott 1999) led to the erosion of diverse viewpoints being tolerated? We could develop surveillance systems *from below*—that monitors Big Brother and blows the whistle on corruption—in order to avert control *from above* and to ensure that local areas do not lapse into so-called 'ungovernable zones' of 'warlordism' (Elliot and Urry 2010).

[7] This approach to ethics is based on considering the implications—social, cultural, political, economic and environmental in the short, medium and long term for all forms of life. The ethical axiom or ideal on which the approach is based is that democracy and governance for a sustainable future needs to support freedom and diversity to the extent that freedom and diversity does not undermine the rights of others or the next generation of life. It requires a very different approach to framing representation and accountability (McIntyre-Mills 2006, 2008, 2010; McIntyre-Mills and De Vries 2011).

In the resource-rich cities of the world, mobile people spend their time rushing from appointment to another. They use mobile technology in ways that can make life even more frenetic, rather than using it to enable more sustainable living.

Digital technology can be used in different ways—not to constantly reschedule meetings but to enable life to be lived at a slower pace. It could be used to enable people to think about alternative ways of living and to 'join up the dots'. The containment of anxiety has been stressed as one of the main reasons for using digital technology by many very mobile workers. Containment anxiety is felt increasingly by overwrought people living very fast-paced lives (Elliot 2010, p. 21) and so digital technology tends to be used to address isolation and rescheduling—but it can be used for transformation.

Cosmopolitanism suggests a different way of using technology, in order to support being rooted in one particular place. Mobility is greater than it has ever been in the past. Powerful decision makers live lives that are mobile and information rich, because they have wide networks. The research in South Australia indicates an increasing awareness of the need to live sustainably, but a sense that people are unable to translate that awareness into practice, because they find it difficult to consider all the different aspects at the same time and then to see how the web of factors impact their choices.

By testing out ideas with people who have lived experience (as well as by people with professional expertise), it is possible to enhance the quality of the decisions and to achieve a better match.

Public Administration Review (PAR) is based on the notion that the complexity of the decision needs to be matched by the complexity of the decision makers. This enhances the robustness of the decision and it is also more likely to be supported politically by those who are affected by the decisions.

The role of the good local citizen who strives to be a steward for future generations is to: (a) enhance wellbeing of communities, (b) support the demographic transition and (c) enhance life chances for all through securing food, energy and water.

She/he builds stocks for future generations and does not externalize the costs, because poverty, pollution and carbon emissions ought not to be shifted to future generations or other people. This requires post-national and post-disciplinary cooperation and new forms of governance.

Could we start to see patterns in the stories? Could we start seeing these as the basis for developing cocreated narratives that become increasingly harmonious song lines for a new society that is indeed post-materialist?

But how can we avoid the danger of imposing one-size-fits-all approaches that deny the fine-grained contextual details?

I argue that multilevel, multi-agency governance is needed to address these challenges. For example, the need for more responsive governance becomes apparent when we consider the issue of the growing gap between the rich and the poor in South Africa. The salaries of mineworkers are way too low in comparison with the enormous salaries and benefits accorded to chief executive officers (CEOs) and managers.

The indebtedness of miners whose wages had been garnished by the law to pay for their debts in a bid to meet basic needs or to acquire just some of the goods advertised in the media. The lack of justice for those who died whilst striking for better pay underlines the importance of always upholding the right to a voice. According to Smith (2013):[8]

> The disaster drew comparisons with the Sharpeville massacre of 1960 and the 1976 Soweto uprising, but this has been bitterly described as the first 'democratic massacre'. The police were serving a black majority government and defending the interests of London-based mining company Lonmin in the world's richest platinum belt. 'Never did we believe that our government would turn their guns on our people in such a brutal and callous manner,' said the Marikina massacre anniversary organizing committee on the worker's behalf. To date, no police officer has been charged, labour relations are in crisis and killings continue in Marikana.... In modern South African history, the prevailing view is that nothing has changed....

Smith goes on to argue that the impact of garnishing the wages of the very poor is desperation. According to Benjamin (2012, p. 2):

> The Marikane riots in Johannesburg can be better understood when we realize that many miners from rural areas with minimal literacy and numeracy bought goods and services that resulted in levels of indebtedness that rendered many close to destitute. Business interests were supported by a legal system that was not in turn supported by a fair, transparent or open administrative system. Errors were made by courts, over worked magistrates approved deductions that sometimes applied to the wrong worker or were erroneous sustained for years after the amount had already been paid·
> We have hundreds of examples of where debt of R 500 became debt of R 5000, 90 % of it due to legal fees.... Debtors signing forms on the same day of signing the loan agreement, consenting to a judgment should they default, despite this being illegal. This robs the debtor the right to fight the amount being charged and ensures it is seen only by the clerk of the court, as a magistrate need not be involved....

Ethical decisions need to be made within context, so how can cosmopolitanism address this criticism?

The response is that the decision needs to be guided by the axiom that freedom and diversity should be sustained wherever possible and that the limit ought to be the point at which the rights of others or future generations are undermined. This requires governance and laws to maintain the conditions for justice, both social and environmental. But the problem is that democracy has been highjacked by the market and by the state.

Corruption extends from Wall Street to boardroom complicity that allows both overt and covert controls buttressed by a corrupt market system that has failed the majority of people and the planet.

I am tired of extensive critiques that end with a sense of hopelessness. A new form of democratic engagement that does not involve immense costs or the ability to command the mainstream print or digital media. Instead, it is possible to work from below, in order to balance the needs of people and the planet. Instead of prefiguring change in an isolated, small community, it is possible to develop exchange

[8] Frustration grows at justice denied after South African Massacre. *The Guardian Weekly*, 23.08.13.

systems that extend beyond the community level to engage with the wider community. This requires accountability for the way in which resources are used.

Complicity extends to the role of elected leaders who play at politics. The role of the senate in the USA, for example, is to slow and delay the passing of bills, according to Burdett Loomis, 2013.[9] In the past, perhaps this stalling tactic provided the context for careful testing out of ideas. But currently it has been used for other reasons, such as the filibustering (asking long questions as a delaying tactic) by Republicans in the senate to delay the processing of decisions.

In addition, the power of social movements has been effectively harnessed by the far right through the so-called tea party movement. Filibustering is the preserve of those who are not elected. It provides an opportunity for participation for those within the senate. But those whom they are supposed to represent—the 99 % that Stiglitz (2012) mentions in his latest book on inequality—remain unaddressed.

The Occupy Wall Street Movement has, to date, had less impact that the Arab Spring. The changes brought about by social movements can be positive or negative. New forms of governance and democracy are required. Existing forms of democracy and governance are no longer effectively addressing the biggest challenges of the day, namely: representation of an increasingly marginalized majority, lack of accountability to the poor, lack of sustainable use of resources and lack of opportunities for effective engagement.

Another cause for concern is the fact that Obama has allowed Manning Clerk to face life in prison at best as a 'traitor', because Manning provided documents to Wiki leaks that were deemed a threat to American security. The issues raised by Snowden about surveillance by the USA of European allies needs to be placed within the context of America in decline and striving to maintain a competitive position.[10]

Glen Grenwald (2012), a concerned blogger associated with *The Guardian* has argued that human rights are compromised when prisoners are kept naked and when their sense of humanity is degraded. Furthermore, the way that the terrorism law is being interpreted in New York by judges is problematic, according to Greenwald. In 2002, a gang member with a Mexican background shot another member and in the process killed a young girl aged 10. Instead of being charged with murder or homicide, he had been charged with terrorism. In the wake of 9/11, 2001 acts of public violence are being addressed through the terrorism law.[11]

---

[9] Loomis, B. 2013 Can we effectively govern ourselves? Public Lecture, Flinders University, March. 'The senate creates a barrier in the USA and roadblocks legislation. He raises the question about the effectiveness of current structures and processes.'

[10] Macskill, E. 2013 'A cold war for the new era? New Snowden leaks tell of bugs at EU embassy.' The Weekly Guardian pg. 1.

[11] Greenwald, G. 2012. 'New York's top court highlights the meaninglessness and menace of the term "terrorism"' A fascinating new ruling unwittingly illustrates the separate system of 'justice' invented for Muslims in the USA after 9/11.

http://www.guardian.co.uk/commentisfree/2012/dec/16/court-terrorism-morales-gangs-meaningless Accessed December 29, 2012.

The so-called fiscal cliff[12] that Americans face has resulted in the poor and middle classes paying for the excesses of the rich through taxes and the limitation of welfare protection for the unemployed. Those who speak out against the state and the ramifications of supporting democracy through violence have faced imprisonment. The identification with Republican conservatism to stop spending has led to a deadlock between Democrats and Republicans. The binary oppositional politics between Right and Left has created a deadlock (29 December 2012 and October 2013). The flow on affects is a cause for concern.[13]

Japan provides another example of the complexities of achieving democracy and sustainable solutions. Although the majority of Japanese expressed concerns about nuclear energy, they voted for a conservative Liberal Democratic Party (LDP) that did not guarantee outlawing nuclear power.[14] Narrow pragmatism guided the voters to vote out and punish the government that they held responsible for the Fukushima disaster. Unfortunately, this has meant that they voted for the other main party on the right. Right–Left politics is far too simplistic and needs to allow for more creative responses to the concerns raised by people.

4.3 A Way Forward: Towards a Post-Carbon Economy?

This section strives to grasp the nettle: Climate change requires not merely adaptation to the consequences of climate change, but addressing the causes, namely the unsustainable consumption of resources by the privileged at the expense of the poor and future generations. This requires addressing the challenge posed by the Earth Charter:

---

[12] http://live.wsj.com/video/everything-you-need-to-know-about-the-fiscal-cliff/EE994540-68DA-4374-81FE-287A76422E5C.html.

[13] Mail and Guardian, on line news,,http://mg.co.za/article/2012-12-29-obama-immediate-action-needed-on-fiscal-cliff Accessed 29/12/2012:
The US faces the fiscal cliff because tax rate cuts dating back to President George W Bush's tenure expire at the end of the year. The pending across-the-board reductions in government spending, which will slice money out of everything from social programmes to the military, were put in place last year as an incentive to both parties to find ways to cut spending. That solution grew out of the two parties' inability in 2011 to agree to a grand bargain that would have taken a big bite out of the deficit. Facing a deadline that was born out of Washington's dysfunction, success was far from guaranteed – even on a slimmed-down deal that postponed hard decisions about spending cuts into 2013—in a Congress where lawmakers grumbled about spending the New Year holiday in the Capitol. If Congress can't reach a broad deal to rein in deficit spending, Obama said Congress should allow a vote on a basic package that would preserve tax cuts for middle-class Americans while extending unemployment benefits for the long-term jobless and working toward a foundation for a broader deal. Republicans and Democrats say privately that any agreement would likely include an extension of middle-class tax cuts that had been set to expire at the end of the year, with increased tax rates at upper incomes—a priority that was central to Obama's re-election campaign.

[14] Japan forges ahead with nuclear power despite protests | News | World | Mail & Guardian http://mg.co.za/article/2012-12-23-japan-anti-nuclear-vote-melts-away.

> Everyone shares responsibility for the present and future wellbeing of the human family and the larger living world (cited by Hayden, 368)

How to bridge individual interests and the collective good through praxis that prefigures change in overlapping regions remains the challenge. The notion of isolated city states with small, static populations is no longer relevant. Democracy and governance needs to develop to respond to current challenges. If the basic premise is that justice requires a recognition that we can be free and diverse to the extent that freedom and diversity do not undermine the rights of others within this generation and the next, then we are able to accept that the ideal of treating others as ends not means can be addressed through thinking about the consequences of political choices in expanded temporal and geographical terms, but also in terms of rethinking the relationships of human beings to the environment and other species of life. The notion that democracy serves the interests of humanity at the expense of the environment is simply unsustainable. The notion that elected governments serve the people who elect them as their agents needs to be expanded to accept that the rights of elected governments and the people they serve need to be expanded to consider the rights of future generations of life. The responsibility of the people (the principles) is to this generation and the next.

This notion can be summed up as strong cosmopolitanism based on the idea of post-national governance in overlapping regions aimed at balancing both rights and responsibilities to others and the environment. The planet is not a credit card to be used to benefit some—whilst others pick up the tab! The responsibility weighs differently on developed and less developed nations and also differently on the rich and poor, this generation and the next.

The architecture of governance (Archibugi 2008) needs to respond to environmental needs that protect the wellbeing of global citizens (Haydon 2010). Sovereign nation states need to consider regional rights and responsibilities in a series of overlapping organizations that apply the rule of law to ensure equitable and fair distribution of rights and responsibilities for food, energy and water. The research is about developing post-national organizations to ensure human rights. Disaster management, movement of people fleeing disaster or injustice and securing food, energy and water are concerns that span boundaries (spatial, conceptual and temporal). We need to solve problems across generations, across disciplines and across nation states to create good neighbourhoods. This requires trust and better communication so that we understand one another better.

The criticism posed by Arendt about the systems approach used to plan the Vietnam War and to consider the implications—as outlined in the Pentagon papers—is very relevant.

We need to ensure that we remain open to the ideas of others in order to test out the consequences of our choices. It is all very well for Luhmann (1995) to argue that global complexity should be the starting point for addressing challenges and that the nation state is inadequate. Nation states will need to work together to address a common threat. If we hope to achieve conscious evolution and we do not wish to rely on chance, then we need to find ways to engage local people in thinking through the implications of their choices.

- To what extent do nations trample on the rights of others by shortening their life span? What midpoint indicators such as decreasing biodiversity and rising sea levels (see Murray et al. 2006, pp. 14–16) can be developed to ensure that we live in ways that do not shorten the life of others and that do not lead to loss of life? The choices for local wellbeing have an implication for the wider region, which is why these choices should be transparent. How could this be achieved? Whistle blowing is necessary before and not only after the horse has bolted. How do we prevent problems through monitoring on a regular basis?
- Could enabling people at the local level (through the principle of subsidiarity) address the concerns for access to information? How do we engage people so that they are willing to act as stewards? If we hope to achieve conscious evolution and we do not wish to rely on chance, then we need to find ways to engage local people in thinking through the implications of their choices. To what extent do nations trample on the rights of others by shortening their life span? What midpoint indicators such as decreasing biodiversity and rising sea levels see Murray et al. 2006, pp. 14–16) can be developed to ensure that we live in ways that do not shorten the life of others and that do not lead to loss of life? The choices for local wellbeing have an implication for the wider region, which is why these choices should be transparent. How could this be achieved?
- Explore the potential for participation supported by decision-making software to match services to need, mitigate the causes of risk and adapt to the consequences of climate change. It makes the case that the following are amongst the greatest challenges facing humanity and that they potentially pose an 'existential risk': (a) representation of the increasingly diverse populations within nation states; (b) accountability to ensure that resources are used fairly, equitably and sustainably; and (c) engagement to enhance the capability of people to understand that attitudes towards consumption have profound implications for social and environmental justice issues.

4.4 Reframing the Future: Implications for Ethics, Democracy and Governance

> Conventional economic growth based on rising consumption of currently prevailing goods and technologies is not tenable. It will leave billions poor and under-consuming, it will leave the affluent unhappy, it will damage finite natural capital that necessary mitigation and adaptation expenditures will be too great to contemplate. A shift to a green economy is inevitable. It is simply a question whether it occurs before or after the world becomes locked into severe climate change and other harm to natural capital. On the assumption that before is preferable, then the following five commitments need quickly to be made and implemented…. (Pretty 2013, p. 20)
>
> According to Pretty, we need to reduce consumption, improve status of women, develop displacement technologies, improve human wellbeing through protecting natural capital, make commitments to limit spending in areas that deplete natural capital, employ taxes

> and market instruments to shift domestic consumer preferences and behaviour in all major economic sectors of energy, transport, building, agriculture, forestry and waste…. (op cit.)

Much of the activity which takes place in the social and natural sciences is in the areas of knowledge that focus on research on others. We need to pause and take time to do some research on our own lives and why we see the world in particular ways.

At a recent conference on creating the future in Melbourne, November 2012, Prof. Susan Greenfield summed up the issue of the plasticity of the brain, meaning that the brain makes neural connections; the more connections the more mindful we become. The making of connections is personal. It is the result of our personal experiences, so even two identical twins will have the potential to develop different connections as a result of their experiences. To what extent can the use of conceptual tools enable us to extend our sense of the world and to enable us to see ourselves as members of a wider group to whom we are responsible and with whom we have solidarity? Can leadership that fosters 'neurogenesis' or making of connections make a difference—or is it all about power and the will to power?

Although activities like playing the piano will help to develop new neural connections, even thinking about playing can develop these connections. So the idea behind this research was that perhaps by getting people to think differently about the way in which they live, and to consider, what if I were to do things differently? Perhaps it will enable the participants who do these mental exercises to transform the way in which they live? I did this research first with people with complex health, housing and social inclusion needs. Many were addressing unemployment and had a range of associated needs and health-related problems—including recovering from drug and other alcohol-related illnesses. Addiction to a way of life can be both a cause and the effect of many other problems, as Stafford Beer (1974) stressed in his research. This is why the approach to research needs to be one of engagement and being the change.

> Arendt (1972, p. 89) stresses that the abolitionists (even Jefferson) did not think that slaves should be afforded space within the nation state. Freed slaves they thought ought to be free to set up their own separate state in Africa—perhaps Liberia (!). The social contract did not extend rights to slaves! So the nation state has always had within it a very limited sense of rights and responsibilities.
>
> 'Systemic racism': discriminatory patterns and practices which involve more than the action of a few individual attitudes, but rather the systemic practices of racism built into society's major institutions (Feagin 2006).[15]

[15] A black entrepreneur in America gives this account of her experiences. They are relevant in the wake of the recent school massacre. Not because the shooter was black, but because it gives an insight into the emotions associated with exclusion and marginalization, as well as the impact on the mental health of the perpetrator: 'We can never be ourselves all around. I think that may be a given for all people, but us particularly, it's really a mental health problem. It a wonder we haven't all gone out and killed somebody or killed ourselves…' (Picca et al. 2011). Strategies for dealing with the pain of rejection: 'I come in here and scream! (laughs) I talk to my friends… she sits and listens to me, I scream and holler. She has even seen me cry because I am so angry til I am to the point of violence, but I know…. I have to be really cognizant of what I am doing…. And I am not going to eradicate racism by knocking off one person. So I just call my friends and get it off my chest with them…. But I can't let it stay in, because if I let it stay in it just makes me angrier and an-

4.4.1 Vignette on Freedom, Slavery, Art and Architecture

The definitions of slave were raised once again this week by Germaine Greer (2013) who discusses the slave labour of poor women who worked in Irish laundries, run by nuns expected to find a way to support themselves and the women who were placed in their care.

She stresses that working conditions were probably on par with other workers at that time. But the bright spot for me is that today people recognize these conditions as abhorrent and that the unreal expectation of celibacy has been recently questioned by cardinals within the Catholic Church.[16]

The value of art as a means to express complexity and contradictions should not be underestimated–the ancient Greeks excluded slaves from their polity, but the playwrights expressed their concerns by allowing slaves a voice in the play as saying:

> One thing alone brings shame to the slaves, the name, says the slave, expressing democratic sentiments. Apart from all of that, a slave is no worse than freemen in anything, if he is good. (Keane 2009, p. 53)

As I walked through Guthenburg, Sweden, in July 2010 I was struck by the architecture of the warehouses along their canals. They reminded me of the Cape Dutch buildings. A visit to the museum enabled me to understand the history of Guthenburg as colonial. The garrisoned city was built by indentured labourers required to work according to contractual requirements. Slavery was no stranger to Sweden, albeit a forgotten part of their past.

The street theatre created by marginalized foreigners made more sense when this was understood and the acting out of slaves led by garrison officers during a lunchtime production outside the train station resonated with the past.

Democracy allows these contradictions or aporias to surface (Keane 2009, p. 53). By enabling a sense of complexity and making connections, we could find our way out of the labyrinth.

External memories in libraries are increasingly accessible now to extend the capacity of human beings to think in terms of multiple variables.

We need to face up to the fact that a capitalist culture that supports excessive consumption and a debased form of democracy is not sustainable. Our limited ability to 'join up the dots' amounts to a 'false consciousness'. We are enslaved by our inability to comprehend the consequences of our choices.

Humanity is dependent on air, water and soil for survival—the global commons and our relationship to it—and needs to be recognized as central to all policy decisions. The implications of policy decisions flow beyond spatial boundaries and af-

---

grier, and every time a little thing happen, it might not even be a racist thing I would take it for that, so that s how I have to let it out to keep that…you know, it is a fine line between that insanity line.'

[16] http://www.theage.com.au/opinion/society-and-culture/dirty-laundry-leaves-a-nation-stained-20130221-2es9z.html.

fect future generations (Ingold 1993). Policy decisions flow beyond spatial boundaries and affect future generations.[17]

Governance needs to be buttressed by new forms of accounting that will enable the market to be monitored in ways that respect and support the environment. Measuring environmental expenditures at the local level and ensuring equitable access and distribution can only occur when the notion of property is reconsidered.

If the constitutions of nation states accept that the global commons needs to include the bases of life, namely water in rivers and oceans, earth and the microbes that support it, seeds and the responsibility to protect seeds and ecological diversity and the right to protect future generations from unsustainable levels of carbon and unsustainable temperature rises, then all nations will need to accept that it is in their interests to protect the common good.

My take on cosmopolitanism draws on the lessons from Indigenous First Nations, based on the idea that as human beings we have the right and the responsibility to care for the land on which we all depend equally by virtue of our humanity.[18]

---

[17] Development is a form of freedom, is the message echoed by Amartya Sen that runs through the praxis of Mamphela Ramphela's work (2012). A review of this research and literature supports the case that we cannot create profit at the expense of others and the environment as it undermines the social, cultural, political, economic and environmental foundations on which we depend. This has implications for the wellbeing of current and future generations. Transformation occurs as a result of 'being the change—or being part of the problem' (Haraway 1991). The choice to move away from the carbon economy or to live increasingly mobile lives that are wasteful will have systemic implications. The social implications of mobility and the carbon economy (Urry, Elliot and Urry) need to be addressed through design and creativity, but also through caring (Mukta 2012) and hospitality to stranger (see Derrida and Habermas in conversation with Borradori, 2003, on hospitality and Bausch on making friends of enemies in McIntyre-Mills 2006 a, b?).

[18] To address complex challenges these days, we need to be able to address issues from many dimensions spanning many disciplines. The rationale for transdiciplinarity (McIntyre-Mills 2000) or 'methodological cosmopolitanism' (Beck and Sznaider 2006) is the need to address social, economic and environmental convergence and 'existential risk' (Bostrom 2011) through ethical governance that is reflected in a new kind of politics (Brassett and Bulley 2007). The book assesses the extent to which consumption and place connectedness are relevant to sustainable responses to climate change. The case study will explore discourses (through focus group discussions) on property and the commodification of the land expressed as resource politics and resource governance. This is a precursor for the next step of the PAR, namely setting up a community of practice (COP) to manage diverse viewpoints on consumption, property and wellbeing.

The independent variable 'participation' is operationalized through attitudes and evidenced behaviour. The dependent variable 'consumption' is measured by the Max Neef (1991) human scale sustainability indicators on which the resilience footprint can be developed.

The dependent variable wellbeing is explored in focus groups to achieve a saturation sample (Romm 2001) based on considering the following prompts: (a) home safety (personal safety social indicators and physical indicators, physical safety of the home and environs); (b) sense of purpose and commitment to self, others and the environment; (c) a sense of connection/belonging to a community and an environment; and (d) rights and responsibilities to this generation as consumers or as caretakers will be used to populate our own software that will be developed through PAR as a community of practice (Wenger et al. 2009) resource by local government service providers and residents.

4.5 Food, Energy and Water: A Planetary Problem for Human Security

In order to support the basic fabric of life, we need to develop a systemic approach.

> Water is a commons because it is the ecological basis of all life and because its sustainability and equitable allocation depend on cooperation among community members (Shiva 2002, p. 24).

But unfortunately, Saul et al. (2012, p. 61) fall into the trap of following Hardin's 'tragedy of the commons' approach. They do not realize that Hardin's approach is in line with John Locke's defence of property and the enclosure movements of the seventeenth century in Britain. Hardin's core argument is that in the absence of private property there would be lawlessness. Hardin's classic argument for nationalism and private property is developed as follows:

> Picture a pasture open to all. It is expected that each herdsman will try to keep as many cattle as possible on the commons. Such an arrangement may work reasonably satisfactorily for centuries because tribal wars, poaching, and disease keep the numbers of both man and beast well below the carrying capacity of the land. Finally, however, comes the day of reckoning, that is the day when the long-desired goal of social stability becomes a reality. At this point, the inherent logic of the commons remorselessly generates tragedy. (Hardin 1968, pp. 1243–1248, cited by Shiva 2002, p. 26)[19]

Shiva argues that this is incorrect. The greatest misuse of natural resources has been by nations and corporations and not by local communities that have acted as water democracies, for example, in Bali, Indonesia and in Gujurat, India, water was sacred and carefully managed:

> Community rights are necessary for both ecology and democracy. Bureaucratic control by distant and external agencies and market control by commercial interests and corporations create disincentives for conservation…. (Shiva 2002, pp. 30–31).

By treating water as a commodity, it is traded and people have to pay for an essential resource. We regard air as free to breathe; water is another basic right.[20]

[19] Each of 10 people own 1 1000 lb. cow, and all 10 cows graze in a common area. If an additional cow is added, then all the cows would eat less grass and they would weigh 900 lbs. But I do not care because I have an additional cow and so have 900 lbs × 2 rather than just 1 cow of 1000 lbs. The health of all the cows is threatened if I continue to introduce more cows, but in the short and medium term I will get richer and more powerful, until the number of cows outstrips the amount of grass for them to eat—then all the cows fall ill and die. Then the rich and the poor cattle owners will suffer as their animals die (adapted from Lloyd 1833 by Hardin 1968).

[20] The terrifying notion of having to work to pay for air was explored in a recent Hollywood film, 'In time'.

4.5.1 The Environment is Eroded to Prop Up the Failing Economy

Biodiversity is threatened by markets that control life, for example, the Trade Related Aspects of Intellectual Property Rights (TRIPS) Agreement of WTO enables the corporatization and commodification of life:

> Parties may exclude from patentability plants and animals other than micro-organisms, and essentially biological processes for the production of plants and animals other than non-biological and micro-biological processes. However, parties shall provide for the protection of plant varieties wither by patents or by an effective sui generis system or by any combination thereof. This provision shall be reviewed four years after the entry into force of the Agreement establishing the WTO. (Article 27.5.3 (b) cited by Shiva 2010, p. xviii)

The work of Shiva (2002) stresses that global markets and mainstream research supported by corporate profits have disempowered local producers and in particular women farmers whose knowledge of plants was challenged by patriarchy and the 'enlightenment' during the witch hunts in Europe and America and then extended through the commodification of seeds through patents that prevent the collection and protection of biodiversity (Shiva 2010, p. xvii):

> The destruction of the self-reproducing character and genetic diversity of seeds was the beginning of seeds becoming a source of profits and control. This was an attack on the feminine principle. The hybrid 'miracle' seeds are a commercial miracle because farmers are forced to buy new supplies of them every year. Hybrids do not produce seeds that reproduce the same result because hybrids do not pass their traits on to the next generation. With hybridisation, seeds could no longer be viewed as a source of plant life; they were now a source of private profit only.

The water management approach is a synecdoche for the challenges for managing the global commons. The laws for water management highlight the challenges, but also the way forward for water management. I will discuss the four theories of water rights raised by Shiva (2002, p. 77):

1. *The first law is the Harmon Doctrine which protects the sovereignty of states and is derived from British private property law. Sharing of water for downstream users is only moderated by the suggestion that good neighbourliness is preferable.*
2. *The second approach is the natural water flow theory based on protecting the rights of up and down stream riparian users. The reintroduction of the hydroelectric power agenda on dams is relevant. The implications of the World Bank's attitudes towards linking with market partners to provide water is increasingly problematic as the commons is threatened by the increased emphasis on the economic bottomland that creates scarcity and a market for selling water.*
3. *The third is the Helsinki principle*[21] *based on the equitable apportionment of water, but as Shiva* (2002, p. 78) *stresses:*

[21] http://www.mpil.de/shared/data/pdf/pdf/8helsinki_rules_on_the_waters_of_international_rivers_ila.pdf downloaded 19 May.

Equitable utility is defined as the maximum benefit accruing to all the riparian states, in light of their differing economic and social needs

4. *Community of interest is closely related to the Helsinki Rules on the Uses of the Waters of International Rivers, 'Each basin state is entitled, within its territory, to a reasonable and equitable share in the beneficial uses of the waters of an international drainage basin'* (Shiva 2002, p. 79).

The complexity of the use of flows, not stocks, also needs to take into account community interests or values that are central to a sense of wellbeing (Shiva 2002, p. 80). Hence, there is the need to critically analyse the work by Stiglitz.

The knowledge that women farmers and as nurturers have developed over millennia we have swept aside as seeds are patented.

TRIPS have to be contested by empowering networks of local people to hold corporations and their political supporters to account. Ann Florini has stressed in a series of books the importance of empowering people from below.

The inspirational work of Donna Haraway stresses that women must not be subject to the design of others; they need to be designers of their own future. It is for this reason that we have worked on technology for monitory democracy and governance to try to give a voice to people and to empower them at the local level.

The liberation potential of the Aarhus convention to enable local people to have access to information and the right to speak out and to be heard on environmental issues provide a means to scale up the principle of subsidiarity. If this is combined with a revised triple-bottom-line (TBL) approach to accounting that develops wellbeing indicators to ensure quality of life within and across national boundaries, then policy could move closer towards addressing social and environmental justice for current and future generations of life.

Development need not modernize the slow, locally based lives of people defined as poor. Poverty is not having time and social relationships. It is not knowing your neighbour and distrusting the quality of the food that we eat. It is competing for a step up the run of status, instead of trying to live lives that support a sense of wellbeing.

Le Monde[22] reported that China has questioned Japanese rule of Okinawa which is a US military base and that "the calls over Okinawa may well revive tensions between Beijing and Tokyo, already embroiled in a territorial dispute over the Senkaku Islands, an archipelago in the south China Sea known by China as the Diaoyu islands".

It is a well-known historical fact that competition for scarce resources should not be underestimated. The current structure of the global economies supported by competitive nation states pose a challenge to food security and to peace, because the carbon economy continues to grow.[23]

---

[22] Le Monde, 'China urged to reconsider Japanese role of Okinawa?' Cited by Guardian Weekly International News. 17.05.13, p. 10.

[23] Carrington, D. 'Global carbon dioxide in atmosphere passes milestone.' Guardian Weekly 17.05.13, p. 13.

4.5.2 *The Social Contract Is Unravelled to Prop Up the Eroding Environment and Failing Economy*

Currently, the social contract is being eroded, in order to prop up austerity measures in a vain attempt to restore the capitalist economic order that depends on profits at the expense of the environment and the social fabric.

Consuming and ability to consume are linked with power and status:

> Ehrlich and Ehrlich (2010) observe this general silence over the relationship between affluence and over-consumption results in consumption of any kind being viewed as an unchallenged good. (Pretty 2013, p. 5)

But ironically, Monbiot raises the point that even those who are part of the 1 % are dissatisfied, because wealth is a 'marker or indicator of status'. Everyone wants to be higher up on the scale, 'money is just a way of keeping score,' according to a banker, cited by Monbiot (2013). He also cites 'How much is enough?' The author shows that money is never enough unless you are at the very top of the 1%. The cost of profit is borne by those who work for the surplus value of corporations and shareholders. He then cites Lauren Greenfield's 'The Queen of Versailles' on the life of David Siegel. The loss of a few assets has led to deep depression. In order to prevent further losses to the rich, the social contract is under further threat:

> In order to grant the rich these pleasures, the social contract is reconfigured. The welfare state is dismantled. Essential public servants are cut so that the rich may pay less tax. The public realm is privatised, the regulations restraining the ultra-wealthy and the companies they control are abandoned, and Edwardian levels of inequality are almost fetishized. Politicians justify these changes with the incentives for enterprise that they create….but the mindless, meaningless accumulation cannot satisfy even it's beneficiaries, except perhaps—and temporarily—the man wobbling on the very top of the pile. The same applies to collective growth…world eating growth is fine, as long as it is growth.[24]

4.6 Systemic Intervention to Protect Social and Environmental Justice

The action to protect the global commons is central for human security (Shiva 2002, p. 28):

> Corporations and laws such as TRIPS and penalties for polluters or trading permits for polluters has shifted the sacred integrity of the relationship between human beings as stewards, to commodifying the commons as a resource, ironically resource actual means regenerate and the extraction of profit runs the risk of bringing existential risk closer to a reality…as stressed by IPPC reports that show the 6 °C rise in temperature is inevitable, given the move

The United Nations Summit in 2015 is the deadline for a 'binding international treaty to curb emissions.'

[24] Monbiot,.G. 2013. Money just makes the rich suffer. The Guardian Weekly. 17.05.13 p. 9.

away from reducing emissions as governments focus on short term austerity measures to try to restart an economy that depends on extraction of time and surplus value.

The challenge is to address the current erosion of the social contract. But the current mainstream labour agendas for social democracy can achieve little unless nation states develop regional shared goals.

The problem is that regional initiatives like the EU are under threat because they are based on the wrong kind of economics. States will remain in crisis until a new way of valuing social and environmental dimensions is achieved, rather than emphasising profit at the expense of the environment. This can only occur through valuing the fabric of life through new forms of accounting and accountability.

The UN is not the organization for Republican government according to Habermas (2005, p. 340). Instead, regional governments need to recognize that managing the global commons requires specific interventions to balance individual and collective needs. This is what the governance architecture that I am trialling attempts to do. It is not based on top-down invention; instead, it prefigures a way to enable people to reflect on their own lives and to try to make changes through self-regulation, in order that interests are not achieved at the expense of others.[25] The bottom-up approach to monitory democracy and governance is the goal of this research. The post-national agenda does not need to undermine strong states; it could build on and extend a social contract, in the way suggested by Habermas. It could provide a way forward to address challenges of food, energy and water security.

The challenge for Europe is to balance this diversity locally. The regional spaces used in regional meetings by world leaders, such as the G8 or G20, whilst relevant for those at the meetings do not enable local people to engage in dialogue which is so important to enable a change in thinking and practice. Electorates need to be in touch with the governments that serve them. Unless a seamless set of conversations

[25] This is what the governance architecture that I am trialling attempts to do. It is not based on top-down invention; instead, it is asking people to reflect on their own lives and to try to make changes through self-regulation, in order that their rights and their responsibilities are secured to the event that they do not undermine the rights of others. Geertz (2000, p. 65) was only half right when he stressed the importance of relativism, in which he suggests: 'Indeed if one cannot face difference one should stay at home.' But now home is diverse and nation states are becoming increasingly diverse. So the challenge is how to balance individual and collective needs. The praxis on which my research is based distances itself from the game theory approach based on the zero-sum approach. Game theory is promoted through the sovereign states. But if sovereignty was softened by a recognition of overlapping regional interests and a recognition of reframed relationships across state market and civil society, through an economics that stewards resources for future generations, then this expanded form of pragmatism, based on testing out the social, economic and environmental implications of choices for this generation and the next, could become the new basis for governance, democracy and ethics that are required to move the vision from us/them to a recognition that the effects of profit are the erosion of both the environment and social relationships. The austerity measures to prop up business as usual, based on saving on welfare and saving on environmental protection, will lead to a descent into chaos. We need to understand that by identifying with others and with biodiversity (Lever-Tracey 2011) we extend the circle of those with whom we feel solidarity and compassion and redefine our identity without hubris—then we may be able to transform the culture (Hulme 2010, 2011) which shapes the planet on which we depend. This requires some space for diversity and freedom and a sense of irony (Rorty 1989).

from local to regional to global occurs through face-to-face and on-line dialogues, that can foster a sense of solidarity.

The solidarity of African unions, EU and Asian groupings need to achieve cross-cutting discussions that focus on food, energy and water.

Top-down approaches to sustainability need to be balanced by bottom-up engagement to ensure that the powerful do not exert power in their own interests.

The vast bureaucracy that can be marshalled by the Vietnamese communist state to address an area of concern such as the attempt to protect the Cat Ba nature reserve was illustrated during the International Systems Sciences Conference, hosted by the Municipality of Haiphong in July 2013.

The top-down potential of telling people to do things, admittedly using a participatory learning laboratory process, has helped to address the level of sewerage in the Cat Ba reserve and the fish appear to be breeding again. This is evident by the returning fisherman who was moved out of the area (to comply with the reserve's new status as a nature reserve).

But the question needs to be asked, how do the fishing families survive outside the reserve? Education and alternative businesses is a key, as is the potential for charging international tourists more to visit. Currently, the cost for locals and international visitors is just AUD 1!

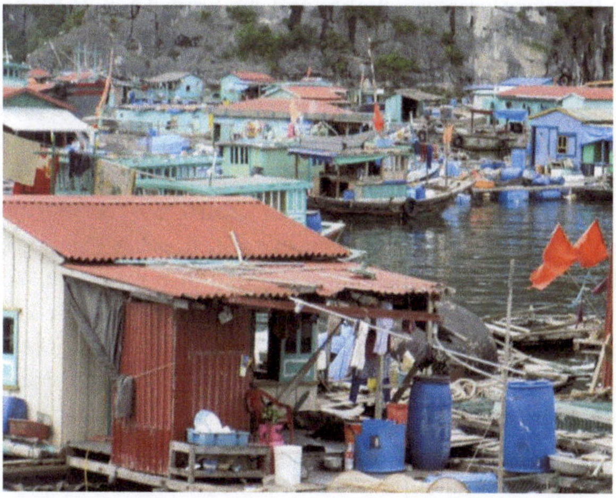

As we left the reserve and moved into the outer harbour, the silence was deafening. Not a single gull called out. During the entire day, I had not seen or heard a single bird! Fifty-eight yellow monkeys continue to exist against the odds. Hunger no longer drives the hunters, because they are being given jobs as nature conservation officers. Can enough jobs be found for the families dependent on fishing?[26]

[26] I hope that the intervention is able to make a difference in time to save the diverse ecosystem and that it is able to support the people who live there, so that they will not have to leave to find work. Finding the balance remains an ongoing challenge.

Food and energy are the bases for human wellbeing and security. Current approaches to international relations and war (Etzioni 2004, 2011) are unsustainable. As the experience of suffering becomes more widespread, the notion of class will become central once again, because 'the poorest people in the world will be the hardest hit' (Beck 2009, p. 37).

4.6.1 Policing and Profiling 'the Other' in Norway

Europe and Africa are borderlands (Balibar 2006), just as Australia and Asia are regional borderlands and Afghanistan and America are borderlands, even if national boundaries do not acknowledge this and populist politics and xenophobia increase as groups compete for limited resources.

Protecting the global commons must be seen as a shared necessity. Fortunately, the plasticity of the human brain is such that we have the capability to redesign our way of life (Haraway 1992, 1994) and governance (McIntyre-Mills 2010a, b). Localized efforts, whilst important for prefiguring change, are insufficient to hold the market to account, unless they are applied regionally and internationally (Giddens 2009). In more equal societies, people consume less and are less status conscious. Thus, the link 'between greater equality and the prevention of global warming involves limiting the consumerism.' The cosmopolitan argument is that we are better off when others are better off—which requires reframing the way we live in post-national, post-colonial regions. In the UK and Sweden, the recent riots are in response to the gap between rich and poor, the young and older generations and the racism expressed towards those from Africa and Asia,[27] for example, in Sweden:

The trigger for the riots—police shooting dead a 69-year-old Portuguese man called Lenine Relvas-Martins—has been dismissed as an excuse. But his neighbours are still incensed. 'They had a bastard-load of police here. You would have thought there was a huge group of terrorists, not a man with a little knife,' complains Milos, 73, Relvas-Martins's neighbour since 1984. 'If he was Swedish they never would have shot him. I'm sure about that.' Martins had been brandishing a knife on his balcony, angry after a confrontation with local youths. Police then broke into his house and shot him in front of his Finnish wife. They say she was at risk. She denies it. The police then inflamed the situation last Sunday, reportedly calling young people causing a disturbance 'monkeys' and 'negroes'. 'They seize people, and strip them and really embarrass them in front of their friends,' complains Yusuf, a young Somali. Yusuf used to live in Birmingham, but says he prefers Husby. And there is no doubt Husby has better facilities than deprived areas in Britain. But it is also more segregated. About 85 % of people here have their origins outside Sweden.

'The politicians are thinking the wrong way. They want to help people, but you never help people when you put 30,000 to 50,000 in one place,' complains the man painting at the library.

---

[27] Orange, R. 2013 'Swedish riots spark surprise and anger', The Guardian Weekly page 10.

Camila Salazar, who works for Fryshuset, a Stockholm youth organization, says: 'For a lot of people who live in segregated areas, the only Swedes they meet are social workers or police officers. It's amazing how many have never had a Swedish friend.'

A third of the 2500 white, ethnic Swedes who lived in Husby 10 years ago have left. 'My children say: "Why don't you leave there? All the Swedish have gone",' complains Milos. 'There's only three Swedish families left in this whole block.'

Just before I left the office on a Friday afternoon, a young person asked to speak with me. He showed me a video on his iPad that he had taken when he was looking out of his flat in Oslo. The video[28] showed a young black man being assaulted by a male plain-clothes police man. He was later assisted by a female officer who followed up the body search for illegal substances. But the ongoing pressure on his neck, whilst probing his mouth with a stick and pinning him on the ground, revealed nothing.

Passers-by did not stop or enquire. They kept walking. Those who saw but did not stop included a woman wearing a headscarf and pushing a pram and several others. This event took place a few metres from where Ang Sun Su Chi won the Nobel Peace Prize. Her speech focused on the importance of kindness and the ripple effects it has in society. The more unkindness, the harder others must work to foster positive ripple effects. I hope this book will provide a positive ripple.

The young man exclaimed: How can Norwegians allow this to happen? Does no one care about torturing another human being for 20 min on the street?

My response was: Yes you care and you are continuing to make a difference by sharing this information and your outrage with others.

His response was: I must, I am the father of a child. What kind of world will it be, if we do not care about one another?

Comaroff discusses 'Law, labour and the contours of contemporary capitalism' in a keynote address at the 'Knowledge and Value in a Globalizing World: disentangling dichotomies, querying unities' (7th July 2011). She stressed: 'Europe is going south.' It could be argued that America has also headed south as indicated by its loss of a triple AAA rating from Standard and Poor's.[29] The time for change—perhaps the great transformation, predicted by many but ignored by most—has arrived.[30] The question is—if it can happen in Europe could it happen in any post-welfare state? What hope is there to achieve social democratic aspirations in Africa and the Middle East?

The question is—if it can happen in Norway what hope is there for other states where the gap between rich and poor is wider? What hope is there to achieve social democratic aspirations in developing countries? The possibilities for 'states in crisis' will need to be achieved through exploring more options in context. I make the

[28] See http://www.circusbazaar.com.

[29] 'Theory from the South: Or how Europe is evolving towards Africa' discusses 'Law, labour and the contours of contemporary capitalism' in a keynote address by Comaroff (2011) at 'Knowledge and Value in a Globalising World: disentangling dichotomies, querying unities'.

[30] We face ongoing social, economic and environmental challenges that are unprecedented. The global economic meltdown needs to be used as an opportunity to change direction.

case in this book that this requires expanded pragmatism in governance and new forms of cosmopolitan politics.

Beck (2009, p. 96) stresses the need for sub-politics from above and below. How to achieve this is the goal of current research on balancing individual and collective needs. The focus is on the local, so that the poor will not be silenced and so that local wisdom can be drawn upon. This enables creative responsive transformation and the emergence of new relationships.

> At the beginning of the twenty-first century, we see modern society with new eyes, and this birth of a 'cosmopolitan vision' (Beck 2006) is among the unexpected phenomena out of which a still indeterminate world of risk society is emerging. Henceforth, there are no merely local occurrences. All genuine threats have become global threats. The situation of every nation, every people, every religion, every class and every individual is also the result and cause of the human situation. The key point is that henceforth concern about the whole has become a task. It is not optional but the human condition. (Beck 2009, p. 19).[31]

4.7 Penal States, the Law and Protection for the Displaced

Justice Julian Burnside stresses that temporary 3-year visas are inadequate to protect asylum seekers:

> TPVs were first suggested by Pauline Hanson in 1996. Her proposal was criticized by Philip Ruddock as "unconscionable". Three years later, TPVs were introduced by the Howard Government; Ruddock was immigration minister. TPVs suffer from a couple of serious vices: not least that they are likely to cause more deaths at sea—something both major parties claim to be concerned about. TPVs provide asylum seekers with three years' protection only, and they deny the visa holder the right to be reunited with their family….
> It is a dismal prospect, considering that allied troops are pulling out of Afghanistan later this year. When they leave, there will be a blood-bath as the Taliban declare open season on Hazaras. Some of them will only have enough resources to head towards Australia, as it is more expensive to get to Europe or America. The Coalition promises to add more misery to their lives….Is this really the Australian way?[32]

Malcolm Fraser on Coalition asylum plans: no limits to the inhumanity, Former Liberal Prime Minister Malcolm Fraser speaks to Guardian Australia about a 'breach of common decency'.[33]

---

[31] Global citizenship ought to become a concept supported by international law and social justice movements (McIntyre-Mills 2000). The four themes of citizenship discourses are: 'inclusion, erosion, withdrawal and expansion'; these 'reflect the foci of contemporary discourses on citizenship' (Kivisto and Faist 2007, p. 13), which are compartmentalist in their assumptions about the world. The book deals with false consciousness. Policy decisions flow beyond spatial boundaries and affect future generations. The refugees from Tunisia and Libya are given the boot on Lampedusa as Italy strives to keep control of the refugees. The attitude towards borders appears to be hardening as the economic climate worsens http://www.watoday.com.au/opinion/politics/we-can-do-better-than-italys-warehousing-on-lampedusa-20091014-gwh7.html.

[32] http://www.theguardian.com/commentisfree/2013/aug/16/temporary-protection-visas-refugees.

[33] the guardian.com, Friday 16 August 2013 13.38 AEST http://www.theguardian.com/world/2013/aug/16/malcolm-fraser-coalition-asylum-policy 19/08/2013.

> …This is a total reversal of some of the values Australia had become renowned for. It saddens me to think that the Liberal party, and as I understand it also the Labour party, are thinking of additional ways to make their policies more brutal…The policies have become so unreal, so inhumane overall; it's very hard to look at just one aspect, which increases the uncaring nature of the opposition. The terrible thing is that the opposition and the government both believe they can win votes by behaving in this way.
> …. Any idea of duty of care to the vulnerable is totally out of the window.

Offshore processing in states whose economy is reliant on Aid could lead to the development of oppressive camps along the lines of convict colonies. The propensity for riots has already been demonstrated along with the reaction of increased control and increased distancing of people as 'other'. Offshore processing of asylum seekers in Nauru and PNG by Australia has been implemented by the Liberal government as a so-called election promise to 'control the boundaries of Australia' and to 'control who has the right to enter'. This is a nationalistic and neo-conservative approach to protecting interests. Instead a regionalist approach that recognises our vulnerability and entangled futures needs to be promoted.[34]

The role of law ought to be to ensure social justice through the fair use and distribution of resources guided by the goal to mitigate and adapt to climate change. Climate change refugees and climate change displacement and migration are raised by Saul et al. (2012) as areas of policy concern for the nation state. But unfortunately Saul et al. (2012, p. 61) fall into the trap of following Hardin's 'tragedy of the commons' approach.

They do not realize that Hardin's approach is in line with John Locke's defence of property and the enclosure movements of the seventeenth century in Britain. Hardin's core argument is that in the absence of private property there would be lawlessness. Hardin's classic argument for nationalism and private property (Hardin 1968, pp. 1243–1248, cited by Shiva 2002, p. 26)[35] is incorrect. The greatest misuse of natural resources has been by nations and corporations and not by local communities that have acted as water democracies, for example, in Bali, Indonesia and in Gujurat, India, water was sacred and carefully managed:

> Community rights are necessary for both ecology and democracy. Bureaucratic control by distant and external agencies and market control by commercial interests and corporations create disincentives for conservation…. (Shiva 2002, pp. 30–31)

---

[34] http://www.theaustralian.com.au/national-affairs/immigration/asylum-seeker-bluff-set-to-be-exposed-by-the-numbers/story-fn9hm1gu-1226686524164 downloaded 28/07/2013.

http://www.theguardian.com/world/2013/aug/15/nauru-transfers-in-doubt-after-fire downloaded 19/08 2013.

http://www.theguardian.com/world/2013/jul/19/kevin-rudd-labor-asylum-border-protection 19/08/2013.

[35] Each of 10 people own 1 1000 lb. cow, and all 10 cows graze in a common area. If an additional cow, is added then all the cows would eat less grass and they would weigh 900 lbs. But I do not care because I have an additional cow and so have 900 lbs × 2 rather than just 1 cow of 1000 lbs. The health of all the cows is threatened if I continue to introduce more cows, but in the short and medium term I will get richer and more powerful, until the number of cows outstrips the amount of grass for them to eat—then all the cows fall ill and die. Then the rich and the poor cattle owners will suffer as their animals die (adapted from Lloyd 1833 by Hardin 1968).

By treating water as a commodity, it is traded and people have to pay for an essential resource. We regard air as free to breathe; water is another basic right.[36] Those who do not have access to essential resources are forced to seek refuge.

4.7.1 Human Rights and Implications for Governance Across States

Human rights within and across nation states seems to be given short shrift as conservative governments strive to balance budgets whilst trying to deliver business as usual. The so-called post-welfare state, discussed by Jamrozik (2001), appears to be a reality. The protection of the vulnerable, the working poor,[37] the unemployed and homeless has deepened and in particular for climate refugees (who will include the displaced victims of fires and floods within nation states), it is inadequate:

Legal category	Protection	Limitations	Comments and adaptations
Refugee	Protects a person from return to a place of persecution	Prosecution is unlikely to encompass victims of carbon pollution, unless discriminatory	The problem is that asylum seekers need to be processed to be recognized as refugees. At this stage they are even more vulnerable
Complementary protection	Protects a person from arbitrary deprivation of life or cruel, inhuman or degrading treatment	It is unclear whether climate-related harms would be recognized as such	Current laws and protocols are outdated
IDP	Rights-based framework to protect all persons displaced within a country	Guiding principles are not binding and cannot be enforced against neglectful government	A cosmopolitan approach to governance would render support of displaced people a constitutional requirement, based on an extension of the social contract

[36] The terrifying notion of having to work to pay for air was explored in a recent Hollywood film.

[37] 'Down in Jungleland', http://www.abc.net.au/foreign/content/2013/s3874510.htm details the working conditions of Americas working poor. The minimum wage per hour is US $ 2.13. Most Americans have seen their incomes stagnate or fall since 2008.

Legal category	Protection	Limitations	Comments and adaptations
Litigation	Potentially offers a binding judicial decision with compensation or other remedy	Foreign governments cannot be sued in local courts; international courts may not have jurisdiction	A new architecture to enable the implementation of social and environmental justice requires management of size of carbon footprint, fines for infringements and incarceration of perpetrators deemed to be undermining the fabric of life for current and future generations

Source: Adapted from Saul et al. 2012, p. 169

If we want to achieve scientific change or we wish to work across conceptual and spatial boundaries to achieve policy changes, we will need to respect complexity and find ways to work with it.

Balibar (2006) highlights some of these challenges and stresses that space for political difference needs to be recognized. Balibar talks of Europe as a 'borderlands', but the starting point for his argument is Eurocentric. We have more options than the following:

- Clash of cultures (see Huntington's 1996) thesis)
- Global networks where goods, services, money and ideally human beings are able to bypass borders
- Centre periphery: a multipolar world with regions
- Crossover model hybrid formations: Euratlantic, Eurasiatic and Euro-Mediterranean

I argue for an alternative approach—namely biospheres across which regional federations overlap.

The mainstream media and elected governments in Western democracies such as the USA focus on the banal. The elected leaders in the USA play at politics. The role of the senate is to slow and delay the passing of bills, according to Burdett Loomis (2013).[38] The filibustering (asking long questions as a delaying tactic) by Republicans in the senate delays the processing of decisions, whilst the power of social movements has been effectively harnessed by the Far Right as the so-called tea party movement. The Occupy Wall Street Movement has to date had less impact that the Arab Spring. The changes brought about by social movements can be positive or negative. New forms of governance and democracy are required. Existing forms of democracy and governance are no longer effectively addressing the biggest challenges of the day, namely: representation of an increasingly marginalized majority, lack of accountability to the poor, lack of sustainable use of resources and

[38] Loomis, B. 2013 'Can we effectively govern ourselves?' Public Lecture, Flinders University, March. The senate creates a barrier in the USA and roadblocks legislation. He raises the question about the effectiveness of current structures and processes.

lack of opportunities for engagement. Furthermore, the way in which educational paradigms and organizations have been segmented, is *both* an effect and a cause of the fragmentation in our thinking and practice. The need for transformation has never been more urgent, because our culture of production, growth and consumption has outstripped the capacity of our planet.

The corporatization of education is part of the problem. Whilst universities need to serve the community and work with industry where appropriate, the emphasis on running education not as a public good but as a business managed along neo-liberal lines to make a profit. Extracting profit from students and staff, just as extracting profit from the labour of other industries in the service sectors needs to be rethought in terms of the wellbeing of current and future generations.

The polarization of politics between the Right and Left in older democracies in response to the hung parliaments is problematic. People versus the planet politics are unsustainable—labour for jobs now and in the medium terms is short sighted.

The binary oppositional politics between the Right and Left has created a deadlock (29th December 2012). The Christmas break was used as an excuse to delay and the Democrats are blaming Republicans for leaving the debate to the eleventh hour. The flow on affects for cuts to welfare is a cause for concern.

Those who speak out against the state and the ramifications of supporting democracy through violence have faced imprisonment. The blogs concerning the human rights of those who incarcerated on charges of treason is problematic. The way in which gang warfare in New York has been classified is also problematic.

This book has attempted to provide an alternative means to address and register concerns raised by people in response to their local and regional concerns. More importantly, it also provides a means to scale up subsidiarity and participatory governance.

To what extent can democracy measure up to the standards of what constitutes ethical behaviour?

Butler (2005) calls for openness and critical reflection as a basis for ethical relationships. This openness requires humility and the assumption that ethical responses are not always clear-cut. They need to be sought within a specific social, cultural, political, economic and environmental context. But we can be guided by principle axioms, namely: Freedom and diversity can and ought to be supported to the extent that it does not undermine the rights of others or future generations of life. This is a guideline for systemic ethics.

Learning about the culture of our neighbours is part of a process of building rapport. This is a basis for transnational relationships.

Bishop (2009) develops an apt argument that a great deal of communication is merely venting emotions without achieving transformation. But emotions cannot be denied when striving for rational, ethical decisions. The emotional triggers need to be understood and respected. The Asian White Paper has been launched by Ken Henry in Dec 2012 at ANU. The Asian Century report contains rhetoric that will need to be funded and applied at all levels of society in Australia. Ross Garnaut launched a similar report 23 years ago.

Some of the measures that need to be introduced are a greater understanding of the cultural achievements and contributions of Asia and Africa. The notion that democracy originated in the West is the first misconception that can be set aside.

The bombing of civilians in the bid to win the war in Afghanistan and Iraq, along with the death of civilians and the ongoing detention of children in Palestine,[39] has led to a sense of outrage that has been fuelled when Islamic sensibilities are affronted through parody or cartoon representations. Civil and social rights are at risk in what could be seen as a shift in the perceptions of what is acceptable to maintain state power. Restraint and compassion are vital dimensions of democracy.

Butler (2006) stresses the continuum of ethical behaviour from those who chose to be sadistic and those who were coerced and prisoners to help maintain the functioning of the camps. The blurring of boundaries may be acceptable when giving an account or self-reflection, but drawing the line is necessary in law and being able to draw the line in one's own moral choices. Being open to critical self-reflection is always important. Expanding pragmatism through testing out ideas helps policymakers to avoid idealistic interventions that could lapse into authoritarianism or fundamentalism. Addressing this tension through dialogue is vital for ethical policymaking. But the challenge is that narratives distort the 'truth' and the different perceptions need to be explored, in order to cocreate a shared truth upheld by the law. Responsibility can be denied by pleading a range of cases.[40]

This is where evidence needs to be brought to bear on a topic. This is where the weaving together of stories needs to move towards making decisions, or cuts to ensure that rights and compassion for individuals does not become the preserve of those who are powerful and heard, because they are part of the 1 % who are articulate and allowed to voice their pain and grievance to others. Compassion is vital. It does prevent our becoming totalitarian, but it is a delicate balance.

[39] Australian Broadcasting Documentary, 2014, 11/02/2014.

[40] See 'Giving an account of oneself' by Judith Butler, Public open lecture for the students of the European Graduate School EGS, Media and Communication Studies department program, Saas-Fee, Switzerland, Europe, 2006, uploaded on 5 May 2007: 'Since in political discourse there is always disagreement about the possible courses of action, the identity of the "we" that is going to be created through a specific form of action becomes a central question. By engaging in this or that course of action we are, in fact, entering a claim on behalf of a "we," that is, we are creating a specific form of collective identity. Political action and discourse are, in this respect, essential to the constitution of collective identities.' http://www.egs.edu/ Judith Butler, feminist philosopher lecturing about 'Primo Levi for the Present'; narrative accounts, forgiveness, holocaust, Auschwitz, victims, execution, war, and crime

Chapter 5
Greed and Complicity

Responsibility to Others and Future Generations of Life

5.1 Who and What Do We Care About?

Mukta (2005) stresses the need for transnational movements to hold governments and international organizations such as the World Bank to account. Mukta (2012) writes an essay 'who or what do we care about in the twenty-first century?' She stresses that instead of the 'gift of life' we are cannibalizing the planet through our greed. Her plea to value life and relationships echoes the plea made by Ramphela (2012) to end corruption and greed.

I will start by addressing current events. One hundred and nine asylum seekers from Afghanistan and Pakistan have sunk whilst trying to reach the coast of Australia. Distress calls were sent out on Tuesday, 19th of June. The search for survivors began today. Over 100 people have drowned in their attempt to escape from social, economic or environmental conditions.[1] How can neighbours think that they live in isolation from one another? How can we turn back those who seek assistance at our borders or 'turn back the boats' at sea in order to 'protect' boundaries?

With whom and with what do we identify as human beings; we are co-determined by one another and the land. We live with creatures and design ways of life for which we are inherently responsible.

More than 200 children and adults are waiting to be transported from Christmas Island, pending a high court appeal.[2] Staff members are afraid to speak out about

[1] Wilson, L. 2012, 'Merchant ships bring salvation for lucky few as boat and friends disappear into sea', Weekend Australian, p. 1 'Most of the 109 survivors, including a 13 year old boy, were last night recovering on Christmas Island after being plucked from the sea by two navy vessels and commercial ships, including JPO Vulpecula. Three were evacuated to a Perth Hospital for urgent treatment with suspected spinal injuries. Others were believed to be suffering from hypothermia and dehydration and at least 10 were transported to the islands small hospital. The latest tragedy has brought renewed calls for an end to the bitter political standoff on asylum seekers and a genuine effort by politicians to find a workable solution that will stop the deaths at sea....'

[2] 'The International Convention for the Safety of Life at Sea is the convention that would be the prime driver in the decision making of the commanding officer', Stewart, C. 2012 Law of the sea versus the dictates of Canberra: there are daunting obstacles to a policy of turning back asylum seeker boats. Weekend Australian March, 11–12, 19.

J. McIntyre-Mills, *Transformation from Wall Street to Wellbeing*, Contemporary Systems Thinking, DOI 10.1007/978-1-4899-7466-2_5,

conditions. As I ended the draft of this manuscript, the containerist approach to nation states within the region had reached its zenith. The four themes of citizenship discourses are: 'inclusion, erosion, withdrawal and expansion', and these 'reflect the foci of contemporary discourses on citizenship' (Kivisto and Faist 2007, p. 13).

Boat people no longer qualify to enter Australia. Although it may indeed 'destroy the business model of the people smugglers', the reasons for people desperately entrusting their lives to smugglers will not disappear.

In a policy, politics and governance sense we are still dealing with decisions (from the Latin to cut) that cut asylum seekers off from the right to entering our country. Quite literally, the asylum seekers on Christmas Island are engaging in acts of self-harm. To my horror, I hear that the workers at the detention centre are cut-off from their right to speak out—they will lose their jobs and that is what people with mortgages and families care about. They care about themselves and their limited family interests. They have little solidarity or compassion with others or sentient creatures—unless when the issues are brought out into the open and then people are ashamed and come forward to speak out against live human and animal transport.

One asylum seeker on Christmas Island has dug a grave for himself and lay in it and another inflicted terrible self-harm—I will not detail it here; these were the news items we heard last night as I watched the ABC (15/08/2011).

These are grim reminders that ontological sanity does not exist and the practice by nation states of protecting their borders, their right to trade in so-called live animal flesh, is reality.

Sixty-five thousand sheep on one vessel were stranded off the coast of Port Adelaide in August waiting to be transported. Inspectors were initially not allowed on board, until protests made it clear that the public were concerned about animal rights.

What is happening to us? New Zealand has banned animal transportation and does not transport children or adults. The ABC news on March 13, 2012, reports that eating red meat has been linked with cancer; perhaps this is yet another reason for living sustainably!

We need to speak out about alternative ways of 'being' and alternative ways of 'engaging in democracy from below'. The concept 'monitory democracy' developed by Keane echoes the theme that the marginalized need to be given a voice, in order to hold the powerful to account.[3]

A PhD student commented on John Keane's 'Life and Death of Democracy' as follows:

> Oh that is a thick book—all on democracy, but what has the West really learned?

[3] See Global citizenship and social movements—creating transcultural webs of meaning (2000) and 'User Centric Policy Design to Address Complex needs (2010)', for example, in which I discuss democratic engagement with marginalized groups—first nations, young people, the unemployed and the homeless, angry people who do not want to hear anything but with the need to implement laws to manage greed.

As a Palestinian, he shared his despair, contempt and anger for the versions of Western democracy that turn a blind eye to the hunger of Palestinians.

Another student and youth leader has described a local government consultant as 'a climate change skeptic' because he questioned whether climate change was caused only by human beings.

Dialogue to explore and cocreate shared narratives is increasingly important.

The local government consultant later explained that he meant that he did not doubt that climate was changing but thought that we 'were going to hell in a hand basket, because the level of carbon emissions was so high'. He stressed that combined emissions from natural disasters such as volcanic eruptions as well as industrial activity were already so advanced as to make disaster inevitable. I asked him whether he believed it worthwhile to try to make a difference and he agreed, by saying warmly: 'It is our only hope!'

We need a transformation and support for the processes to make it possible to protect human rights.

The life chances for those who leave as asylum seekers to enter Australia has been eroded through bipartisan narrowly pragmatic announcements about 'turning back boats' or 'destroying the business plan of the people smugglers'.

The 'us–them' mentality supported by domestic and international politics is unsustainable. This book develops an argument as to why systemic ethics provides an ethical and rational way forward to enable people to extend compassion to others, the environment and themselves.

The argument begins where Caney (2008) ends, namely those sovereign states per se are not necessarily the best option for defending the rights of this generation or the next. The case he makes rests on three points: the moral arbitrariness of the state boundaries, the incompleteness and conservative nature of rights and their inadequacy. The notion is that distributive principles such as equality ought not to be limited by narrow readings of the social contract. I make the case in this book that to address social and environmental injustice, global humanitarian and environmental governance is needed. The challenge of food, energy and water distribution and redistribution requires new approaches to representation, accountability and sustainability.

It discusses the need for valuing different dimensions of life in a post-materialist society and the need for a new form of governance architecture that is capable of balancing individual and collective needs to prevent excessive toxic luxury and greed.

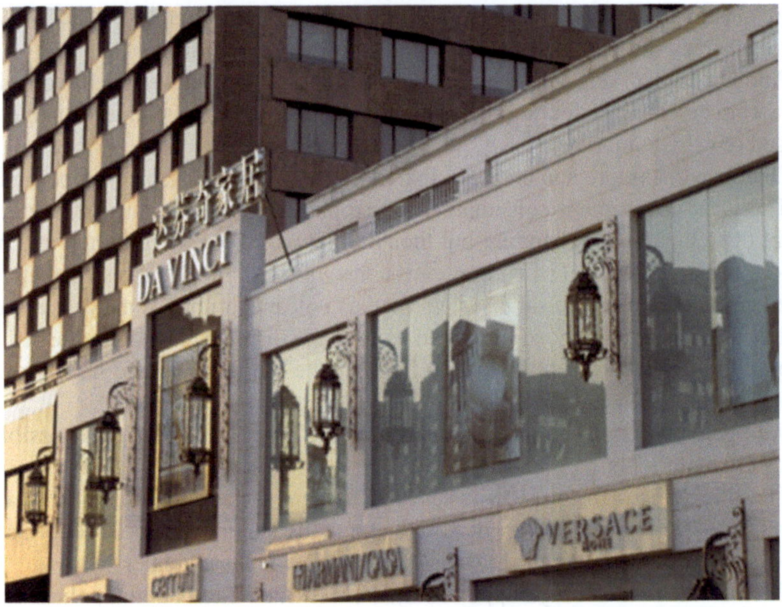

The shops near Tiananmen Square could be on Wall Street

The prior problem is that people either: (a) have the capacity to understand the implications of greed and do not care about the lack of responsibility for others and the next generation of life or (b) they do not have the capacity to understand the implications of their choices or (c) that the more people become accustomed to better living standards; the more attached they become to this way of life, the more they deny responsibilities to others.

The challenge of enhancing representation, accountability and sustainability remains an ongoing challenge for all who are concerned about preventing hunger and war.[4]

The argument developed in this book is that we need to value the environment in order to provide for human beings in the medium and long term.

So why should an argument for more global humanitarian and environmental governance be an argument for social or environmental justice?

---

[4] This involves reframing the state to address a new role. We have exported the notion of the state as we have colonised and globalised. 'What is a state if it is not sovereign?' is the question posed by Clifford Geertz (2003).

Independence has been fiercely fought for by past colonies, or subsections of marginalised groups who wish to splinter away from dominant centralised control of authoritarian governments. The powerful economies of the world have been built upon exploitation and the lack of representation.

The meanings that people attribute to their sense of self and self-worth are important. A study of a map provided by Wilson[5] (2011, p. 21) shows that the incidents of rioting and looting were highest in areas with the highest level of unemployment, namely above 10 % of the population. To feel disrespected leads to anger. Bauman (2011, p. 8) published an article which in many ways anticipates the riots in London:

> In Britain for instance, the share of the top 1 per cent earners doubled since 1982 from 6.5 to 13 % of the national income while chief executives of the 100 FTSE companies have been (up to the recent credit crunch' and beyond) earning not 20 as in 1980, but 133 times more than the average earners.
>
> This is not, however, the end of the story. Thanks to the network of 'information highways', rapidly growing in its extension and density, all and any individual—man or woman, adult or child, rich or poor—are invited, tempted and induced…to compare one's own individual lot with the lot of all *other individuals,* and particularly with the lavish consumption of public idols…and to measure the values that make life worth living by the opulence they brandish….

These are 'unrealistic aspirations' which are 'toxic' according to Bauman (2011) who cites Oliver James' (2008) article in the Guardian (3 January 2008).

5.2 Addressing the So-called Limits of Democracy and Governance

The problem with moves towards any form of world governance is who governs the governors? World governance per se is not the answer. Could a set of overlapping and cross-cutting appointments ensure that the global commons is protected? Could this sort of architecture: (a) protect the vulnerable and voiceless within the region, (b) support hospitality and care for those in need and (c) provide the right to a home for those who are without a home?[6]

I suggest that it does not mean that citizenship within nation states is necessarily undermined. It merely provides another overlay to a multilevel and multi-agency approach. Derrida (2005b) stresses that hospitality does not always go far enough to protect others.

West Churchman (1982) stressed that we need to look both inwards and outwards by 'unfolding our values' and 'sweeping in' social, cultural, political and economic ideas. If the 'the systems approach begins when first we strive to see the world through the eyes of another', as he stressed, then it is developed through

[5] Wilson, P. 2011, Moments of madness amid calculated rage. *The Weekend Australian* August 13–14, p. 21.

[6] The disjunct between weak cosmopolitanism and strong cosmopolitanism is no longer feasible (given that we need to protect the basis of life). This has conceptual, spatial and temporal implications for the design of governance and a new form of democracy that rests on a scaled up form of subsidiarity that enshrines the rights of global citizens to secure stocks for the future protected by local and international governance. This section addresses the issue of whether it is possible to scale up democracy and governance and whether it is advisable to do so—in order to ensure a sustainable and socially just future.

striving to turn the lens upon oneself and through exploring issues in terms of both rational and emotional dimensions.[7]

That is why we need to draw on West Churchman's questioning approach 'the design of inquiring systems'—before 'making a cut' (the Latin for decision) we need to 'unfold' our values and to 'sweep in' the social, cultural, economic and environmental considerations. Yes, we need passion and compassion; for the latter, we need to realise that decisions are both rational and emotional. The past is understood by reviewing archives and through reflecting on genealogy. The present is comprehended through watching news footage and documentaries and through thinking about our own genealogical location in past, present and future. We can watch events unfold, in order to try to comprehend the values of diverse stakeholders and to gain an understanding of the ways in which emotions play out. Why did the London riots happen? Shaming people—the sense of lack of status is evident in the statements made by young people who said that they were stopped and searched regularly by police in ways that made them feel disrespected. Young people carry the sense of being disrespected and the rage of seeing ways of life which are paraded on the television or in street parades boil over.

5.3 Excessive Luxury Is Toxic

The riots in London after the royal wedding euphoria had subsided are easily understood when we remember that the gap between rich and poor is wider in the UK than in other Organisation for Economic Co-operation and Development (OECD) countries. Lack of status and emotional feelings of disrespect are central. According to Wilson[8] (2011, p. 21):

[7] According to Abbot (2007, p. 66), lyrical sociology is different from narrative sociology: 'I oppose to narrative sociology, by which I mean standard quantitative inquiry with its "narratives" of variables as well as those parts of qualitative sociology that take a narrative and explanatory approach to social life. Lyrical sociology is characterized by an engaged, non-ironic stance toward its object of analysis, by specific location of both its subject and its object in social space, and by a momentaneous conception of social time. Lyrical sociology typically uses strong figuration and personification, and aims to communicate its author's emotional stance toward his or her object of study, rather than to "explain" that object.' I continue to draw on West Churchman because he makes a plea for questioning those taken for granted through considering logic, empiricism, idealism, dialectic and pragmatism. But he also stresses the importance of values and emotions which enables us to think about the lyrical meanings. Balancing individual needs and the common good—without resorting to closed systems which deny the right to question—this is the challenge we face: 'In the realm of totalitarian kitsch, all answers are given in advance and preclude any questions. It follows, then, that the true opponent of totalitarian kitsch is the person who asks questions. A question is like a knife that slices through the stage backdrop and gives us a look at what lies hidden behind it…' (Kundera 1984, p. 254). 'Kitsch causes two teas to flow in quick succession. The first ear says: How nice to see children running on the grass! The second tear says: How nice to be moved, together with all mankind, by children running on the grass! The brotherhood of man (sic) on earth will be possible only on a base of kitsch' (Kundera 1984, p. 251).

[8] Wilson, P. 2011. Moments of madness amid calculated rage, The Weekend Australian August 13–14, p. 21.

> The sense of corruption being pervasive is not difficult to understand. The Prime Minister, Cameron is tainted by the ongoing investigation into phone hacking. His own media adviser was one of the employees who are currently mentioned as being aware of—if not implicated in the practice of phone hacking in order to secure access to information for news stories to sell newspapers for the Murdock News of the World Company. The feeling is—look at how they live—look at how we live.

Wilson goes on to cite some of the perceptions of young people as follows:

> The people whose shops got smashed up will get compensation from the government or from insurance. It's not really their money that we robbed.
> It's just anger at the police for everything. They do everything to humiliate young people. My brother got punched in the face for objecting to a stop and search, and he had nothing on him. They just try to make you feel small. This has all been our chance at revenge….

5.4 The Challenges

The greatest challenges are the *consequences of inaction* that will potentially pose an existential risk to humanity. These challenges include *representation* of the increasingly diverse populations within nation states along with a*ccountability* to ensure that resources (e.g. water, food, and energy) are used fairly, equitably and sustainably in local and regional biospheres. The book addresses the convergence of social, cultural, political, economic and environmental challenges that together pose an existential risk. Complexity requires more than attempts to manage risk. It requires transformation of our relationships to one another and the land on which we depend. It requires a transformation in the way economies are framed, but most importantly it requires a change of heart.

Better forms of *engagement* are needed to enhance the capability of people to understand that attitudes towards consumption have profound implications for social and environmental justice. The continuum of nature and the natural have been brutally shaped by the digital. If we accept the continuum across all life forms from the human to the animal and the earth and air to which we return, then we accept that all social responses need to be inclusive, to the extent that they do not undermine the rights of others and future generations of life. So if we accept the continuity of life as reflected in the new physics, it has implications for our thinking, our practice and the way in which we teach and learn. It also has implications for ethics.[9]

This requires cultural transformation, but of course cultural transformation is needed to create the will to do things differently. This is the terrible paradox in which we are trapped. We spend so much of our energy just treading water. The massive and unsustainable administrative minutiae required by bureaucracies leave little room in existing organizations for doing things differently.[10]

---

[9] But the digital is more limited than being the change from moment to moment in the way we choose to live our lives. Perhaps we are part of the transition; we are just looking at a very short time in human history.

[10] This is why learning communities although important need to be sustained by new learning organizations that foster the capability and confidence to work in groups with people who share the same concerns, but have different cultural frames of reference.

Since the commission on wellbeing that was requested by Sarkoszy and the book that resulted from it, called '*Mismeasuring our lives*' (Stiglitz, et al 2010), the global financial crisis has escalated to a social and environmental crisis that continues to unfold. Leading economists and development theorists, such as Stiglitz, Sen and Fitoussi (2011, p. 5), stress:

> We are also facing a looming social and environmental crisis,[11] especially associated with global warming. Market processes are distorted by the fact that there is no charge imposed on carbon emissions; and no account is made of the cost of these emissions in standard national income accounts. Clearly, measures of economic performance that reflected these environmental costs might look markedly different from standard measures.

The essence of the commission's findings is that wealth needs to include stocks for the future. These are social, economic and environmental. Leisure should also be given a price. If all measures consider wellbeing in terms of median households, then consumption, wealth and income could be compared with rich and poor households.[12]

5.5 Transdisciplinarity and Working Across Domains of Knowing

The Australian Public Service Commission 2007 report entitled 'Tackling wicked problems[13]' needs to be critically analysed in terms of the unexamined policy discourses. What are wicked problems? What are the so-called tame problems? Why is

[11] Wayne Swann (2012, pp. 3–4) discusses the gap between the rich and poor in Australia and America. The so-called rise of the 0.01 % of the wealthy has led to protests: ' Today the gap between the rich and the rest in the US is around twice the size of outs: in 2008, the top 1 % in the US received around 17.7 % of all income, while the figures is just (!) 8.6 % in Australia…. The catch cry of Wall Street's Zuccotti Park and the Occupy Movement "We are the 99 %" has shone a spotlight on the top 1 %. Between 1979 and 2007 in the US, the top 1 % saw their after-tax incomes rise 275 %, while the middle two thirds saw their after-tax incomes increase by less than 40 %.'

[12] It is possible for measures of average to disguise the fact that a high income does not enable exhausted workers to enjoy the same kind of leisure that a lower income family enjoys that has access to the safety net of capital, a home that is not mortgaged to the hilt and the security that loss of income will not lead to a loss of their home or their social networks.

Conservative economists argue that consumption can be modified by those with an income to build up wealth. The difference in this report is that consumption refers to stocks that are usually not included in economic measures. The most important point made is that by contributing to the public good, individual households could enhance their wellbeing.

[13] http://www.apsc.gov.au/publications-Accessed 8/01/2013 Rittel, H. and Webber, M. 1984, *Planning problems are wicked problems Developments in Design Methodology*. New York: Wiley. Wei-Ning Xiang 2012, Editorial: 'Working with wicked problems in socio-ecological systems: Awareness, acceptance, and adaptation', *Landscape and Urban Planning* 110, pp. 1–4. *Wellbeing and existential risk: engagement to address the policy and governance challenges of mitigation and accountability*, McIntyre, J. (School of Social and Policy Studies, Flinders University, janet.mcintyre@flinders.edu.au presenting author, De Vries, D. (Computer Science, Engineering and informatics, Flinders University, denise.devries@flinders.edu.au, paper delivered at CASS Research Conference *Sustainable Environmental Policy and Global Governance*, Beijing, China, 18–19 September 2012 and submitted to the journal of convergence, China.

it problematic to think of taming or tacking problems as opposed to recognising our need to live in harmony with others and the environment?

How can governance protect the global commons and the collective good? How can complex social, economic and environmental challenges that are perceived differently by different stakeholders with different values be addressed?

John Keane's book (2009, p. 877) on the rise and fall of democracy stresses that democracy will need to become more monitory if it is to prevent too much control by political masters.

Some of the arguments against a more systemic approach can be countered by arguing that the big challenges of the day—climate change and poverty—require working across conceptual and spatial boundaries. This requires working in a transdisciplinary and open manner:

> ...a holistic and process oriented approach that is by nature adaptive, participatory, and trans disciplinary (APT for short). By examining a wicked problem as a whole through a panoramic social lens rather than a scientific microscope, and working with it through an open and heuristic process of collective learning, exploration, and experimentation, the APT approach promises to be efficacious in fostering collaborative behaviour, reducing conflicts, building trust among all stakeholders and communities involved, and ultimately producing better and more satisfying results.... (Wei-Ning Xiang 2013, p. 2)

But Sen (2009, pp. 140–141) argues in the idea of justice that it is impossible to scaleup the social contract at a global level. Scaling up the social contract has received the thumbs down from all but a few strong cosmopolitans who are described as unrealistic. The objection is that it is illogical to try to apply notions of good out of context and without the participation by those who are to be affected by the decisions. But instead if a form of nested governance was developed, it would address some of the very legitimate concerns for world government coming about in the guise of a scaled-up form of democracy that becomes more powerful that the worst nation state. World government could become a leviathan, unless monitory democracy and governance is developed within and across overlapping federalist republics. So in political and governance terms, the logical next step would be to scaleup the social contract through applying the principle of subsidiarity through monitory democracy and governance. This would enable the testing out of ideas and consequently it would enrich the vision, the narrative and the accounts of those who will be affected by decisions in this generation and the next.

The Design of Inquiry System (DIS; inspired by the work of West Churchman) provides the means by which individuals and groups can think about the way in which an area of concern is framed. What is the case from the point of view of diverse people about the way in which we consume and waste food, energy and water? The notion of leaving food on the plate, throwing away excess leftovers and not redistributing them, is cultural and perhaps associated with lack of time. The time taken to deliver food to people in need at a distance socially and spatially may simply make it appear easier to make a donation. The notion that resources are infinite however is being increasingly challenged and one of the greatest will be to find ways to get resources relocated to where they are needed. The cost of distribution could be borne by taxing those with resources. This would be a way to address poverty and climate change, by reducing waste through redistribution. But the transport of resources remains the problem.

A design solution could address this more effectively, spanning governance codes that ensure that daily food redistribution collection points within each local government area are setup. Garbage collection could be replaced by food, clothing, white goods, furniture and packaging redistribution. The DIS is a means to address so-called wicked problems. It is based on considering the many kinds of knowledge that need to be brought to bear on an area of concern. These include an appreciation of logic, empirical data (both qualitative and quantitative), idealism, based on thinking about what ought to be done, dialectical engagement to explore one argument or thesis, antitheses and also synthesis and then most importantly thinking about the consequences for ourselves, others (including sentient beings, the voiceless, the disabled, non-citizens) and future generations of life on the planet.

How can we extend our horizon of solidarity? The horizon always seems as a perfect circle centred on the viewer. But other viewers in other places will have different horizons.[14] Banathy also stressed this in his book on conscious evolution. Imagine if we could enhance our capability to think and practice by extending our vision? The DIS is not a solution to complex challenges; it is a process that helps to honour many ways of seeing an area of concern. Importantly, it also enables an exploration of the values associated with the different views. The DIS to human inquiry can enable many stakeholders to give an account of the way in which they see the world. Values after all—along with emotions—are filters that need to be taken into account. The more we can think about our thinking and the way in which we view the world, the more connections we can make—quite literally

[14] We are human animals and have both rights and responsibility to the voiceless as caretakers and advocates. The emphasis on anthropocentricism could be said to be killing us, because we cannot see that in modifying the food chain, using pesticides widely has affected the bee population (Mathews, 2010) which affects food production and killing top predators leads to the proliferation of other species that can place pressure on the ecology which leads to further degradation of the land on which we depend for food. This is arguably unravelling the fabric of the planet. Just as the telescope helped us to see in the distance and the microscope helped us see in detail that which was beyond our comprehension with the naked eye, the use of external digital software could enable us to hold in mind many variables and to find agreed pathways towards a sustainable future. According to De Grasse, it is thought that the universe is 14 billion light years. The light from 15 billion years ago has not yet reached us. We are unaware of it. We do not know if the entire universe is finite or not. This is just one example of our lack of understanding—limited to our intelligence at the moment. Human beings cannot fly and they cannot smell as well as many animals. But the microscope has helped them to see in depth and the telescope has extended their vision. But this is not enough. We all evolved on the plains of Africa to escape lions. Brains were shaped by natural selection. Those who collaborated and competed survived. The ability to think in terms of the big picture and the long term and to support those beyond our immediate family needs to be developed. We need to understand that the zero sum or us–them approach is not the answer to survival. Meat is no longer killed and shared just with the immediate kin and those with whom we want an alliance. Now, we may need to think in terms of how to support large numbers of people in cities. According to De Grasse, as we develop tools, so we evolve to the next level.

neural connections—so that we are capable of seeing the world in terms of a bigger picture.[15]

So the chapters of this book constitute a series of essays that attempt to grapple with the human condition—the will to power, the will to achieve individual success and the desire to connect with others and with the environment on which we all depend—as animals (including human animals), birds, insects and reptiles. We need to acknowledge our hybrid nature and realise that design is not merely about control, it is about stewardship. Once we accept with humility our role as stewards, we can protect future generations of life. Realistically and ethically, it is in our own interests. Once the linear approach of cause and effect is replaced with a respect for two-way feedbacks and feed forwards or interconnectedness, we will comprehend that flow is a matter of physics and governance. Similarly, once the overlaps are recognised, the notion that the social contract cannot be scaled up will appear less convincing!

How can transdisciplinary research help us to address the challenge of mitigating the causes of climate change and adapting to the effects? This question addresses business and consumer discourses, habits, range of behaviours and associated emotions (Hogget, 2010) shaping dualistic attitudes towards rights and responsibilities and denial of responsibility for unsustainable consumerist culture.[16]

We need to address the Australian Public Policy position paper on wicked problems[17] and current research in Australia to work across disciplines and sectors. Local government representatives from the metropolitan and regional could be invited to both these workshops. To what extent does understanding the social or environ-

[15] The neuroscientist Baroness Professor Susan Greenfield (2000) stresses that consciousness is a result of making connections. When we are out of our mind, as a result of rage, joy or drugs, we are less likely to make rational decisions. Emotions will rule our decisions or at least our behaviour—as we may act without even knowing what we are doing. I could list many examples of this sort of behaviour by those in power: traders, bankers and political leaders who are in the thrall of their own will to power based on the emotions of greed and desire for the trappings of a powerful and so-called successful life.

[16] *Personal, interpersonal and public transformation*: Systemic governance in terms of this argument refers to working across: conceptual boundaries of professional, discipline-based and lived experience, networks, interest groups and organizations, cultures and identities and socio-geographic arenas locally, nationally and internationally, in order to achieve sustainable social, economic and environmental futures. The massive and unsustainable administrative minutiae required by bureaucracies leave little room in existing public, private and many mainstream non-government organizations for doing things differently. This is why learning organizations although important need to be sustained by new learning communities, projects that prefigure change and social movements that foster the capability and confidence to work separately and with people who share the same concerns or who have different cultural frames of reference.

[17] According to Wei-Ning Xiang (2013, p. 3), '…is also noteworthy that the tone in which people describe their relationship with wicked problems has become progressively softer, from "tame," "deal with," "handle," "tackle," to even "work with" (Australian Public Service Commission 2007, p. 11, 17, 35),"live with" (Norton 2012, p. 460), and "embracing" (Raisio 2010), reflecting a greater degree of acceptance of wicked problems as sustained social reality that human society has to live with.'

mental consequences of decisions affect business and consumer choices? According to Wei-Ning Xiang (2013, p. 3):

> …is also noteworthy that the tone in which people describe their relationship with wicked problems has become progressively softer, from "tame," "deal with," "handle," "tackle," to even "work with" (Australian Public Service Commission 2007, p. 11, 17, 35),"live with" (Norton 2012, p. 460), and "embracing" (Raisio 2010), reflecting a greater degree of acceptance of wicked problems as sustained social reality that human society has to live with.

5.6 Making Connections Based on our Shared Sense of Vulnerability

Contextual detail based on the recognition of the power of both emotion and reason (whilst mindful of the need for federalist legal and governance systems) needs to be held to account by a watchful, open and monitory democracy (Keane 2009a, b) that could puncture spin and hyperrealism (Baudrillard 1994). It is possible to strive for both emotional connection and rationality through testing out ideas but also ensuring that people have the right to be free to the extent that they do not undermine the freedom of others. Kundera is critical of sentimental narratives that are both imposed and which overemphasise the obvious.

> In the realm of totalitarian kitsch, all answers are given in advance and preclude any questions. It follows, then, that the true opponent of totalitarian kitsch is the person who asks questions and who listens to narratives about people's experiences. A question is like a knife that slices through the stage backdrop and gives us a look at what lies hidden behind it…. (Kundera 1984, p. 254)
> Kitsch causes two tears to flow in quick succession. The first tear says: How nice to see children running on the grass! The second tear says: How nice to be moved, together with all mankind, by children running on the grass!
> It is the second tear that makes kitsch, kitsch. The brotherhood of man on earth will be possible only on a base of kitsch. (Kundera 1984, p. 251)

For Kundera, a sense of shared meaning is important, without crude sentimentalism or imposed values to underline meaning. Narratives need to be cocreated, but through open discursive dialogue that includes questioning and respect for those who participate in making meaning. But Kundera has not considered the gendered nature of language and thus more questioning is clearly needed, by both so-called experts and non-experts—if knowledge is to be developed through lived experience (Wynne 1996). The feminist arguments about 'false consciousness' and 'liberation from patriarchy' would not have progressed without rallying for 'emancipation from oppression'—albeit mediated by diverse culture and class positions. Similarly, the emancipation of young people who do not have the vote, but who are required to live with the results of oppression, require recognition of false consciousness about rights and responsibilities that are supported by current systems of governance. Most importantly, the false consciousness of anthropocentricism which denies the pain of sentient beings shapes our culture and language. We have built nations on 'horse power' and the labour of people who 'work like dogs', even if 'beasts of burden' are now mechanized.

Pathways out of oppression need not be totalitarian or universal, provided the pathways are guided on the maxim that we can be free and diverse to the extent that freedom and diversity does not undermine the future of others. This is the point of a form of expanded pragmatism—not idealism—because it enables those who are to be affected to be part of the conversation—or at the very least represented by stewardship processes. The focus for participatory democracy and governance needs to be on *the local,* so that *local knowledge of the land* can inform decisions. This could enable creative, responsive transformation and the emergence of new, non-anthropocentric relationships that respect our symbiosis with other living creatures. Food supplies depend as much on bacteria as they do on the bee for pollination (Mathews 2010).

5.6.1 Recognising both Overlaps and Diversity Within and Beyond Regions

Wellbeing requires the desire for transformation, based not only on power expressed in totalitarian systems but in recognition of the 'disarray' (Caudill 1997) that we face when we do not analyse the implications of our choices. This has profound implications for the way we practice democracy and governance, in order to protect the biosphere on which we depend for food security. People within society compete for resources that are unjustly governed and distributed which impacts on social, economic and environmental resilience and wellbeing. Now certain questions still arise.

According to Rorty (1989), if we are able to identify with the suffering of others, we may have more solidarity with them. But *the will* to respond with compassion can be resisted or rationalised in terms of human security for the nation state versus 'the other'.[18] In the past, 'the other' was considered in racist, sexist, ageist or in species terms. The notion of structuring reality which is 'out there' in 'us–them terms' is a political response that allows for winners and losers. This is why agency needs to be fostered through enhancing the capability to shrug off 'false consciousness'.

[18] Why do *voters* think in the short-to-medium term and not the long-term impact of their decisions on vital issues such as food and energy security? This is arguably a result of the way human beings have evolved. It is as much a product of nature as it is a product of nurture. Thinking about strategies for the survival of this generation makes evolutionary sense. But survival and liveability *do not* have to be achieved at the expense of long-term resilience. Rational arguments have not been able to convince people. Emotions play a vital role in the way people think about themselves, others and the environment (Hoggett 2011). Linked with the current way of life in democracies is an expectation that rights need to be preserved in social and economic terms. These are achieved at the expense of the environment. Why do *politicians* pitch their policies to respond to the short and medium term? The answer is surely to ensure re-election every 3 years. This is a function of the short-term *design* of democracy and governance. Democracy and governance need to balance rights and responsibilities to the environment. The notion that governments are the agents of the people should be reframed. Instead, governments are the elected stewards of resources for future generations.

According to Baudrillard (1994), representations of reality have become confused with the real.[19] According to his argument, commodification of people and the environment becomes the reality—which now confronts us in the form of problems in which the market is complicit. For many people, image becomes more important than anything else, because their identity is shaped by advertising images.

How do we find our way out of the hyperreality we have created? Perhaps by realising that although the simulations are created by the powerful, it is possible for the less powerful to redesign our futures—rather than accept the current simulations. The analogy of the Mobius band helps us to understand that we shape and are shaped by nature (McIntyre-Mills 2008; Hulme 2010).

Just as party political sectarianism has the potential to divide, rather than to create solidarity, religious denominations and religious dogmatism can undermine the spiritual potential to create shared narratives. Similarly, the compartmentalism in primary, secondary and tertiary learning undermines holistic creativity and appreciation that we are part of a continuous cycle of life. Policy and legal constructs need to reflect an understanding of this interconnectedness (see also Rittel and Webber 1984) because design choices that shape governance decisions can create and destroy this web. The concept 'property' is a product of this misplaced commodification of all things. Caretakers return to the land when they die. They are the ancestors of the land. Our understanding of who we are and how we relate to one another is a starting point for exploring the points made by Rose Bird (1996, 2004) about identity, research and alienation.[20] Bird argues that building capacity to understand our role as caretakers requires recognising the colonial mind-set as a first step. This is vital without adopting a naïve approach that indigeneity has all the answers. The Eddie Mabo Land Rights case in the Torres Straits extended over 10 years, whilst he made the case that people who cared for the land as gardeners had as much right as those who declared property rights. Mabo, a gardener, had stressed the importance of gardening and caring for the land as part of his case for land rights in the Torres Straits.[21] The legal construct can be redefined and reconnecting with the land can be relearned.

---

[19] We have created visions of lifestyle through the media that represent how life ought to be lived and now we confuse these visions with reality. News is edited and presented to us as reality. Governments make decisions that simulate taking responsible caretaking decisions. The spin then becomes a form of hyperreality.

[20] I am trying to develop a response to this alienation by applying an approach to research that decentres the researcher and empowers participants to address wellbeing and the implications it has for our identity and 'being in the world' and the way we are consuming resources. By drawing a line or 'mastering' disciplines, we are fragmenting ourselves and denying that 'we are the land' (Getano Lui 1993; Nazarea 2006) and that we return to the elements of life when we die. In turn, we become the ancestors and nurture the land from which new life grows.

[21] Mabo v Queensland (No 2) [1992] HCA 23; (1992) 175 CLR 1 (3 June 1992) HIGH COURT OF AUSTRALIA MABO AND OTHERS v. QUEENSLAND (No. 2) [1992] HCA 23; (1992) 175 CLR 1 F.C. 92/014: "The groups of houses were and are organised in named villages. It is far from obvious to the uninitiated, but is patent to an islander, that one is moving from one village to another. The area occupied by an individual village is, even having regard to the confined area on a fairly small island which is in any event available for 'village land', quite small. Garden

Bridging capital does not go far enough to span differences (Putnam 2000) because it starts with the assumption that connections are a form of capital. Instead, this research begins with the assumption that connections are a sine qua non of wellbeing. Recognising *space for diversity* needs to be guided by an axiom that: *diversity is vital provided the diversity does not undermine the wellbeing of others.* But wherever possible, overlaps across cultural diversity need to be recognised and created—through both respectful dialogue and emotional narratives within 'post-national constellations' (Habermas 2001).

Policies and processes need to protect the rights of the voiceless. These include young people (who will have to live with the results of current policy), asylum seekers (who flee from climatic disaster) and sentient beings (who cannot speak for themselves).

Stewardship praxis is a process resulting from thinking and practice based on an understanding that what we do to others and to the environment, we do to ourselves and to our children. The land is placed first by First Nations internationally (Rose 1996). Post colonialism and indigenous knowing is important in understanding what stewardship entails. It runs the risk of being debased by irony and cynicism if it remains at the level of ideology or window dressing. An international legal framework needs to make respectful dialogue in post national constellations (Habermas 2001) a precursor to wide ranging transformations. But the place of emotions needs to be recognised as central and ways to enable the expression of grief and anger (through narrative) at the local and post national level will be vital in communities facing loss of livelihood as a result of a changing environment.

The collective good requires recognition of common needs and legislation. So the iconic symbols of interrelatedness, such as the symbolic mandala, the Mobius band or Mandelbrot set (see McIntyre-Mills 2008)—if not the kitsch—could be

land is identified by reference to a named locality coupled with the name of relevant individuals if further differentiation is necessary. The Islands are not surveyed and boundaries are in terms of known land marks such as specific trees or mounds of rocks. Gardening was of the most profound importance to the inhabitants of Murray Island at and prior to European contact. Its importance seems to have transcended that of fishing… Gardening was important not only from the point of view of subsistence but to provide produce for consumption or exchange during the various rituals associated with different aspects of community life. Marriage and adoption involved the provision or exchange of considerable quantity of produce. Surplus produce was also required for the rituals associated with the various cults at least to sustain those who engaged in them and in connection with the various activities associated with death. Prestige depended on gardening prowess both in terms of the production of a sufficient surplus for the social purposes such as those to which I have referred and to be manifest in the show gardens and the cultivation of yams to a huge size. Considerable ritual was associated with gardening and gardening techniques were passed on and preserved by these rituals. Boys in particular worked with their fathers and by observations and imitations reinforced by the rituals and other aspects of the social fabric gardening practices were passed on.' 'It seems that before European contact social cohesion was sought by the combined operation of a number of factors. Children were inculcated from a very early age with knowledge of their relationships in terms of social groupings and what was expected of them by a constant pattern of example, imitation and repetition with reinforcing behaviour. It was part of their environment—the way in which they lived….' The findings show that Meriam society was regulated more by custom than by law."

used to mobilize solidarity, rather than exclusion[22] of 'the other', because they symbolize that what we do to others, we do to ourselves as we are part of one cycle of life.

As global stewards, we need to consider our complicity in commodifying our relationships with others and with the environment (Binkley 2000; Newton 1997).

Our mirror neurons 'fire in sympathy' (Turner and Whitehead 2008) with hyperreal characters on the news and in the media. Instead of being connected with others or with the land at the local level in real time, we are distracted by digital connections. We repress our feelings and deny ourselves and others the time that is needed for building rapport and relationships, because 'time is money'. This in turn breeds hurt and resentment (Eisenbergerger and Lieberman 2004) because we 'know the cost of everything and the value of nothing' (Oscar Wilde 1892). Humanity is spending more time being connected with digital representations of others, rather than giving full attention to those with whom we come into contact.

The environmental crisis is a result of unsustainable living together with the unfolding economic crisis (triggered by bundling the debt which flowed from non-repayments of the subprime mortgages and the bungling by Wall Street). This affects the lives of people on the streets—from Madrid to Manila and from Tahirir Square to Hindmarsh Square in Adelaide, South Australia. The disenfranchised in Australia include farmers who are losing their livelihood as a result of water shortages and workers and the unemployed—who are not the beneficiaries of the mining boom—form part of the 'fall out' from the so-called two-speed economy. The Hindmarsh Square organizers in Adelaide, for example explain their protest as an extension of the Occupy Wall Street movements. The challenge is to:

- Build the capability[23] to resist 'false consciousness' not only in the sense in which Marx used it, but in order to understand the impact of the market on labour and the land. Resource stewardship needs to be governed by the overarching federations.
- Ensure that people who are to be affected by decisions can play a role in developing the indicators of wellbeing in an ongoing manner with the caveat that individuals and collectives have the right to be free to the extent that their freedom does not undermine the rights of others or the next generation of life. Stiglitz et al. (2010) stress that citizens feel cynical about the way in which current governance systems operate. Not only are current governance systems

[22] Historically, religion has always provided a 'way to make the unbearable, bearable'. 'It is the opium of the people' (Marx 1843; Spivak 1998; Eyerman 1981). Religion along with 'morality, politics and aesthetics' can be seen as *human values* which *filter* our understanding the world (West Churchman 1979,1982)—these values (and linked emotions) are vital to cultural transformation.

[23] People spend less and less time exploring complex ideas. Reading books and thinking about concepts—imagining the symbols and thinking through complex narratives—is lost when children give up reading (Greenfield 2008). Hyperreality is encouraged through computer games; the game becomes more real than the real. New kinds of media engagement need to build the capability of local people to think about complexity.

outdated, they also do not support the wellbeing and resilience of the planet (Leonard 2011, McIntyre-Mills and De Vries 2011). International law and ethics need to be reframed to address issues of representation, accountability (Beck 2009) and resilience defined as 'adaptive capacity…of the physical environment' and the capacity of members of a community to act together…. (Hulme 2009, p. 167).

The basis for change lies in transformations that flow from the potential of subsidiarity (see McIntyre-Mills and de Vries 2011) to enable local people to have a say in local affairs within overlapping regions for sustainable governance. The debate about where to draw the line is fraught and has consequences for human lives. The demise of social democratic platform is evident in Australia and in other welfare states. Needham (2011) stresses that self-harm of detainees has increased. There were:

> 1100 incidents last year and 54 incidents the first week of July alone…. The immigration Department said it was working with a mental health advisory group to "examine self-harm and suicide trends across the network.

Hospitality to those who flee disaster—drought, famine or conflict—needs to be supported through corridors that protect biodiversity. The Nagoya Biodiversity Summit (2010) on biological diversity has recognised that the containerist argument is inadequate. Nagoya, Japan, 29 Oct:

> History will recall that it was here in Nagoya that a new era of living in harmony was born and new global alliance to protect life on earth was established….

Little has eventuated from these proceedings because discussions have faltered on the same concerns raised by Charlton (2011), namely that humanity continues to polarize progress on poverty versus protecting the planet—rather than understanding that systemic 'both and' thinking is vital for a sustainable and politically acceptable future. But Charlton's creativity is largely focused on technocratic interventions, rather than on wide ranging sociocultural transformation. Multidimensional responses are needed ranging from direct action by individuals, households, communities, nations, regions and post national regions to subsidies to foster research and new Green responses aided by market response that taxes carbon in ways that send a strong message to polluters. Laws need to ensure sustainable approaches are applied globally within federalist responses that ensure that regional areas co-operate and do not compete for resources. Direct action without subsidies and a price on carbon—that is supported by post national international laws and implemented widely—could be inadequate. International law entails: (a) recognition that global citizens need to protect the global commons and (b) the collective good based on stewardship for this generation and the next. Thus, cocreated narratives need to develop to protect the biosphere through extending the process of democracy and governance at the local level (McIntyre-Mills and De Vries 2011, 2012).

5.7 Grasping the Nettle: The Role of Monitory Democracy and Governance in Designing and Directing our Future Development

Where have we come from and where are we going in our evolution or preferably revolutionary transformation based on ethical choices?[24] We have the capacity to design our future. Accepting our role as stewards, rather than as extractors of profit is the challenge!

Can cosmopolitan politics address the criticism raised by the Left, namely that politics needs to strive for debate that ensures the pseudo-politics of right and left in a capitalist society leads to a transformation of the neoliberal market?

Emotions need to be acknowledged when striving to think and act ethically, but they need to be tempered with empirical evidence. This was the strength of the first-hand account by Carboni, who wrote the following at the outset of his narrative on his participation in the Eureka Stockade:

> I undertake to do what an honest man should do, let it thunder or rain. He who buys this book to lull himself to sleep had better spend his money on grog. He who reads this book to smoke a pipe over it, let him provide himself with plenty of tobacco—he will have to blow hard.

Just as the quotation is dated by the unselfconscious references to tobacco and grog, perhaps our future narratives will reveal the extent to which our complicity and our thinking is a reflection of society today!

A new architecture for democracy and governance needs to be designed. We need to learn from capitalism, anarchism and communism when developing a new form of monitory democracy and governance. Anarchism echoes the larger attack on the state. Neoliberalism has said that the state is the problem and that instead we need to '…let us do it ourselves in small local communities'. This is not practical if we wish to avoid isolated warlordism in a new medieval age! I recognise that aspects of cosmopolitanism (if not communism) is something that we should work towards as the horizon. We need production by and for the common good. But this requires open systems.

The most pressing challenge is food security through overlapping regional domains and systemic accountability supported by monitory democracy from above and below.

Utopian agrarianism is irrelevant because current elites and middle classes are increasingly mobile. Current forms of transport are part of the problem, but not mo-

[24] US team creates synthetic life By North America correspondent Craig McMurtrie Updated Fri May 21, 2010 9:37am AEST A bio-technician demonstrates the beginning of the sequencing procedure (Reuters: Larry Downing, file photo). Scientists in the United States have announced they have developed the world's first synthetic living cell…*the Maryland-based research team says it is the first time synthetic DNA has been in complete control of a cell*…. His research team inserted watermarks in the synthetic DNA to be decoded, including a James Joyce quotation: 'To live, to err, to fall, to triumph, to recreate life out of life.' http://www.abc.net.au/news/stories/2010/05/21/2905396.htm?site=news.

bility per se. The notion that we need to move from mobility to localization stressed at the 'Economics of Happiness Conference'[25] raises issues about energy and the power to transform the economy so that the rich do not continue business as usual whilst encouraging a new proletarianisation of the 99 %.

Humanity has been both mobile as hunter gatherers and parochial as agriculturalists. The challenge is to find alternative forms of energy and to enable agricultural land to be protected. Food security needs to be regarded as vital for human security.

New regional approaches to food security will require transnational approaches that place security and protection of the global commons at a post national level. This does not mean that the state ought not to play a role in federalist regions. But the local, national and international domains will need to be seen as integral or part of a systemic whole.

According to Morton (1998, p. 6):

> The concept of 'think globally and act locally' underlines the importance of local government involvement in environmental management. Local government operates at the local level not only as a service provider but also as a planning, regulatory and coordinating agency. This multi-functional role provides a capacity to combine both economic instruments and regulatory provisions to achieve specific environmental management objectives in an efficient and effective manner. The principles of Ecologically Sustainable Development (ESD) are also an important element of local environmental management, typically underpinning the land use planning and control functions delegated to local authorities. The location, intensity and form of human settlement within an area tend to pose threats to the environment which need to be addressed….

Morton (1998, p. 6) does not address the additional and systemic issue which is the security of human settlements from disaster. Instead, he focuses on the threats to the environment as:

> Wasteful use of scarce natural resources; loss and/or pollution of natural habitats and associated water and reduced biodiversity; production of greenhouse gases and associated global warming; air and noise pollution through factors such as excessive use of private vehicles and poor settlement planning and location.
>
> In 1993 the United Nations published a handbook describing the conceptual basis for implementing an Integrated System of Environmental and Economic Accounting (SEEA). SEEA is a comprehensive framework which outlines a range of potential and monetary measures of the environment/economy relationship which could be used to support integrated social, economic and environmental policy and planning. SEEA outlines a number of possible accounts and sub-accounts which relate to different aspects of the interactions that occur between the environment and the economy. The ABS has based its environmental accounting program on the accounts outlined in SEEA…. (Heycox et al. 1997 cite UN 1993, p. 3)[26]

How can we move from polarising politics in democracy to approaches that explore the potential of discursive democracy? How can we find the potential in many di-

---

[25] http://www.youtube.com/watch?v=Mmg_MMGCxXI&feature=youtube_gdata_player.

[26] Summary of the SEEA accounts relevant to local government. Cited by Heycox et al. 1997: p. 3 cite United Nations (1993) Integrated Environmental and Economic Accounting: Handbook of National Accounting: Studies in Methods, Series F. No 61, Department for Economic and Social Information and Policy Analysis, Statistical Division, United Nations, New York.

verse ideas and cocreate meaning in ways that protect diversity and freedom to the extent that it does not undermine the diversity and freedom of others and future generations of life?

The crisis we face in current democracies stems from polarised debates that do not draw on many diverse ideas or allow for developing new paradigms and responsive praxis that could address the current challenges.

The danger of top-down intervention is not the preserve of nations who are 'part of the axis of evil'. We need to face up to our own complicity. The approach detailed in *Identity, Democracy and Sustainability* (McIntyre-Mills and De Vries, 2011) and developed in this book addresses a means to operationalize environmental protection through engaging members of the public in the process of developing appropriate measures of wellbeing. This is a vital step in cultural transformation as it raises awareness. It also requests contracting at a household level as to the trade-offs they are prepared to make. Nevertheless, detailed accounting and accountability ought not to create a legalistic environment where attempts are made to find ways around the letter of the law. Sanctions can never replace ethical responsibility. Values, not law, are the most vital consideration for cultural transformation. Furthermore, the funding of environmental protection activities needs to be supported by all levels of government[27] and by the private sector.

The users of services, the providers of services and the beneficiaries all need to make contributions. The problem with neo-conservative communitarian arguments is that the burden of responsibility ought not to be shifted to locals without the private sector, welfare sectors and all levels of government playing an equal role.

Unlike the approach suggested by Heycox et al. (1997), the UN 1993 approach and the approach developed by Stiglitz et al. (2010) to accounting and accountability, this design reframes governance and develops a suite of measures that enable participatory design and governance by every resident within a region. It builds on and applies the policy suggested in the Aarhus convention (1998) but extends it to social issues.

This approach does not attempt to disaggregate; instead, it allows for and works with overlapping domains in order to maximize changes towards a more sustainable future. The crisis we face in current democracies stems from polarised debates that do not draw on many diverse ideas or allow for developing new paradigms and responsive praxis that could address the current challenges.

Clearly, the Asian Century has not really been fully appreciated by Australia or by America. Africa is aware that aid is more forthcoming from Asia than from elsewhere. The largest developments in a small town of Port Elizabeth in South Africa

[27] According to Heycox et al. 1997, p. 4: 'Data published by the ABS on the environmental protection expenditures by the public sector, including local government, is derived from the public sector finance collection which is based on an international Classification of the Functions of Government (COFOG). The problem arises due to the structure of COFOG was designed long before collecting data on public sector transactions does not enable the environmental component of transactions…to be separately identified". But separation or disaggregation is quite the wrong way to approach the problem. This is why a systemic approach is vital and why the research supports the promotion of well-being as an integrated measure for a sustainable future.

are by Chinese investors. A casino that dwarfs the rest of the landscape along the coast illustrates that Africa is seen as a place for expansion.

The indebtedness of America[28] mirrors the indebtedness of other nations to China. It raises questions about democracy and globalization and the direction for the future. Politicians driven by so-called realist politics could argue that cosmopolitanism is absurd when 'national advantage' is the name of the game. But the zero-sum approach will not achieve a sustainable future.

In some ways, governance from above could bring about change very rapidly. Some would argue that we have too much freedom and that the right to pollute and exploit has been taken too far.

Facing the hard truth, rather than running election campaigns in the media with all the attributes of personality politics, rather than debating the hard issues, is the core problem that needs to be addressed by the people who are going to have to live with some hard choices in the future. Already people are saying we have had enough of the phony politics of neo-liberalism.

The suburban lifestyles of the middle and lower middle classes is funded on debt and limited sleep. People want a change, but it will need to be created through transforming what we care about and what we value. Everyone at some stage of their working life jokes that they would like to retire to a Greek Island and to spend their time looking at the far horizon and enjoying long lunches. In particular, Ikaria seems like a good place to live. Despite 40% unemployment, the people who have a largely socialist outlook as the majority identify with the communist party. They live a communal life in which working in their vegetable patches, walking up and down the steep inclines of the village, communal meals and a strong sense of local identity play a role:

> We simply do not care about the clock here. Pointing across the ocean toward the neighbouring island of Samos…. Just 15 km over there is a completely different world. There they are much more developed…. In Samos they care about money. Here we don't. For the many religious and cultural holidays people pool their money and buy food and wine. If there is money left over they give it to the poor. It is not a *me* place. It's an *us* place…in the late 1940s, after the Greek Civil War, the government exiles thousands of Communists and radicals to the island. Nearly 40 percent of adults still vote for the local communist party…. (Beutner 2013, p. 22)

Many factors could play a role in longevity; the combination of diet, physical exercise and commitment to one another in a less unequal and less uncaring community seems to play a role. The empirical evidence of Ikaria seems to support the research of Wilkinson and Pickett (2009) who argue in their book '*The spirit level: Why more equal societies almost always do better*' that the health of people in equal societies

---

[28] Clearly, America's fiscal debt is such that it too should realise the implications of business as usual. In Obama's accession speech, he stresses the importance of a cultural change. He stressed the respect for diversity and the need to acknowledge the unions of gays as having equal merit. He also stressed the importance of moving towards a green economy. But the rhetoric was expressed in terms of American leadership. The cost of the so-called democratic election in America was US$ 2 billion. One has to ask, is this necessary? Apparently, in a single month the Obama campaign garnered US$ 114 million. Conrad (2013, p. 14) asks if this is indeed the way forward.

is much better than the health of people in less equal societies. Beliefs, time to spend with others and eating food that is locally grown is good for the health of people and the planet. Slow living and limited numbers of food miles play an important role. I wonder if the zombie mind-set could be set aside by helping people to realise that we are asleep while walking over the cliff.

This book is my contribution to a wakeup call.

The democratic electoral system and the notion of freedom are under threat. The cost of electoral politics in Western democracies (particularly in America) threatens wellbeing because democracy has been captured by the market. Monitory democracy (in the sense used by Keane 2009) is vital in order to hold the market to account.

Fenbyt (2013) estimates that there are more than 150,000 protests each year in China and that the Pew Institute has recorded the number of people concerned about food safety in China has risen from 12 % in 2008 to 41 % to date. In pursuing good neighbourliness, however, we need to stress more than a desire for trade.[29] Both sides of politics in Australia are in agreement that our future is Asian, but we need to develop conversations about our relationships and our responsibility to future generations.

Not only competition for scarce resources fuel tension but also fears for the future.[30] In Japan, 340,000 people have been displaced by the Fukushima disaster. The reaction of the electorate was to vote the incumbent government out of office. But ironically, they elected Prime Minister Abe who is keen to rely on nuclear energy and to change the Japanese constitution to allow it to take a more active role in its defence.

According to Malcolm Cook, the world looks a fairly dangerous place from Tokyo, with less-than-amicable relationships with its neighbours. It faces a debt burden that ranks amongst the third highest in the world in 2013. This tension between China and Japan over the islands is a synecdoche of the tensions within the region for power and rights to resources. The tensions are repeated between Japan and Korea over islands called Takeshima or Pokto.[31]

Ironically although nationalist concerns were expressed by Rudd (2013),[32] he has acted in a nationalist manner in declaring that all asylum seekers arriving by boat will be sent to Papua New Guinea. The challenge to address complex social, economic and environmental issues could be assisted through regional dialogues that enable the consideration of options in 'if-then' scenarios. I am not so naïve as to imagine that the reasons for the tensions would be remedied so simply because of-

[29] Van Onselen, P. 2013 Beware the dangers of fawning on untamed China Weekend Australia, April 13–14, p. 20.

[30] The regional disasters within nations range from tsunamis and storm surges in Japan as well as regular seismic instability to regular flooding in Australia and fires, earthquakes and landslides in China. In Indonesia, all these disasters pose a challenge. According to the head of the Torrens Resilience Centre, Professor Paul Hare, 'Indonesian officials claim that for those concerned about disaster, Indonesia provides all the examples…it is a supermarket of disasters….'

[31] 24th August 2012. Malcolm Cook reports on Australian Broadcasting.

[32] Rudd, K. 2013. Asia's own Balkans a tinderbox; China's tensions with Japan and Vietnam should urgently be defused. Inquirer Feb 2–3, 19.

ten they are the result of political power plays for the home electorate, as in the case of the official approval of the Chinese nationalist sentiment of burning the Japanese flag. But it could help to enable conversations that could prevent further escalation.

Similarly, the tensions between Vietnam and China are expressed through fears expressed by Vietnam is associated with being economically indebted to China.

> It is also clear that the Chinese today possess considerable leverage over Vietnam, to the extent that one senior Vietnamese official candidly remarked recently that China could simply wreck the Vietnamese economy if it so chose. It would be wrong however, given ancient resentments, to assume that economic dependency would automatically constrain Vietnamese diplomatic or even military action in relation to the South China Sea.... Whilst Rudd quickly stressed that he believed 'a pan-Asian war extremely unlikely'. Nonetheless, for those of us who live in this region, facing escalating confrontations in the East China and South China seas, Europe is a cautionary take very much worthy of reflection....

The demographic transition appears to be a prerequisite for a less fierce competition for resources. Education and a rise in living standards need to be achieved in ways that ensure food security. In the first instance, we need to consider that the shorter the chain between production and consumption the less problems there will be in the quality of the food. In large societies where face-to-face connection breaks down and where profit rules, the notion of reciprocity and relationship breaks down. A case in point is the way in which children's milk powder was contaminated and the way in which diseased pig carcasses have been dumped in the river so that Shanghai's water supply has been threatened.[33]

The need to address ethics in relation to food security is a case in point. We need to consider the cultural, legal and social issues.[34]

5.8 Recognising Overlapping Biospheres to Protect Systemic Flows and Food

How can we move from polarising politics to approaches that explore the 'liberative potential' (Gouldner 1971) of discursive democracy? How can we find the liberative potential in many diverse ideas and cocreate meaning in ways that protect diversity and freedom to the extent that it does not undermine the diversity and freedom of others and future generations of life?

[33] Davidson, N. Dead pigs threaten Shanghai's water. Guardian Weekly 05/04.13.

[34] Upton (2013, pers.comm) stressed the importance of the China reform proposal paper: Zhou, Tianyong, Wang Changjiang and Wang Anling, 2007. In English: 'Storming the Fortress–China Political System Reform Research Report after 17th National Congress'. See http://chinadigitaltimes.net/2008/02/elite-china-think-tank-issues-political-reform-blueprint/ 'But the 366-page report give a strikingly detailed blueprint of how some elite advisers see political relaxation unfolding, with three phases of reform in the next 12 years, including restricting the party's powers and expanding the rights of citizens, reporters, religious believers and lawmakers.' http://www.guardian.co.uk/world/2008/feb/19/china.pressandpublishing.

According to Upton: Professor Kerry Brown has several references to the report in his book *Ballot Box China.* 2011, Zed Books London and New York.

We cannot rely on the state-based social contract to protect the collective good or the global commons. For example, the sea is a source of food, a place where waste has been dumped and it provides a contested space for power plays over boundaries to resources and access to nation states by those who seek asylum or refuge. River systems are also part of this contested space. The competition for power over water supplies in the Mekong River requires attention.[35]

'The Mekong River runs through or border six nations: China, Myanmar (Burma), Thailand, Lao PDR (Laos), Cambodia and Vietnam. The Mekong River Commission (MRC) was established with the signing of the 1995 Mekong Agreement by the governments of the Lower Mekong Countries—Cambodia, Lao PDR, Thailand and Vietnam—to ensure the sustainable use and management of water and related resources of the Lower Mekong Basin.'

The construction of dams in the upper reaches of the river in China will affect the flows of water and also affect the migration of fish. This has implications for food, energy and water security within the region. The increase in the supply of energy needed by the region will lead to the scaling of hydroelectric power use. China could affect the downstream wellbeing of the river if too many dams are constructed and if the migration of fish is affected. How the river is governed will be very important for the region. Attitudes towards neighbours will be expressed in the way in which water is managed and the way in which maritime fishing rights are managed.

The issue of fishing rights is problematic for Australia. Minister Burke banned the super trawler Margiris, cynically renamed Able Tasman, from fishing in Australia. The owners of the super trawler are engaged in a law suit with the Australian Government and has sailed to South America where no doubt it will aim to ply its trade. The global commons and the rights to food security need to be protected by overarching laws to ensure that overfishing does not occur:

> The ship, which was banned from fishing by Mr Burke last year, is being prevented from operating as a factory-freezer mother ship to be supplied by smaller trawlers ....The 9500-tonne fishing boat, formerly called Margiris, came to Australia last year to fish an 18,000-tonne quota that operator Seafish Tasmania holds for mackerel and redbait.[36]

Similarly, the standoff over whaling between Japan and Australia is just another part of the same challenge of the right to resources versus the need to protect the global commons.[37]

---

[35] Lee, G. and Scurrah, N. 2009. Power and responsibility: the Mekong River Commission and Lower Mekong mainstream dams. A joint report of the Australian Mekong Resource Centre, University of Sydney and Oxfam Australia.

[36] Abel Tasman has been banned from fishing in Australian waters by federal Environment Minister Tony Burke. See: http://www.theage.com.au/opinion/political-news/burke-rejects-second-bid-to-use-super-trawler-20130213-2ebvw.html#ixzz2NYkL2raw, http://www.theage.com.au/opinion/political-news/burke-rejects-second-bid-to-use-super-trawler-20130213−2ebvw.html.

[37] Black, R, 12 July 2011 Japan '*to continue 'Antarctic whaling* http://www.bbc.co.uk/news/science-environment-14132320 Australia-Japan talks: development, regional security, and whaling. Media release 13 January 2013 Foreign Minister Bob Carr and Japan's Foreign Minister Fumio Kishida today held talks on regional security, development and whaling, in Sydney. The talks come less than a month after the election of the Abe Government in Japan on December 16, 2012 and are

Both Australia and Japan have filed detailed written arguments in the Court, which will set the case for oral hearing in The Hague. The case is likely to be listed for hearing in the latter half of 2013. Regionalist approaches within the nation state are becoming more prevalent to address risk. According to Wear (2012, p. 469):

> The establishment of regional Management forums was an experiment in collaborative governance. Similar governance structures were also established in other jurisdictions.

Garnaut cites Senior Colonel Liu Mingfu, at the People's Liberation Army's National Defence University:

> Within two decades the United States will be forced out of the western Pacific, says a senior Chinese military officer, amid concerns that increasingly militarized great power rivalry could lead to war.

The Chinese Academy of Social Sciences Institute in China hosted the sustainability conference at a time of the orchestrated protests against the Japanese. The tensions in China over islands and fishing rights were evident when I was in Beijing in September 2012 for a conference on environmental sustainability at the Chinese Academy of Social Sciences.[38] The orchestrated protests had just been tidied up when I went for a walk with colleagues through Tiananmen Square. The posters protesting the Japanese use of the waters in Senkaku also known as Diaoyu for fishing are indicative of the tensions around food and energy.[39] Our delegation to the conference on the 3rd Sino Australian delegation on Sustainable Policies and Global Governance started the day after the state-supported protests against Japan

part of Minister Kishida's first overseas visits as Foreign Minister. Security: On security matters, Ministers agreed on the need for the UN Security Council to deliver an effective response to North Korea's rocket launch in December 2012. Security discussions also included Afghanistan, Syria, the Middle East peace process, Iran and conflicts in Africa including piracy off the Somalia coastline. It was agreed that Australia and Japan would further strengthen their cooperation in United Nations activity related to peacekeeping, nuclear non-proliferation and the advancement of an Arms Trade Treaty to reduce the flow of illicit weapons to rogue states and terrorist groups. Australia and Japan also agreed to continue cooperation on the need for Security Council reform. Australia reaffirmed its support for Japan's permanent membership of the UNSC. Minister Carr reiterated Australia's strong position against so-called scientific whaling by Japan. Australia is pursuing action in the International Court of Justice on the issue and considers Japanese whaling to be contrary to its international obligations.

[38] September is the time of year when wind is most likely to blow away pollution. Pollution was also limited by the decision to ban all large trucks from travelling into town as attempts were made to clean up the city prior to the National People's Congress at the Great Hall. Recently, the levels of pollution have reached alarming levels that have led to people questioning whether growth at the cost of the environment is a worthwhile economic agenda. See http://www.smh.com.au/environment/beijing-barely-suitable-for-life-as-heavy-pollution-shrouds-chinas-capital-20140226-33ghq.html.

[39] In Japan, 340,000 have been displaced by the Fukushima disaster. The reaction of the electorate was to vote the incumbent government out of office. But ironically, they elected Prime Minister Abe who is keen to rely on nuclear energy and to change the Japanese constitution to allow it to take a more active role in its defence. According to Malcolm Cook, the world looks a fairly dangerous place from Tokyo, with less than amicable relationships with its neighbors. It faces a debt burden that ranks the third highest in the world in 2013.

ended. The posters displayed prominently demonstrated the support of the Chinese government for displays of national protest.

This tension between China and Japan over the islands is a synecdoche of the tensions within the region for power and rights to resources. Similarly, the tensions are repeated between Japan and Korea over islands called Takeshima or Pokto.[40]

Nationalist concerns are raised by Rudd (2013)[41]: the challenge to address complex social, economic and environmental issues could be assisted through regional dialogues that enable the consideration of options in if-then scenarios. I am not so naïve as to imagine that the reasons for the tensions would be remedied so simply, because often they are the result of political power plays for the home electorate, as in the case of the official approval of the Chinese nationalist sentiment of burning the Japanese flag. But it could help to enable conversations that could prevent further escalation.

Similarly, the tensions between Vietnam and China are shown through fears expressed by Vietnams associated with being economically indebted to China.

> It is also clear that the Chinese today possess considerable leverage over Vietnam, to the extent that one senior Vietnamese official candidly remarked recently that China could simply wreck the Vietnamese economy if it so chose. It would be wrong however, given ancient resentments, to assume that economic dependency would automatically constrain Vietnamese diplomatic or even military action in relation to the South China Sea.[42]
> Concerns about China's strategic ambitions have grown since last year's Chinese occupations of islands administered by the Philippines in the South China Sea and, particularly, China's continuing brinkmanship with Japan and its security guarantor the US, in the East China Sea.

According to Garnaut at the East Asia Summit, China blocked discussion on maritime security issues. He cites Hugh White as saying 'it is the most dangerous strategic crisis that the US has faced that the world has faced since the end of the Cold War'. In 'White Papering over the Cracks', Hugh White (2013) points out that the current Labour government is not planning adequately for Australia's role within

---

[40] 24th August 2012. Malcolm Cook reports on Australian Broadcasting.

[41] Rudd, K. 2013. Asia's own Balkans a tinderbox; China's tensions with Japan and Vietnam should urgently be defused. Inquirer Feb 2–3, 19.

[42] Whilst Rudd quickly stresses that he believes 'a pan-Asian war extremely unlikely. Nonetheless for those of us who live in this region, facing escalating confrontations in the East China and South China seas, Europe is a cautionary take very much worthy of reflection…', it is not by chance that the Weekend Australian has been running articles about the educational aspirations of Chinese parents who make great sacrifices to give their children the best possible education and who require their children to excel. Lewis, L. 2013 Born to be dragons, but not free: Chinese families pay tutors to teach children before they're even a year old. Should Australian parents worry? The Weekend Australian January 26–27, 11 '…the boy will have more responsibility to shoulder. We may only let him have 60 min free time every day….' This highly competitive mother (a successful entrepreneur) stressed the importance of being competitive locally and internationally:

"…. Western parents should feel concern at the single mindedness of their Chinese counterparts…."

the region. Nor is Australia acknowledging that our neighbours are Asian and not American. He stresses that the Asian Century will decentre America as power broker and that geographically Australia needs to recognise that America will not be calling the shots. Hugh White (2013) argues that the policy direction of both Australia and the USA fails to recognise the shift in the power dynamics to Asia and that Australia should recognise that geographically it is Asian and that policies should not strain Asian relationships. White does not follow through with any alternative policy suggestions.

> After permission was refused by Mr Burke last November, it was…. The company's managing director, Joe Pirrello, announced a plan last month to use a fleet of smaller vessels to catch the fish and deliver it to the Abel Tasman for freezing and storage.
> 'The Abel Tasman will not put a net in the water', Mr Pirrello said. Conservation groups opposed the plan…. Independent MP Andrew Wilkie queried whether it was an attempt to circumvent the ban.
> Mr Burke said on Tuesday that he was concerned about the same environmental consequences as the first proposal, and that he had halted the process under national environmental law.
> 'This declaration will prevent the super trawler from operating in the manner proposed for six weeks while the company responds,' Mr Burke said.
> The standoff over whaling between Japan and Australia is just another part of the same challenge of the right to resources versus the need to protect the global commons.[43]

Hugh White stresses in 'White Papering the cracks' that the Asian century will decentre America as power broker and that geographically Australia needs to recognise that America will not be calling the shots.

---

[43] Black, R, 12 July 2011 *Japan 'to continue' Antarctic whaling*

http://www.bbc.co.uk/news/science-environment-14132320 'Australia-Japan talks: development, regional security, whaling' Media release 13 January 2013 Foreign Minister Bob Carr and Japan's Foreign Minister Fumio Kishida today held talks on regional security, development and whaling, in Sydney. The talks come less than a month after the election of the Abe Government in Japan on December 16, 2012 and are part of Minister Kishida's first overseas visits as Foreign Minister. Security. On security matters, Ministers agreed on the need for the UN Security Council to deliver an effective response to North Korea's rocket launch in December 2012. Security discussions also included Afghanistan, Syria, the Middle East peace process, Iran and conflicts in Africa including piracy off the Somalia coastline. It was agreed that Australia and Japan would further strengthen their cooperation in United Nations activity related to peacekeeping, nuclear non-proliferation and the advancement of an Arms trade Treaty to reduce the flow of illicit weapons to rogue states and terrorist groups. Australia and Japan also agreed to continue cooperation on the need for Security Council reform. Australia reaffirmed its support for Japan's permanent membership of the UNSC…. Australia is pursuing action in the International Court of Justice on the issue and considers Japanese whaling to be contrary to its international obligations. Both Australia and Japan have filed detailed written arguments in the Court, which will set the case for oral hearing in The Hague. The case is likely to be listed for hearing in the latter half of 2013. Regionalist approaches within the nation state are becoming more prevalent to address risk. According to Wear (2012, p. 469), 'The establishment of regional Management forums was an experiment in collaborative governance. Similar governance structures were also established in other jurisdictions'

The recent power plays over the resource-rich islands claimed by Japan and China could escalate as a way to draw a line between the USA and China. Will Japan, Australia and India together develop a balance as suggested as an alternative to closer links with the USA? Shinzo Abe has suggested forming a 'democratic security diamond'[44]..."

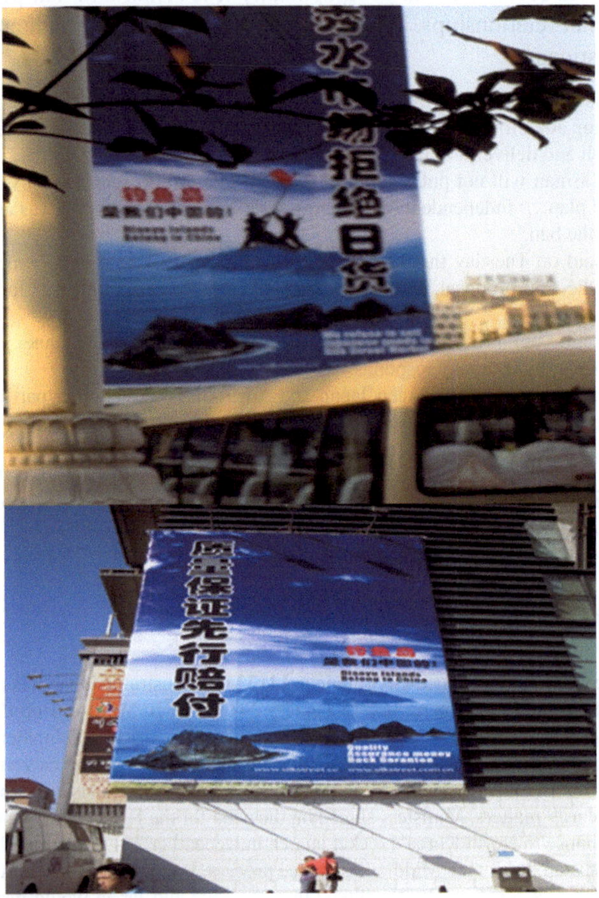

[44] 24th August 2012. Malcolm Cook reports on Australian Broadcasting.

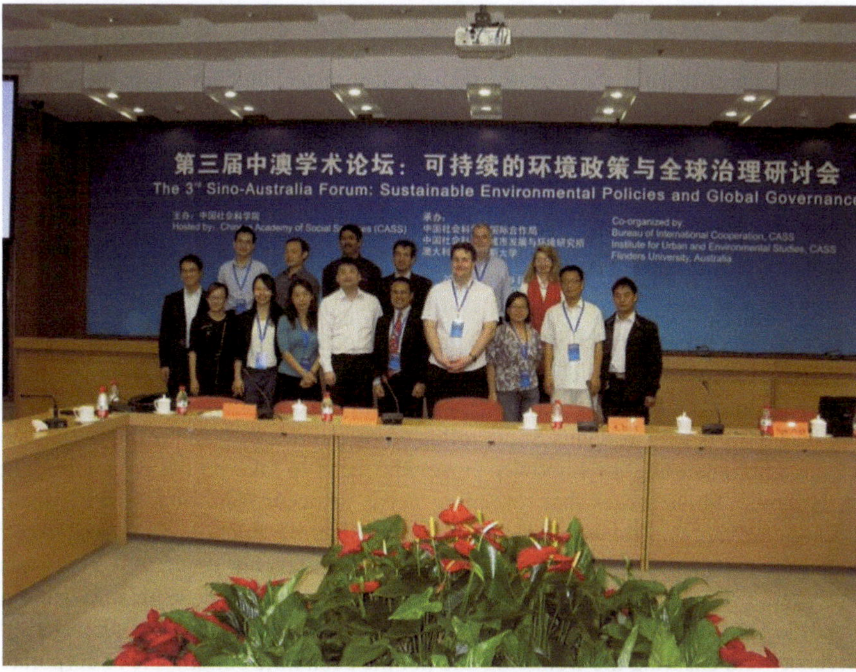
第三届中澳学术论坛：可持续的环境政策与全球治理研讨会
The 3rd Sino-Australia Forum: Sustainable Environmental Policies and Global Governance
Co-organized by
Bureau of International Cooperation, CASS
Institute for Urban and Environmental Studies, CASS
Flinders University, Australia

Although the conference was opened with a speech praising the work of Kenneth Boulding and closed with a speech about how we all shared the same desire, namely to live on a sustainable planet, some points raised during the conference need to be explored:

The first is that the current plans for the needs of populations in cities underestimate the needs of the residents because the illegals from the rural areas (internal migrants) are excluded. The other challenge is the resentment of Hillary Clinton's comments about the management of the Mekong River. According to Le Monde (cited by the Guardian),[45] The People's Daily, a Communist Party News Paper, publishes articles by Cass academics. It stressed the territorial rights to Okinawa (part of the Rryukyu archipelago) whilst informally academics stressed that American commentary by Clinton was not appreciated.[46]

A well-meaning lawyer discussed the global commons, namely water, air and stressed pricing fresh air…would help people to value it…the issue of course being who will pay?

The regional disasters within nations range from tsunamis and storm surges in Japan as well as regular seismic instability to regular flooding in Australia and

[45] Le Monde cited by The China urged to 'reconsider Japanese rile of Okinawa?' Cited by Guardian Weekly International News. 17.05.13, p. 10.

[46] Hilary Clinton made the comment as she stepped down from office that she thought that the many tensions internationally were cause for concern. But as a counterpoint to the concerns about competition and the zero sum approach, others are moving towards a more compassionate way of life.

fires, earthquakes and landslides in China. In Indonesia, all these disasters pose a challenge. According to "Paul Hare, of the Torrens Resilience Centre, Indonesian officials claim that for those concerned about disaster, Indonesia provides all the examples.... it is a supermarket of disasters"....

5.9 Transformation Through the Right Praxis at the Right Time

The most important challenges of the day are food energy and water, these will be the focus for 'we the people' and a focus of future governance concerns.[47]

By finding just the right praxis at the right time the principle of leverage can be applied. This is why Vandana Shiva reflected on the role of Gandhi and his choice of the spinning wheel to empower those who wish to take on the colonial might of Britain.[48] Shiva writes that reframing needs to occur from outside the system through Satyagraha. Resistance is based on passive mass action. She stresses that the space for change needs to be created at the local level in small, powerful ways that prefigure other wide-ranging changes. Shiva stresses that systemic intervention needs to focus on small powerful interventions from below, such as protecting seed diversity and ensuring the wellbeing and not the economic bottom line of corporate companies. Shiva did not stress that India is now likely to be one of the few countries internationally to have a growth economy because in fact growth is not what is needed. We need a transformed economy.

The shift from producing local goods to controlling profit through anthropocentric trade is a central concern.

[47] Lee, G. and Scurrah, N. 2009. Power and responsibility: the Mekong River Commission and Lower Mekong mainstream dams. A joint report of the Australian Mekong Resource Centre, University of Sydney and Oxfam Australia.

[48] http://www.youtube.com/watch?v=UOfM7QD7-kk.

Chapter 6
Conclusion Towards a Non Anthropocentric Stewardship Approach

6.1 Choosing to Be Stewards of Current and Future Generations of Life

If we are prepared to recognize our mutual vulnerability, it provides a basis for stewardship. We are all reliant on others and need to be able to depend on our connections with others.

What if we could recognize our vulnerability and what if we could foster a sense of caring for others?[1]

If we move away from situated knowledge and accept that by listening to diverse viewpoints we are more likely to see wider perspectives. The horizon changes when we listen to narratives told by those who have different perceptions and experiences. Instead of idealism and essentialist categories, this book makes a case for why we need to extend our vision to take into account the views of diverse others in order to make more informed policy decisions that take into account the social, economic and environmental consequences for future generations of life. We live in interesting times and 'we face a perfect storm'.

Arendt (1963, 1969) stresses that evil is comprehensible. It results from the way in which policy is made and practiced through the architecture of governance. Arendt stresses that lying in politics occurs in democracies and in totalitarian states. The implications—as outlined in the Pentagon papers—are very relevant to this research.[2]

Arendt has criticized the systems approach for imposing change through ABC-type scenarios that pose a false dichotomy or an oversimplification of options and then encourage a compromise through option C. Whilst the criticism is fair for closed systems and operations research, it does not apply to the work of critical heuristics or open systems that cut through the governance game and the minutiae

[1] http://unpresentable.wordpress.com/2010/05/13/toward-a-post-human-political-theory-deleuze-guattari-and-disability-studies-%E2%80%93-pt-4/.

[2] The sociologist Hannah Arendt (1969) criticised the systems approach used to plan the Vietnam War in her book '*Crises of the Republic*'.

J. McIntyre-Mills, *Transformation from Wall Street to Wellbeing*,
Contemporary Systems Thinking, DOI 10.1007/978-1-4899-7466-2_6,

of bureaucracy that is pervasive, banal and part of the wicked problem. So many people say that they want to be the change, but how?

The greatest challenges of the day comprise: (a) representation within and across increasingly diverse nation states to address cosmopolitan justice for the common good; (b) accountability to ensure food, water and energy equity; and (c) engagement to enable the silenced a voice and a seat at the table. This chapter discusses an alternative form of governance and democracy and grapples with ways to address wellbeing. How should wellbeing be defined? Should we follow a definition based on:

> …contentment and experienced wellbeing, in a Benthamite hedonic utility sense? Or do we care about eudaimonia or life purpose, in an Aristotelian sense? Particular individuals will value one more than the other depending, in part, on what they are capable of. While scholars surely can measure both, from a societal and policy perspective, which dimension of happiness should policy aim to maximise? (Graham 2011, p. 121)

The right to equal opportunities versus equal outcomes is a core policy and political consideration. The responsibility to ensure that some do not prosper at the expense of others is a core challenge. I have used the concept 'Wall Street' to symbolise economic rationalism and 'wellbeing' to symbolise a reframed approach to 'being interconnected' and through treading lightly, rather than slashing pathways that are turned into highways.

The provision of food, energy and water are the three major concerns for people and the planet. How can Archimedes lever be applied to addressing these concerns?[3]

- By concentrating on the preservation of biodiversity (such as diverse seeds that are water and salt resilient), we can take a step in the right direction, according to Shiva.
- By respecting diverse ways of knowing and diverse relationships.
- By caring about children at risk and sentient creatures we can change the size of our carbon footprints.
- By means of a new architecture for global covenants to we can protect the global commons and hold the corporatisation of the planet at bay.

[3] Food and energy are the bases for human wellbeing and security. Current approaches to international relations and war (Etzioni 2004, 2011) are unsustainable. As the experience of suffering becomes more widespread, the notion of class will become central once again, because 'the poorest people in the world will be the hardest hit' (Beck 2009, p. 37).

Chapter 7
Post Script: Responding to Existential Risks

7.1 Implications for the Way We Live Our Lives

> all the indications are that the universe is at its simplest at the smallest and the largest scales…. One can draw further parallels with the selfish, individualistic behaviours that are often the root cause of our environmental and financial crises. Within physics I see the idea of a "multiverse" as a similarly fragmented perspective, representing a loss of confidence in the prospects for basic science. Yet I believe all of these crises will ultimately be helpful if they force us, like the quantum physicist, to remake our world in more basic and far sighted ways…. If we can only link our intelligence to our hearts, the doors are wide open to a brighter future, to a more unified planet…to quantum technologies that extend our perception… (Thurok 2012, pp. 256–257).

The problem with integrated approaches is that they need to preserve space for doubt, diversity and disagreement. But the axiom that needs to guide this freedom is that we should not allow freedom and rights of some to undermine the rights and freedoms of others and future generations of life. This is where transformation is needed. Much of the activity which takes place in the social and natural sciences is in the areas of knowledge that focus on research on others. We need to do some research on our own lives and to reflect on the consequences of our choices. Instead of idealism and essentialist categories, we need to extend our vision to take into account the social, economic and environmental consequences for future generations of life.

The future is quantum and fluid,
not
digital and compartmentalised
The only constant is
change
This has implications for science, democracy, ethics and governance
Change needs to be fostered
by open responsive systems
guided by designs
underpinned by the ethical axiom:
We can be free and diverse

J. McIntyre-Mills, *Transformation from Wall Street to Wellbeing*,
Contemporary Systems Thinking, DOI 10.1007/978-1-4899-7466-2_7,

To the extent that freedom and diversity does not undermine the rights of others—
Including future generations of life
Closed, fragmented systems
Lead to
Entropy

7.1.1 Being the Change

Competition is not the only basis for survival or the only basis for evolution as stressed by De Waal (2009) and discussed in 'Identity, Democracy and Sustainability' (McIntyre-Mills and De Vries 2011).

We can evolve through co-operation.[1]

The 'both and' possibilities[2] of expanding pragmatism is based on considering the consequences of choices within context and with future generations in mind.

The continuum of nature and the natural to date has been brutally shaped by the digital. But we could use digital technology in ways that support our evolution towards sustainable living.

If we accept the continuum across all life from the human to the animal and the earth and air to which we return, then we accept that all responses need to be mindful of others and future generations of life. So if we accept the continuity of life as reflected in the new physics, it has implications for our thinking, our practice and the way in which we teach and learn. It also has implications for ethics.

Capitalism needs to be transformed in terms of what it values and it needs containment by collaborative efforts buttressed in law and governed by a shared 'global covenant' (Held 2004), in order to address the mitigation of the causes of climate change.[3]

Do we wish to live in a world where we do not want to help one another and in which we deny the pain of sentient beings?

---

[1] I rebel with every fibre of my being to the 'either or' logic of the zero sum game of profit and loss—zero versus 1. The competitive logic that plays out between human beings in competition for jobs and resources is unsustainable.

[2] As a result of being reintroduced to the work of Hirschman by Adelman's lecture, I feel vindicated in advocating this approach. *States in Crisis Conference*, 2013, Society for the Advancement of Socio-Economics June 27–29.

[3] Thus I start where Stiglitz et al. (2010) end in 'Mismeasuring our lives' in which they argue that we need to build well-being stocks for future generations based on valuing the social and environmental factors that support life as we know it. This is vital if we have a hope of redressing the worst effects of climate change. This book explores a number of interrelated themes and uses a range of methods—where appropriate to enable an understanding as to why the containerist or compartmentalist argument is unacceptable for human survival. If democracy is to survive into the next century, we need to emphasize both rights and responsibilities to address interrelated concerns:

- Increased natural disasters; for example, Cyclone Irene bore down on the US East coast and New York.
- Increased pressures on communities as food becomes costly and scarce as a result of higher-energy costs, drought and floods.

Social and environmental justice needs to be addressed through social movements that are buttressed by international law that is supported by regional courts.[4]

Change requires necessity, desire and will (see Bogue 1989 on Delueze and Guattari). Entangled social, economic and environmental challenges posed by the food, energy and water shortages require a revision of compartmentalist or containerist approaches limited to the nation state and informed by failed enlightenment agendas (McIntyre-Mills et al. 2006a). As Eyerman (1981, p. 55) stressed, false consciousness refers to:

> *an experience* in society, ideology to a proposed or offered *explanation of that experience*. One however that only further distorted real understanding. As these questions developed within the Frankfurt School during these years of emigration and exile, the problem of *how real understanding* was at all possible, became the central one.

Human beings are not digital genes that switch on or off. They are able to respond to complexity in ways that are unique and based on their ability to think and feel. This perspective does not need to be essentialist in the sense used by Somerville and Frankl who consider this the essential difference between human beings and animals and that this gives human beings more rights than other sentient creatures. Instead, I argue (drawing on Haraway, Butler, Deleuze and Guattari) that appreciation of our connections with others can help us to emerge from our fixed identities and help us to recognize our interconnected rhizomatic connections.

The need to reframe governance is essential. Social change through exploring interdisciplinary frameworks to address environmental politics, ethics and legal frontiers is a necessity for human security and food security.[5] The goal is to foster an understanding that 'We *are* the land' (Getano Lui 1994). Given that humanity is dependent on air, water and soil for survival, the global commons and our relationship with it need to be recognized as not merely entangled but co-determined. Food and energy are the bases for human wellbeing and security. Current approaches to international relations and war (Etzioni 2004, 2011) are unsustainable. Protecting the global commons must be seen as a shared necessity.

Social change frameworks to address greed and the commodification of the powerless and the environment need to be informed by debates on ethics, human reasoning capability, environmental politics and the role of the market in achieving a sustainable future for the next generation.

---

[4] The biologist Rayner (2011) argues that all life is interconnected. The strong cosmopolitan argument is that the basis for categorical or containerist thinking is fallacious. Global citizenship ought to become a concept supported by international law and social justice movements (McIntyre-Mills 2000). The four themes of citizenship discourses are: 'inclusion, erosion, withdrawal and expansion'; these 'reflect the foci of contemporary discourses on citizenship' (Kivisto and Faist 2007, p. 13), which are compartmentalist in their assumptions about the world. But we do not live in separate compartments or containers; we live in interconnected, overlapping regions

[5] In Paris, the precursor to the G20 summit highlights the challenge of starvation in Africa and parts of the Middle East. Ironically, our foreign minister is extolling the agricultural merits of Australia. The reality is that our current approaches to farming are being challenged by the Wentworth Group.

Franklin, M. and Wilson, L. 2011. Government pushing for action at G20 Food Security Summit. Hunger driving trade reform. The Australian June 22, p1.

The elephant in the room is that human beings are animals—primates who need to relearn our vulnerability and interdependency with nature. Cultural narratives that foster sustainability are a starting point for democratic transition.[6]

The New Jerusalem could be a world in which we identify with other human and sentient beings.

7.2 Representation, Accountability and Sustainability Based on Communication, Consciousness and Appreciation of Signs

Communication develops as a result of responsiveness, reciprocity and the trust that flows from these interactions that can transform data into information and knowledge. Communication has evolved through developing signs in context with responses that are consistent. In contexts where signals are used often between human beings or humans and animals, the signalling can develop into shared symbols with particular meaning.[7] The communication between sentient beings is only part of the ecosystem. The signs shared by the land with human beings and animals also need to be given more attention. The vibrations are felt long before a tsunami hits the land. Following the migration of animals to higher ground is one of the ways to develop resilience (Shanor, Kanwal et al. 2009, pp. 120–121; Sharpe 2005; De Waal 2009). More importantly, reading the landscape signals in order to prevent further deterioration is vital. The signals of melting ice, rising sea levels and temperatures that are unseasonal need to be read. Just as we develop rapport with one another or with sentient animals with which we develop a caring relationship, we need to read the signs from the land. Signs are merely signals, whereas symbols develop through shared meaning and a sense of reciprocal relationship. If we ignore the signals from the land—in the same way as we can choose to ignore the signals from animals—then we will be unable to communicate or commune with nature. Often, communing is regarded as a spiritual act. Today, we have created a simulacrum—an

[6] Green buildings roofed and walled with earth and shallow rooted plants breathe and produce photosynthesis. They are also cool and require less air conditioning. Walls made of wire, with spaces filled by means of recycled plastic bottles, filled with soil and planted with shallow rooted plants or tyres filled with rammed earth provide alternative ways of building. The notion of community reciprocity enables new forms of economy based on trust. But narratives that remain translated into equitable governance destroy trust and lead to cynicism. Our research strives to translate narratives into accountable governance to transform and manage the size of our social, economic and environmental footprints. Well-being requires identifying with nature. It requires limiting growth through living responsibly. If we reuse, recycle and live locally, perhaps we can regain a sense of community. In the ghettos, we find lessons in survival.

[7] A tail movement accompanied by particular tones of sound can be understood as annoyance. Blinking eyes and purring can be understood as friendship or gaining attention when accompanied by weaving through ankles and herding by running ahead towards the location of food. Communication breaks down when there is no trust.

artificial world in the media that we are beginning to believe as real (Baudrillard 1994) and which guides the toxic consumption of resources. Human beings are in the thrall of digital media. A case could be made for using computing as a means to escape the matrix or simulacrum of false consciousness and toxic desires. This has implications for identity, democracy, governance and ethics.

Most traditional religions bind together the people and the land and establish a sense of hierarchy in which the land is prior. Communication is both verbal and nonverbal. The pandemics of disease associated with swine flu, bird flu and mad cows disease are another signal. There are so many human beings that food security cannot be maintained through intensive farming that ignores the quality of life of sentient farm animals and undermines our own health. We do not have the right to intensively farm creatures. We are ignoring the signals. James Lovelock has said all this before (2006, 2009). Dawkins is misrepresented to a certain extent—genes evolved because they survived and looked after their interests, but this should not be confused with culture; we may survive because we compete or collaborate, this has been stressed by De Waal (2006, 2009). We are ignoring our part within the Gaian system. We communicate with one another and with sentient creatures and with the land—we write our stories on the land and design the land in response to our dreaming.

Participation for monitory democracy is not just about ensuring that resources are used fairly and equitably. It is to enable people to think more deeply about the consequences of their choices and to enhance their consciousness.

The governance gaze from above and monitory democracy 'from below' need to achieve a balance, and some develop humility to avoid the dangers of hubris. Lessons from nature, science, religion and art/design help restore a respect for the need to nurture biodiversity and a realization of our place within it. It also enables human beings to appreciate the extent to which we are designers of our future and the extent to which we are limited by our unfolding circumstances. The global commons need to be supported by laws to protect the collective good. According to Brown (2012)[8]:

> There's a growing resistance—particularly among young Bali locals—to rampant development on the island and tourism at any cost so they're mobilising. They're angry about the environmental and cultural impact of millions of international visitors, the staggering hotel and commercial development that's gobbling up their island, and they're uneasy about a creeping "Kuta cancer" that's spreading, they fear, from the Bintang boulevards of the island's busiest beach all the way to the spiritual heartland of Ubud up in Bali's high country….

Finding ways to reconnect to the land and creating ripples to achieve a wave of change is vital to protect wellbeing and to secure food, water and energy supplies.[9] We have enough to pay for 'the needs of all, but not the greed of all', to draw on Shiva who cites Ghandi.[10] Sanctions need to be applied to international organizations

[8] Matt Brown, They Paved Paradise, Broadcast: 15/05/2012see Foreign Correspondent http://www.abc.net.au/foreign/content/2012/s3503493.htm?site=centralwest.

[9] http://www.rolefoundation.org/index.php/environmental-assistance-projects/.

[10] http://www.navdanya.org/news/229-awesome.

that try to extract profit from labour, the land and now, through patenting, life.[11] The core challenge is not only that these resources will need to meet the needs of rising populations. In developed nations there is a negative population growth rate. It is a fact that higher levels of education and better quality of life lead to lower numbers of children. The demographic transition can be achieved through building capability (Nussbaum and Sen 1993; Crocker et al. 1995; Sen 2000). A negative birth rate is achieved in many developed nations. Shiva (1989)[12] could have also included an explicit argument for gender mainstreaming policy to enable men and women to work together in agricultural and other development initiatives. Enabling quality of life begins at the household level and is then scaled up to enhance equality at the local, national and post-national level (Kabeer et al. 1999; McIntyre-Mills and de Vries 2011). The demographic transition will occur—provided enhancing quality of life is focused on meeting needs—as opposed to encouraging the greed and lavish lifestyles that are enjoyed by the minorities. The value of agricultural production needs to be promoted, rather than increasing the intensive production of farm animals such as pigs, cattle and chickens for slaughter. Not only is the erosion of their quality of life unconscionable but it also leads to their ill health, and leads to epidemics and possibly pandemics of diseases such as bird or swine flu or Creutzfeldt–Jakob disease (commonly known as mad cow's disease). But most importantly, the approach to meat production is flawed, not only because of the erosion of quality of life because the amount of meat required to feed the large numbers of people living in urban areas is unsustainable, given the amount of water required to sustain them.

[11] We need to beware the leviathan state and the leviathan global state. The way forward is multilaterism, but not at a state level. The new multilateralism is of regionalist federations, in other words, post-national biospheres. A single global parliament makes me shudder, but a series of post-national parliaments in overlapping regions would be able to hold one another to better account. We may even be able to achieve three overarching parliaments which negotiate, but one global parliament would surely be unwise. Brown (2012): 'There are just 23 million Australians among 7 billion equal earthians. Unless and until we accord every other citizen of the planet, friend or foe, and regardless of race, gender, colour or other characteristic, equal regard, we like them, can have not assured future…The political debate of the 20th Century was polarized between capitalism and communism. It was about control of the economy in the narrow sense of material goods and money. A free market versus state control….in this 21st century the political debate is moving to a new arena. It is about whether we expend earth's natural capital as our population grows to 10 billion people in the decades ahead with average consumption also growing…. Earths citizenry is already using 120 per cent of the planet's productivity capacity….'

[12] Empowering women requires gender mainstreaming through working with both men and women so that men understand the advantages to their households. Literate, numerate women can produce beyond the household and this provides a way out of poverty. Then it may be possible for progress to be achieved. Women and men who have other means to survive are more open to understanding that more children does not mean prosperity because eventually there will not be enough resources to maintain their health. This is quite different from the autocratic controlling of population that would be a negative sanction on the poor. Instead of negative sanctions, better quality of life needs to be achieved through development and education. This approach has better results in achieving a demographic transition.

7.3 Personal, Political and Planetary Wellbeing

As I get older and I look around me, I begin to understand the notion that we write the landscape in our daily choices and we create the world around us with every word we utter and every action we take. The joy of living and the life-giving energy as we create rapport with one another can contrast with the negative energy or deathly silence or coolness towards one another which creates distance. When we die, who we are and how we live as individuals and as groups are written in the landscape and a memory trace is carried by those with whom we made a connection. For some, the memory trace is carried at the local level by their grace and their stewardship of the land which they touched gently and with care. For others, the memory trace is carried through their words written on paper from trees that have been felled and carried in digital waves through highly developed internet systems that generate landfill and toxins. It seems to me that living lightly and designing renewable forms of communication will become increasingly important.

The work of Yoland Wadsworth and Rose Bird stresses the importance of human praxis. Our bodies are part of the environment when we are alive and when we die. The connections we make with other sentient creatures and with the land are part of this understanding of the interconnectedness of life. We need to think of the human body as connected to the air we breathe and to the land or air to which we will return. Perhaps we will donate our organs to others and traces of our learning will be shared in this way? The notions of Eros and Thanatos are always at play in politics. Protecting human rights and a life of dignity should be uppermost. But human rights have rested on the rights of other species, just as some human beings have wrested power over other human beings and commodified them.

> We are of the land,
> We are the change,
> We write the future,
> What will it be?

Time and containerist constructions of organizations are unsustainable. But in a practical sense, those who work long hours will find little comfort in 'new-age' admonitions to enjoy work and to achieve work–life balance. Global transformation in post-national confederations needs to enable the state-market and civil society to protect the overlapping regional biospheres that constitute the planet.

7.4 Vignette: Flying to Jakarta in the Wake of the Rift Between Australia and Indonesia

We fly en route to Jakarta on November 22, where I am invited to meet with three ministries to discuss ethics and to give workshops to staff. Following a lecture last year entitled 'from Wall Street to Wellbeing' at the University of Indonesia to education students, I am reminded of the lessons from my mentors.

Australia remains a small player in the Asia Pacific as underlined by a realization that respectful dialogue with neighbours is vital. The attitude towards revelations of spying and the role of Pine Gap in Alice Springs in implementing the surveillance policies of the USA were underlined by terminating the Indonesian and Australian government-to-government relations on military and migration issues at the end of November, 2013.

As a colleague in Indonesia stressed whilst I was visiting their organization on November 24:

> …even Obama apologized to Merkel after the snooping revelations…. We know who is responsible for the snooping….

The issue appeared to be used to galvanize a sense of national pride prior to an election, even though it was acknowledged in the Jakarta Post that spying was indeed a two-way process, but that being respectful is vital.

The science-fiction movie that I watched as we flew to Jakarta focused in my mind the worth of governance, democracy, ethics and education for transformation. The film entitled 'In time' takes the commodification of time as a theme and develops the notion of gated communities where the rich ration time and space to ghetto dwellers. They are programmed to die at the age of 26, unless they can earn credits by working. The rush hour becomes quite literally a rush to buy time credits. Life is commodified so that the rich can enjoy a quality of life at the expense of the majority

The notion of accounting and accountability needs to be made clear and transparent through systems of governance and democracy that are governed by laws to protect the global commons.

People need to be free and diverse to the extent that their freedom and diversity do not undermine the next generation of life. This maxim needs to be upheld locally, regionally and globally in overlapping biospheres.

If we hope to achieve conscious evolution and we do not wish to rely on chance, then we need to find ways to engage local people in thinking through the implications of their choices. If *Homo sapiens sapiens* is capable of conscious evolution and is in fact a creator of the landscape through design choices, then we need to be mindful of the plasticity of the brain and the power of thought and consciousness on the landscape. Sociologists and social anthropologists such as Donna Haraway and Rose Bird understand that as designers we can be stewards or destroyers—we are hybrids and our intersubjectivity needs to be appreciated, rather than denied. The limited horizons of humanity could be compensated by drawing on the very *different and diverse horizons* of humanity. People with different experiences as a result of their life chances, their age, gender, culture, class or level of education or ability see the world differently. It is also undeniable that they share common a web of basic needs, although to list them as a hierarchy in the way Maslow did could be simplistic. Values play a role in the way they are ranked. Life and safety may not always be a priority. A human being (and some sentient beings) may choose to be altruistic in order to rescue another.

Perhaps the new radio telescope will help us to see further. To paraphrase de Grasse: ‘we do not know if the universe is expanding or contracting, because we cannot see beyond 14 billion light years or so! The light from the beginning of the universe has not reached us yet.’ Certainly we are about to extend our understanding of the nature of the universe—perhaps it is expanding—perhaps it is contracting? Perhaps—if we were able to look far enough—we would see cyclical phases. I think this is also a possibility worth considering.

West Churchman’s work on open systemic approaches to the philosophy of knowledge develops a coherent argument as to why we need ongoing processes of critical review based on considering many viewpoints and many forms of knowledge in order to move closer to achieving social and environmental justice through policy and governance decisions. His work on a ‘Design of Inquiring Systems’ could be extended to include further ways of knowing—created through acknowledging the praxis knowledge associated with reading the environment and living systems of which we are part.

The human–animal connection and the human–environmental connections need to be understood in far more depth. This sort of insight was developed further by Gregory Bateson and many first nations have a deep systemic understanding of the ecology of mind. The human machine connection could perhaps enable us to extend our powers of understanding by holding in mind multiple variables. Just as the microscope or telescope can help us to extend our depth of view, the ability to make more neural connections could perhaps enable us to create new forms of knowledge (see McIntyre-Mills and De Vries 2011) for a discussion of ‘Identity, Democracy and Sustainability’. Will we achieve further levels of conscious evolution when we are capable of creating more neural cascades and more connections? Some early thoughts along these lines are discussed in ‘Wellbeing, Mindfulness and the Global Commons’ (McIntyre-Mills 2010).

Dialogue is the basis for democracy and weaving together strands of experience. This is the basis for enhancing consciousness, which results in making connections or holding in mind many ideas through recognizing connections and perhaps also appreciating that connections can be made and disconnected, just as cells open or close or neural connections are made or rerouted for reasons of survival. We can be free and diverse to the extent that our freedom and diversity do not undermine the rights of others. This is a core axiom based on the idea that not all diversity is good. By virtue of our humanity, we need to take into account our values, which could filter the way in which we see the world. These values are ‘the enemy within’. West Churchman wrote of G.O.D. as the generator of diversity. Sensibly, he did not confuse social and natural systems and he stressed that decisions (cuts) are made on the basis of considering many kinds of knowledge, asking questions and considering the consequences for others and the next generation of life. This approach to knowledge, based on critical heuristics, enables a greater openness to ideas and a greater willingness to reframe ideas on the basis of new perspectives. This openness to testing out ideas is essential for science, democracy and ethics.

7.5 Vignette: Reflection on Art and Diverse Virtues

The highlight of the Anthropology conference on 'Knowledge and value in a globalizing world' in Perth (June 2011) was a concert held in the University of Western Australia Art Gallery on sacred music and art. The gallery displayed paintings by Aboriginal artists from around Australia. One of these was by Dorothy Robinson, winner of the Telstra award.[13] She made sense of the complexity by displaying it on a black canvass on which appeared myriad acrylic white dots—to me they are stars. Some are distinct, some appear to blur as one looks at the canvass. Throughout history, we have tried to make sense of the world we live in through art or music. Consciousness and sense making is continuous with other species and with nature. From our origins as dinosaurs, we had sculls designed to make sounds that resonate. Making music by means of repeating basic sounds, such as the vowels between consonants a, e, i, o and u, creates a sound like a didgeridoo—or throat singing—by Buddhist monks. The same sounds express myriad emotions—the patterns can be varied infinitely—but there is an underlying structure. Ethical literacy is needed to develop the capability to think reflexively and to match responses in context. This requires not only the phronesis of Aristotle but also the contextual considerations of power.

Transformation needs to find a way to bridge the divide between monist or Universalist approaches and extreme forms of diversity. The bridging process can be achieved through constitutions to uphold a priori axioms, such as freedom and diversity (to the extent that the rights and freedoms of others or the next generation of life are not undermined). This requires reflexivity and the capability to take into account many kinds of knowledge within context. But social and environmental justice requires monitoring from above and below—within and beyond the nation state—in post-national federations. Transformation through extending capabilities to think differently is vital—this willingness to co-operate will come about, as a new form of monitory democracy becomes global.

As I edited this manuscript, many graduate students celebrated the end of Ramadan.

> The world of early Islam emphasized as well the importance of shared virtues such as toleration and mutual respect among skeptics and believers in the sacred, and the duty of rulers to respect others' interpretations of life. During this phase Muslims' belief that human beings were bond to treat nature with compassionate regard, as if it was their equal, because both were divine creations, also surfaced. That imperative would later come to trouble all democracies.' (Keane 2009, p. xvii)

I do not agree with Russell (1952)[14] or Dawkins (2006) that religion is necessarily an impediment to seeing more broadly, provided we understand that religion can and does play a role in filtering our perceptions.

---

[13] https://www.google.com.au/search?q=dorothy+robinson+napangardi&client=firefox-a&hs=Tr&sa=X&rls=org.mozilla:en-US:official&tbm=isch&tbo=u&source=univ&ei=7CwpU5v7OMuWkQXOs4HoCA&ved=0CDgQ7Ak&biw=1920&bih=910 Images. Accessed 19 March 2014.

[14] Religion and Morals, 1952, in 'Why I am not a Christian', Russell (1957). 'Intelligence is impeded by any creed, no matter what; and kindness is inhibited by the belief in sin and punishment (this belief, by the way is the only one that the Society Government has taken over from orthodox Christianity)….'

The system's approach begins when we strive to see the world through the eyes of another (Churchman 1982[15]).This requires critical reflexivity and humility. It also requires the capability to join up the dots and to realize that the horizon shifts depending on where one is standing.

The only constant is change. So if quantum physics is the way forward, we are being shaped and determined by the wrong paradigm (Thurok 2012[16]).

The implications of realizing that the future is quantum and not digital are profound. Genes are digital, but human beings respond constantly to the environment based on their own thinking and their own interpretations which go beyond an either/or approach, as new approaches can be created out of blended options, depending on the context. They are capable of remaking and reframing choices (albeit shaped or limited by our genetic heritage and capabilities).

Simplistic binary oppositional or 'either or' logic is outdated as is 'the zero sum' game of profit and loss.

Competition is not the only basis for survival nor is it the only basis for evolution—as stressed by De Waal 2009 (see the argument in 'Identity, Democracy and Sustainability', McIntyre-Mills and De Vries 2011). Co-operation and compassion also help our survival.

What we do to others and the land, we do to ourselves. The plasticity of our human brains can either develop greater capabilities for stewardship or we can delude ourselves that the current economic system is sustainable.

The plasticity of the human brain is increasingly accepted by educationalists such as Arrowsmith-Young (2012) who trained her brain to address learning difficulties, despite many hurdles. The more we are able to think about our thinking, the more aware we become. This is what I mean by expanding pragmatism.

[15] This is why hope for democracy rests in the ability to think about our human values, Churchman's (1982) so-called the enemies within (religion, morality, politics and aesthetics) and also the ability to rise above sectarianism through developing greater understanding through considering the consequences for ourselves, others and the environment.

[16] When human beings understood that the world is not flat, but it is spherical, it had profound implications for explorers. When human beings understand that the universe is not finite or infinite, but instead, it is a continuum—perhaps a Mobius band that results in flux and flow (see McIntyre-Mills 2008). I am wading out of my depth, as I am not a physicist. The challenge of course is that political decisions must be decisive. So where do we draw the line and how? The answer is perhaps to ensure that the decisions are as inclusive as possible. Thus, diversity of thought is as important as biodiversity is for human survival (Shiva 1989). Freeman Dyson anticipates the limitations of relying on access to digital information, whilst making the case for learning to think about ideas and to engage with others, rather than merely collecting information, which is quite different from generating new knowledge based on critical analysis. Human beings are able to shape their lives through critical thinking and thus they are not completely determined by genetics. (See Dyson, F http://www.edge.org/3rd_culture/dyson_ad/dyson_ad_index.html downloaded 11/3/2013. Dyson is professor of physics at the Institute for Advanced Study, in Princeton. His professional interests are in mathematics and astronomy. Among his many books are 'Disturbing the Universe, Infinite in All Directions Origins of Life, From Eros to Gaia, Imagined Worlds, and The Sun, The Genome, And The Internet'.

7.6 Concluding Thoughts

In Scientific American, the article 'Limits of Intelligence', by Fox (2011) summarizes the contributions made by neuroscientist Simon Laughlin about brain size, diminishing returns and the speed of neural connections:

> …if our body and brain got much bigger, there would be costs in terms of energy consumption, dissipation of heat and sheer time it takes for neural impulses to travel from one part of the brain to another. The human mind, however, may have better ways of expanding without the need for further biological evolution. After all, honeybees and other social insects do it: Acting in concert with their hive sisters, they form a collective entity that is smarter than the sum of the parts. Through social interaction we, too, have learned to pool our intelligence with others….[17]

Paradoxically, we need to rely upon others and co-operate if we are to pool our intelligence. Competition could at this stage of our evolution pose an existential risk!

We lose our way if we think of computers as robots controlling us because we have allowed them to shape us. We have to take responsibility to design tools that are a means to an end, namely caring for others (including sentient voiceless and the environment). But ethical discussions based on being the change 'moment to moment' are central to sustainability.[18]

The future is quantum, not digital.

[17] Simon Laughlin, professor of neurobiology, said 'We have demonstrated that brains must consume energy to function and that these requirements are sufficiently demanding to limit our performance and determine design. Far-reaching powers of deduction demand a lot of energy because for the brain to search out new relationships it must constantly correlate information from different sources. "Such energy demands mean there is a limit to the information we can process." Other scientists claim that the brain's wiring or network of fibres linking different areas to one another cannot get any better. They found that the smartest people have…messages carried very quickly between different parts of the brain…but the wiring request vast amounts of extra energy to become more efficient' (Borland 2011).

[18] The implications of realizing that people are humans and not digital are profound. Genes are digital, but human beings are able to make choices (albeit shaped and limited by genetics) but nevertheless they respond to the environment based on their own thinking and their own interpretations. Human living systems at best are capable of responding to their environment and constantly evaluating their thoughts and actions. The only constant is change. So if quantum physics is the way forward, we are being shaped and determined by the wrong (digital) paradigm (Thurok 2012). The future is fluid and quantum; it is not predetermined. Although the engagement software is digital, it is only a *means* to enable people to be responsive to climate change. It provides a means to record patterns of responses, in order to assist better mitigation and adaptation responses, based on up-to-date empirical evidence. We could develop localized living in regions that support appropriate technology and use solar or biofuels to run digital systems that monitor from below and enable alternative forms of democracy and governance based on the principles of subsidiarity (Schumacher 1973) that support local face-to-face engagement supported by other forms of digital communication. We need to foster a new approach that ensures that communication for science, democracy, governance and ethics is based on many forms of engagement and many ways of knowing (including quantitative numbers, qualitative experience of taste, smell intuition, imagination and emotions as well as perceived, sounds and images). The notion of trying to develop approaches to risk governance from above or from local government needs to be balanced by engagement with those who have lived experiences.

It requires a transformation of our values and the way we relate to one another and the environment. Technological design needs to be based on considering not whether we can design an intervention, instead we should consider: 'ought we to do this?'[19]

My concern is that a digital as opposed to quantum future could lapse into control and surveillance from above.[20]

Steven Hawking argues for a direct connection between brain and computer—hybridization in other words—but this argument needs to be looked at carefully. He warns that

> we must develop as quickly as possible technologies that make possible a direct connection between brain and computer, so that artificial brains contribute to human intelligence rather than opposing it' (Greenfield 2003, p. 46).

But the core issues are not technical; they are ethical and systemic in nature. The challenge is also that we are part of our subject matter. The education system to support our understanding of systemic social, economic and environmental challenges is lacking.

> Our education system will need fundamental reform to develop the capabilities required to ensure that the millennial generation becomes the solutions generation (Black 2008).... Black highlighted the distinctive capabilities that society will need to develop. The development of core curriculum that develops skills—including inter-systems thinking, good judgment abilities, adaptive leadership skills, network mobilizing skills, a developed meaning and emotional intelligence and solid global ethics—is imperative if we are to address current and future complex challenges adequately (Black 2008; Helfetz 1994; cited by Connell 2012, p. 316).

The absurd education systems force science and social sciences into different tracks, purely because there is less effort made to develop the capabilities of all students through recognizing their strengths and using the strengths to help develop

[19] The scenarios outlined by Greenfield (2003, 2008) of a change in the nature of humanity through becoming increasingly public in the way in which they live is worth considering as designers of our future. Greenfield stresses that we risk our own subjectivity if we start to erode the boundaries between self and others—the challenge remains to balance individual and collective needs. If we become hybrids (human machine) as a result of linking too closely with the digital divides that we use as extensions of our memory (iPads and mobile phones that could not only be miniaturized by hybridized to become part of our own bodies – so that we become carbon and silicon. This is already the case with artificial parts and organs. Similarly, the issue of human animal hybridization becomes important to be raised. As the use of machine technology and machine culture and biological research changes our way of life, it may lead to changes in our own human nature that shift our understanding of rights and responsibilities. The need for more forms of energy could also lead to our recycling our own energy supplies and monitoring our own use of energy. This is potentially a scenario where the carbon-poor could compete with the carbon-rich, who live in the digitally controlled and climate-managed equivalent of domed and gated communities, serviced and/or controlled by the carbon–silicon enriched. But it does not have to look this way!

[20] But this is not inevitable as is illustrated by the Arab Spring and the ways in which social media and wiki leaks have changed the face of democracy and governance. What are the options for social democracy? The Participatory Action Research is based on the axiom that freedom and diversity ought to be fostered to support wellbeing and creativity, but only to the extent that the rights of others and the next generation of life are respected.

their potential. It may require some remedial teaching, but with education systems becoming increasingly open to a range of digital media (in the developed world), this could be redressed. Similarly, aid budgets will need to stress food, energy and water supplies for all, so that children and adults have access to broadband media and are able to concentrate because they are not hungry and thirsty. It is all about distribution and will. The resources do exist. One-off events such as Band Aid rock concerts need to be replaced with governance and democracy architectures that are participatory and monitory in style. They need to ensure that those in power are held to account and moreover that those who aspire to power are held to account too.

Governance and democracy will also have to deal with three options pertaining to truth (McIntyre-Mills 2000; Crowder 2003): (a) One truth responses defended by grand narratives or conflict, (b) no truth (postmodernist) approached defended by relativism, (c) mediated (harmonized) responses based on stewardship. The book makes the case for social change through exploring interdisciplinary frameworks to address greed, the commodification of the powerless and the environment. It drew on the debates on ethics, human reasoning capability, emotions[21] and environmental politics and the practical implications for social democracy (Judt 2010). This appears to be a long leap from neural research. But it is not.

This work builds on the previous research to enable people with complex needs to consider the consequences of continuing to live the same way as before or the consequences of making changes to the way that they live. It is hoped that this research could make a contribution to resilience and wellbeing. People face increased risks associated with climate change, such as rising food, energy and housing costs.

Part of the inquiry involves a study on emotional connections to particular kinds of life.

Wadsworth (2010, p. 28) cites Winston Churchill's phrase: 'We shape our houses, and after that they shape us' and draws attention to the way in which sociologists such as Giddens (1986) understood the way in which societies are shaped by people and then they shape us. Similarly, she cites the work of neuroscientists (Doidge 2007) and makes the connection with the way in which society is made up of a series of nested systems writ large. They are a reflection of who we are.

The social boundaries shaped by current socio-economic systems between 'us and them' and the poverty endured by the majority[22] are unsustainable.

The case is made in this book for making connections with many ways of knowing and with many cultures. It is vital to develop these connections rather than to emphasize only one approach to understanding the world. Climate change will lead to migrations of people and this will require rethinking the way in which the contained nation state is replaced with porous states that are part of regional, republican federations. This requires moving from weak cosmopolitanism to strong cosmopolitanism. Thus, limiting hospitality to strangers becomes a core issue.

[21] The pain of rejection and unemployment based on categories such as age, gender and culture including religion, ideology or physical or mental abilities also trigger anger.

[22] The minority are able to live lives of luxury at the expense of current and future generations.

Even if the nation state continues to exist, it will require new forms of regional governance. This is the context for developing post-national monitory democracy and governance.

To what extent are human beings essentially different from other sentient beings and machines? What are cyborgs? What are chimeras? What are the implications for disability studies? The human being who survives because of an organ transplant from another sentient creature or because they are connected to a dialysis machine?

The so-called hard problem (Chalmers1995) is 'what is consciousness?' Is it the preserve of human beings? What do we have in common with other sentient beings?

I argue that the connections between organic and inorganic life are a matter of life cycle or stage, not one of separate category. In accepting our non-essentialism, we need to avoid abandoning a sense of the sacred.[23] Drawing the line is still vital to ethics, but where and how to draw the line depends on who is involved in the ethical conversation and whether we are acting as stewards for biodiversity.

The sense of the sacred should not be undermined in the bid to squeeze profit out of the increasingly hollowed-out middle classes in developed nation states or to tempt/lure the rising middle classes in developing nations to emulate the mistakes of so-called developed nations.

We can choose or ignore the sacred, depending on our will to power. Human beings can choose to rise above difficulties as did Victor Frankl (1955) who survived the atrocities of a prison of war camp by his capability of thinking about the future and by making sense or meaning out of what was going on around him. It was his choice to believe and not to be crushed. He discusses the importance of making meaning and on the ability of human beings to choose because of their human spirit. This ability to show compassion and humanity is not however an entirely human capability, nor should it be used as a terrible justification of being cruel to others species. Being a member of a particular race was used as an excuse for racism or slavery. Being a member of the human race ought to constitute responsibility to other forms of life. Frans de Waal, a primatologist, argues in 'The Age of Empathy' that survival is based on not only competition but also the ability to co-operate. Thus, emotions and not rationality also play a significant role in evolution and emergence. It thus provides a challenge for Dawkins who I argue confuses genes and dualism/digital either or thinking as the basis for enlightenment and rationality. Knowledge is based on many ways of making sense—informed by all our senses—feeling, emotions and intuition are as important as sight, sound, touch and taste. The commodification of sentient beings—workers, animals and the land—cannot continue. The rent seeking behaviour of CEOs and bankers do not add, create or produce—they simply demand a larger slice of the existing pie (Stiglitz 2012).

The sense of entitlement has led to profit being extracted from those who can be excluded from contractual rights, such as non-citizens who do not vote or are incapable of voting. It also means that non-human sentiments can be treated as objects.

[23] The ironical argument developed by Donna Haraway in a 'Cyborg manifesto', 'Promises of monsters' and 'Speculative fabulations' (1991, 2010) makes this point the danger of some essentialist identity categories.

Transportation of slaves has been banned, but we still debate the transportation of asylum seekers—'turn back the boats' has been used as a slogan. The trucking/shipping and railing of so-called livestock erodes not only the quality of life of sentient non-humans but also our own quality of life because the costs to our carbon footprint are unsustainable.

We need to understand that by identifying with others and with biodiversity (Lever-Tracey 2011), we extend the circle of those with whom we feel solidarity and compassion and redefine our identity without hubris—then we may be able to transform the culture (Hulme 2010, 2011) which shapes the planet on which we depend.[24]

This requires some space for diversity and freedom and a sense of irony (Rorty 1989).[25] We are the designers of our future and we can create hybrid designs (Haraway 1991, 1992) which respond to 'Beck's (2009) world at risk'. This requires rescuing the 'enlightenment from itself' (McIntyre-Mills et al 2006), rather than extending the myth of so-called risk management and resilience and recognizing

[24] The goal of this book is to foster an understanding that 'We are the land' (Getano Lui 1994). Humanity is dependent on air, water and soil for survival. The global commons and our relationship to it need to be recognised as not merely entangled but co-determined.

[25] Relationship between the press and governments at the national and international level Freedom of the press is no longer a given in democratic society. The press freedom in UK was called into question after journalists hacked into phones in order to obtain information. The freedom to make fun of others through cartoons or posting videos has also been questioned, given the extent of violence it can unleash. But surely the response to provocation through art is to counter the insult through art or through an essay, one may argue. But the level of anger felt by those who identify with injured civilians in the so-called war on terror makes me think that some restraint is required. The freedom to make a hoax call on the hospital where a pregnant member of the royal family was undergoing tests, in the name of the queen, and the subsequent death of a nurse who committed suicide needs to be considered with restraint. Clearly, the prank call had disastrous results, but it was an ill-considered prank. The governance of the hospital, the health of the nurse and the relationships to hierarchy need to be unpacked. The freedom of climate change skeptics to denigrate the science of climate change is a requirement of all enlightened societies, provided that their right to the freedom to express their views does not undermine the right of children to a safe future. Existential risk is so great that it is wise to take measures to protect the planet through innovative design that makes use of renewable energy supplies. But science and progress cannot be built on silencing criticism. The use of force by individuals or nation states needs to be the last resort and avoided if at all possible. Emotional outrage can be an appropriate response to outrageous events. The attempted assassination of a young girl who protested her right to study in Afghanistan and the gang rape of a girl in a bus in New Delhi: 'The calls for calm came after the Indian woman who was gang raped on a New Delhi bus died in a Singapore hospital early on Saturday after suffering severe organ failure. People across India have started coming out to mourn the death of the 23-year-old student, whose death has already sparked mass protests. Police said they would allow people to hold peaceful demonstrations only in some areas and hundreds of policemen have been deployed to prevent any violence on the streets. Indian Prime Minister Manmohan Singh also said he was deeply saddened by the death, and the protests that were sparked by the case were "understandable".'

Read more: http://www.news.com.au/breaking-news/world/police-urge-calm-after-rape-victim-dies/story-e6frfkui-1226545025294#ixzz2GQEnBfda.

our vulnerability and interdependency.[26] They will also need to have the right to be whistle-blowers. This legislation in Australia is only in place at a state level, not a federal level. Could the Aarhus Convention be used to support the United Nations Convention on Corruption and European 'Whistle Blowing legislation' (see Brown 2008)?

The argument developed in this book is that social democracy has failed because it has veered too far in the direction of rights and has paid insufficient attention to responsibilities.[27] I do not argue that social democracy needs to be abandoned—only that it needs to be reformed through participatory governance within overarching biospheres that are subject to global laws to protect the environment and the fabric of life based on the careful weighing up of the consequences for current generations and future generations of life. This is the law of the land which is sacred and which most indigenous and first nations understand. But the argument developed in this book should not be confused with the closed system's arguments that allow for the idealism of totalitarian World Government. The architecture detailed in Chaps. 1 and 2 could support wide-ranging engagement for monitory democracy in which people are required to think through the implication of their choices for others and the next generation.

How can local engagement be encouraged without fear, unless a form of local engagement also provides disclosure protection.[28] The problem is that members of

[26] If the details of the Biodiversity summit 2010 in Japan were actually addressed, it would require intersected, nested transnational policies and law to make it possible for local people—local residents to have a say—irrespective of whether they are citizens of a nation state. Governance structures ought to provide corridors enabling movement from place to place. As Beck (2009, p. 190) stresses, Kantian normative hospitality is insufficient. People have a right to live on the planet. In 'World Risk Society', competing risks will become a way of life. People will need to be able to move to escape fire, flood and to find water during droughts.

[27] The notion of austerity and elegance are key themes—not in order to live a life that is not worth living, but instead to live a life that is meaningful and that is guided by a sense of arête that spans generations. The convergence of social, economic and environmental issues is clearly evident. The gap between rich and poor today is the widest it has ever been in human history. The argument used for apologists of extreme capitalism a decade ago was to say that the overall standard of living was better than in the past. Today, that argument no longer holds. The majority of capital in the form of wealth and ownership of the means of production is concentrated amongst the elites. But the extent of concentration leads to the inability of the masses to consume—in order to maintain the economy—unless they borrowed. Their ability to borrow has now reached its limit because they are unemployed and because the surplus value extracted by capital has not taken into account the so-called social, spiritual, cultural and environmental externalities on which it depends. Stiglitz, a World Bank economist and now whistle-blower on extreme capitalism, argues that we need to factor well-being into all sustainable living calculations. We need to think of the implications of economic choices for others and for the environment in this generation and the next. This is a form of expanded pragmatism, an approach to ethical living which needs to become widespread in order to ensure human survival.

[28] http://www.aph.gov.au/house/house_news/news_stories/news_whistleblowers_Feb2009.htm The House of Representatives Legal and Constitutional Affairs Committee has released its report on whistle-blower protection for the federal government public sector. The report recommends that the federal government introduce new dedicated legislation to facilitate the making of public interest disclosures and strengthen legal protection for whistle-blowers in the Commonwealth

the public are also not given protection to the whistle-blower as well as a requirement to follow up on the disclosures. Unless this is in place, people will not be able to engage in stressing that accountability become central in a society that requires austerity. Three options exist for transformation: centralist interventions, anarchist and negotiated discursive dialogues with a focus on expanded pragmatism. Expanding policy pragmatism is a process to address the context and consequences of human decisions. Let us start with the formula that addresses the implications of polarising *people versus the planet.*[29]

Accounting and accountability at the local level need to be fostered by means of monitory democracy and governance. Our research applies this philosophy at the local level and advocates for its extension to post-national regional biospheres. The notion espoused by policy thinkers that representation needs to be carefully controlled (to support democracy) is fallacious. If people are required to participate and to engage in 'if then scenarios', they are likely to be able to understand one another's viewpoints better and more likely to make connections, provided that the axiom is maintained and that we can be free and diverse to the extent that our freedom and diversity do not undermine the rights of others. Perhaps 1% of the people will realize that their right to consume indiscriminately needs to be curtailed so as not to limit the freedoms of others. This is the point raised by researchers such as Murray et al. (2007) in the Tuvalu Test to address the use of resources equitably within the region. How to apply the freeware to enable the self-management of a carbon economy is discussed in McIntyre-Mills and de Vries (2011) in 'Identity, democracy and sustainability'.

Can dialogue contribute to balancing short-term liveability and long-term sustainability? Greenfield stresses that if we spend too little time developing the conceptual skills needed to understand abstract concepts (such as identity, greed or consumption), then we run the risk of reducing the size of the conceptual assemblies (or connections) that we are able to make (Greenfield 2009, p. 127). This is because we are not thinking through ideas and drawing analogies. Consciousness involves 'making connections' (Turner and Whitehead 2008, p. 45) across larger assemblages of ideas and thinking about the implications of our potential decisions for governance. Rosenberg's research (2002) on political decision making confirms that 'either or' thinking is responsible for contributing to dualistic policy and

public sector.The Chair of the committee Mark Dreyfus QC noted that specific Commonwealth legislation on public interest disclosures is overdue. 'The Commonwealth is the only Australian jurisdiction that does not have legislation to encourage public interest disclosures,' Mr Dreyfus said. 'While some limited protections are available to whistle-blowers employed by Australian Public Service agencies, evidence to the inquiry indicates that those protections are grossly inadequate.' 'The current legal framework and organisational culture discourages public servants from speaking out against what they consider to be illegal or improper conduct in the workplace. People who raise allegations of misconduct could be exposed to serious criminal or civil liability.'

[29] E (Emissions) = Population × Consumption per person × Energy Efficiency × Energy Emissions. Reducing waste, reusing resources, saving resilient seeds and recycling wherever possible need to become the litmus test for households and local development in order to redistribute resources to that in need and as a means to limit the misuse of scarce resources. The loss of insects, the unbridled greed and hubris will impact food security just as it will jeopardise seed security.

governance decisions in the USA, rather than a careful consideration of complex viewpoints. This could be developed by means of more thought-provoking democratic processes (Banathy 2000; Christakis and Flanagan 2010; Dryzek 2010) that inspire discussion based on considering the consequences of people's decisions for themselves, others and the environment. It will establish whether people are able to extend their understanding as a result of critical systemic engagement on the ramifications of unequal consumption (Guddemi 2006; Hulme 2009). Dualist thinking, where two opposing types of views are set against each other (e.g., climate change believers vs. climate change sceptics) may pervade consciousness and be reflected in the current social contradiction between capitalism and sustainability (Chase-Dunn 2010; Hulme 2009, pp. 301–302).

A nested form of representation would ensure that those elected to represent regionalist concerns would sit at regional government and negotiate within the limits prescribed in transnational labour and environmental law.

Just as a cell is both open and closed, the biosphere approach will need to determine when it is possible to expend more and when it is necessary to expend less. Global wellbeing standards defined in trans-national law developed and set out by Regionalist Biosphere Protection Agencies could ensure that food security for all is placed at the heart of all governance decisions.

This volume attempts to explain a way forward by arguing that social democracy can be redesigned to place greater emphasis on participatory governance within responsive biospheres that respond to the environment.[30]

The Age newspaper provides a space for the cartoonist Leunig's view on the world. In cartoons, he expresses his sense of the absurd.[31] A poignant cartoon represents a crowd of sad hurried urbanites off to work. They scowl and look down at the pavements. No one raises their heads to look at the towering skyscrapers that loom

[30] The means to achieve this change already exist. Bartley (2011) has argued that governance across nation states can 'layer rules' that 'intersect public and private standards'. His approach is based on an understanding of open systems, but his paper does not explain how to translate this idea into practice. Kolben's (2011) paper delivered at the same colloquium does not hold out much hope because he bases his argument on an understanding of closed self-reinforcing subsystems, without understanding that all systems rely on the environment and are thus always reliant on it. The notion of the Mobius band takes into account the idea that systems are open and closed, depending on the context (McIntyre-Mills 2008). Biosphere regulation will need to determine the extent to which we have a responsibility to use fewer resources and when we have the right to use more. The notion that this could lead to dictatorship would need to be carefully addressed, given the argument that Michels developed in 'The iron rule of oligarchy', namely that even in the most democratic trade union, those who hold leadership positions can and will abuse their rights. Transparency to all will be a sine qua non, as well as rotation of the leadership position, in much the same way as the European Union leadership has functioned. Lessons from their mistakes need to be learnt. The European Bank has lent to those who could not pay back their loans. The credits given out by the biosphere regulator will need to be carefully accounted. How can this be achieved? What implications does the biosphere approach have on our sense of identity? Can we reconstruct identity and move beyond the sort of national xenophobia that I have already described elsewhere?

[31] Published on http://www.leunig.com.au/index.php/recent-cartoons/97-breakfast Saturday 23rd of February,2013.

above. One little human being looks up and notices a sign post saying 'Freshly laid, free range eggs, served with organic wheat brown toast'.

The human turns around and follows the sign. It is hoped that this book can act as a sign post to another and happier way of life.[32]

[32] When will we realize that the big issues of the day are not whether the sporting hero of the moment has cheated or committed acts of violence, distressing though this is, because those on pedestals are held in high regard for success to which others aspire. When we discover that their achievements are the result of bending the rules or breaking them, it leads to a sense of distrust in the order of things.

But much worse is the way in which we pay attention to the trivial in order to avoid facing up to the bigger issues, such as the inability to manage the size of our cities and the burgeoning populations.

When will we realize that dualistic thinking that polarises people and people versus nature—and other species—is not only misguided but also leads to the undermining of our collective wellbeing? This question explores whether dialogue enables research participants to identify with others and whether dialogue could reshape attitudes towards the right to consume versus the responsibility to conserve natural resources which constitute the global commons (Bakker 2007). Dialogue could enable the better match of development responses to context, thus enabling evolutionary development and policy adaptation (Giddens 2009), rather than 'development for growth' that is unsustainable because it does not account for economic externalities or the opportunity costs of consumption to the next generation (Hulme 2009, pp. 124–126).

Chapter 8
Executive Summary

8.1 Stewardship Praxis: Towards Ethical Democracy, Governance and Stewardship

So many people say that they want to be the change, but how? The ongoing research makes the case that stewardship requires transformation of the way that we live. Being the change from moment to moment requires reflection on the way we choose to live our lives and the implications these choices have on others and on the environment.

The software is only a means to an end, namely to enable people to reflect on their lives. It provides a way to enable people to explore the question: how should we live and what constitutes wellbeing?

Participants are invited to consider the following: what material and non-material conditions are important to them by viewing their lives in terms of the Max Neef Human Sustainability Index (1991) *of being, having doing and interacting.* This approach shapes the design and analysis of the research and illustrates the need to be the change through rethinking the way in which we place human beings above our responsibility for the land.

Our sense of identity as citizens of nation states needs to be transformed to take into account the needs of our neighbours and future generations of life. The research attempts to enable people to think through the 'if-then' scenarios, not merely to 'unfreeze' (to cite Lewin's concept) but to work towards sustainable praxis, based on an understanding of our interrelatedness. Creativity is needed to underpin the transformation from 'Wall Street' to 'Wellbeing'.

Participants are asked to reflect on what they have, what they need and what they perceive to be the social, economic and environmental turning points for the better or the worse in their lives and what they perceive to be the barriers. They are also asked to consider the services that help them meet their needs.

J. McIntyre-Mills, *Transformation from Wall Street to Wellbeing,*
Contemporary Systems Thinking, DOI 10.1007/978-1-4899-7466-2_8,

The exercise of 'thinking about their thinking' is an attempt to build new neural pathways in the mind—to rehearse a different way of 'being in the world', based on thinking about the consequences for themselves, others and the environment.[1]

The software updates as it is used and the idea is that it will help people to make better decisions to address complex needs. Excel sheets are provided that give cross tabulations of socio demographic details and the choices they make. The idea is that by thinking about their lives, they will be able to consider the consequences of their choices for their own wellbeing and the wellbeing of others. To use the software, please enter your user name as 'test' and enter your password as 'test'.The starting point is to listen to the three scenarios. The pathway address for local government is https://wellbeing.csem.flinders.edu.au/.

The book reviews work in progress to date and makes the case that using a computer-aided model could enhance data collection, analysis and ongoing engagement to address complex social, economic and environmental issues associated with climate change. But it is only one of the approaches for engagement and will never be sufficient. Nor will it make a difference, unless it is implemented more widely. So at best, it provides an alternative architecture that has some potential for prefiguring change and enabling people to think about their lives and the consequences of their choices.

The software is loaded onto the Flinders Website, in the first instance, but has the potential for links with local governments elsewhere at a sub- and post-national level within the region.[2] A diverse range of values, emotions and opinions are associated with wellbeing, quality of life and climate change. These can be regarded as a wicked problem, in the sense that it has many diverse and interrelated variables that are viewed differently by people with different values (see van Gigch and McIntyre-Mills 2006).

This book discusses an alternative form of governance and democracy based on a new paradigm. Creativity guided by humility and the willingness to care for others is needed to underpin the transformation from 'Wall Street' to 'Wellbeing'.[3]

The concept 'Wall Street' symbolises economic rationalism and 'wellbeing' symbolises a reframed approach to 'being interconnected' and through treading lightly, rather than slashing pathways that are turned into highways. Wellbeing today does not need to cost the planet. So how do we hold the 1 % in check? How

[1] The notion that the more we are able to think about our thinking, the more conscious we become, underpins this research. As we make more and more neural connections, our ability to address complex challenges increases. The work of neuroscientist Baroness Professor Susan Greenfield as thinker in residence in Adelaide, South Australia, helped to inspire this work (Greenfield 2000).

[2] Part of the rationale for trialling the software was to establish to what extent computing per se is a useful way to engage different interest groups and whether it could be useful to enable managing large data sets spanning many diverse interrelated variables about which residents have strong values.

[3] It makes the case that using a computer-aided model could enhance data collection, analysis and ongoing engagement to address complex social, economic and environmental issues associated with climate change. But it is only one of the approaches for engagement and will never be sufficient.

can whistle blowing be achieved? How can we be the change when dollars and cents and not wellbeing are the bottom line?

The problem with operations research is that it sought to control humans and nature as human and natural resources for development. The mechanistic- and systems-oriented approach however was not intended by West Churchman who understood the importance of contextual human values when considering an area of concern. Thus, he called his approach an 'open systems approach' and was open to criticism. For this reason, the starting point for this book is that design interventions need to become part of a way of life.

Expanding pragmatism is a process to address the context and consequences of human decisions. Let us start with the Intergovernmental Panel on Climate Change (IPCC) formula that addresses the implications of polarising people versus the planet.

$$\begin{aligned}&\text{IPCC formula, } E(\text{Emissions})\\&= \text{Population} \times \text{consumption per person} \times \text{energy efficiency} \times \text{energy emissions}\end{aligned}$$

Existential risk has implications for representation, accountability and sustainability. Consumption is very unequal and the gaps between rich and poor become wider and wider.

The root cause of consumption is power without responsibility—so whoever comes to power needs to be held to account through mechanisms to develop social, economic and environmental indicators that secure the wellbeing stocks for the future.

Rights to consume need to be balanced by the responsibility to consume in ways that impact the life chances of others (including future generations of life). Thus, the rule of law needs to be post national and global supported by a covenant to protect all life. This needs to be secured by overlapping federations of biospheres buttressed in law and supported by a judicial system. Hence, the axiom for expanding pragmatism—we can be free and diverse to the extent that our freedom and diversity does not undermine the rights of others or future generations of life.

Appendix 1: User Guide for Engagement to Address Climate Change Through Participatory Democracy and Governance

How to Use the Site
http://prezi.com/mmfaghm40kdf/pathway-to-wellbeing/
https://wellbeing.csem.flinders.edu.au/

1. Log on as User Name "*test*" *Password* "*test*" on the top right corner, if you wish to have a quick peek through the system.

Otherwise in the "New User" area, create your own *username* and *password*, write it down and complete the relevant details and press "Create Account".

All personal or identifying information collected through this tool is stored and used confidentially to ensure participants remain anonymous.

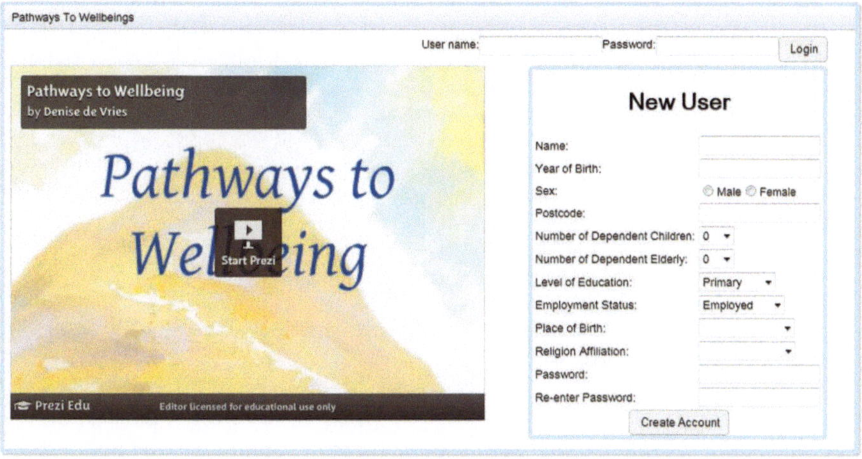

J. McIntyre-Mills, *Transformation from Wall Street to Wellbeing*,
Contemporary Systems Thinking, DOI 10.1007/978-1-4899-7466-2,

2. This is your second screen once your account has been created. Simply move to the next step by selecting "Create new Pathway"

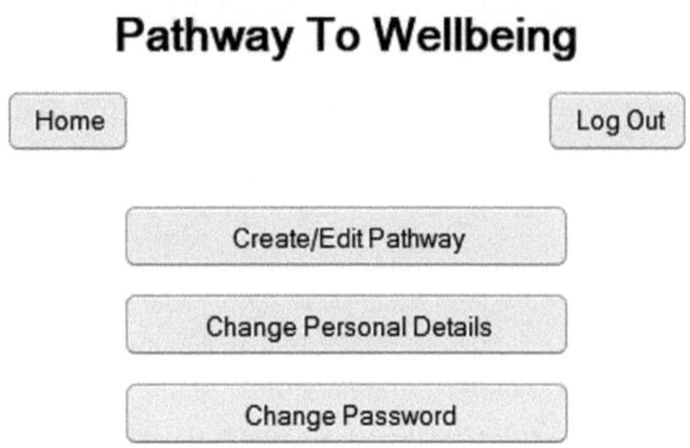

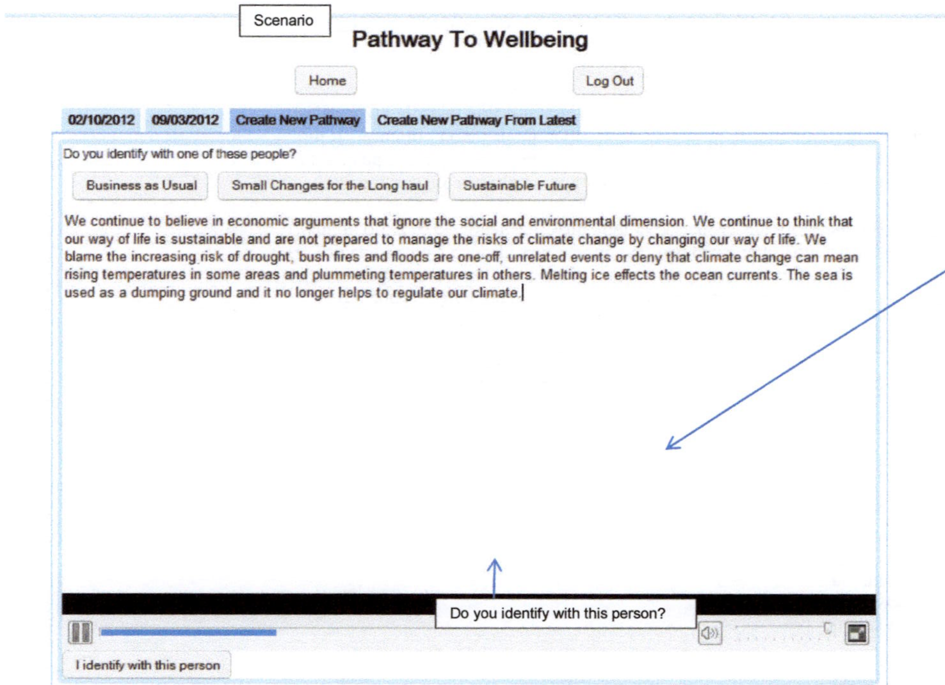

3. Please listen to audios of the scenarios;

Please choose one that you most identify with by clicking the button in the bottom section

The audio tool at the bottom of the section will allow you to listen to the recording of the text. The appearance differs from computer to computer depending on what you use for your web browser.

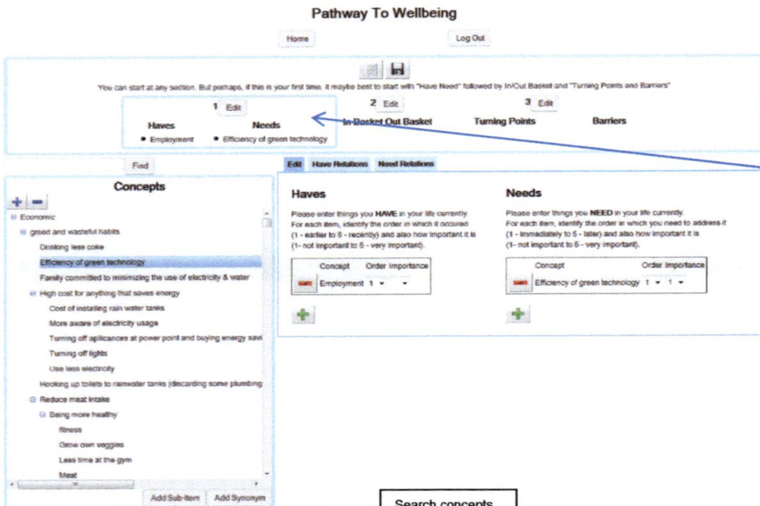

4. After completing step 3, you will arrive at this screen. The top section lets you navigate between the 3 sections "Have Need", "In Basket, Out Basket" and "Turning Points and Barrier".

It is perhaps best to start with identifying what you have and what you need in life. Select the have and need section if it is not already selected.
Here you will be able to personalise your pathway by selecting the items in "Concepts" section on the left.

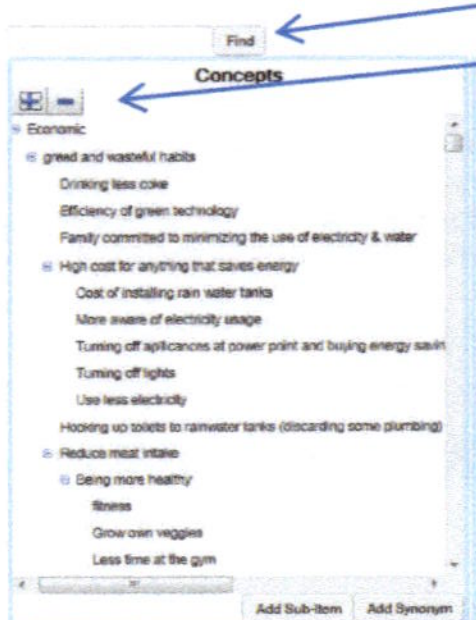

5. In the concept area the blue plus symbol expands the concept trees. If you see a concept that you agree with,
You can also search for the concept in the find box by typing a word in and press "find".
If you can't find a concept you would like, you can add in your own words to the social, economic and environmental as a sub item, in order to personalise it with your experiences, emotions and perceptions.

If something is not there, then add your own ideas to the drop-down lists under social, economic and environmental tabs, e.g. I want to add to In Basket 'improve insulation'. I will add it to the list by placing it under "Social", as a subsection of "home". But if I want to I could add it under Economic as "I cannot afford to insulate my home. The subsection you decide to choose depends on whether you consider an item to be social, economic or environmental.

6. Personalise your profile by using *the green plus sign* to add your highlighted concept and using *the red minus sign* to delete items that do not apply to you.

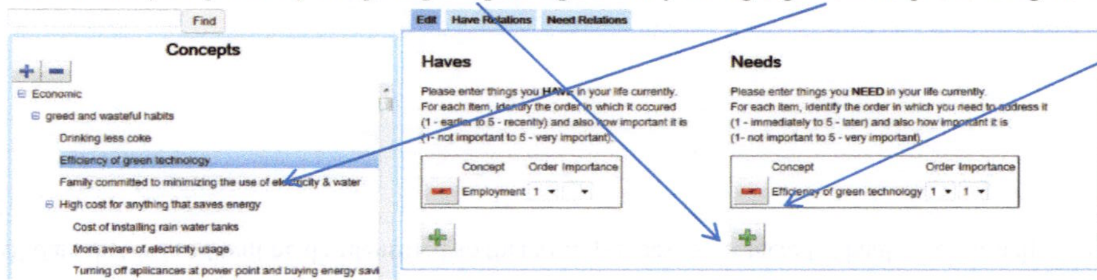

7. Save each step by clicking on the save button if you would like, however this is done automatically.

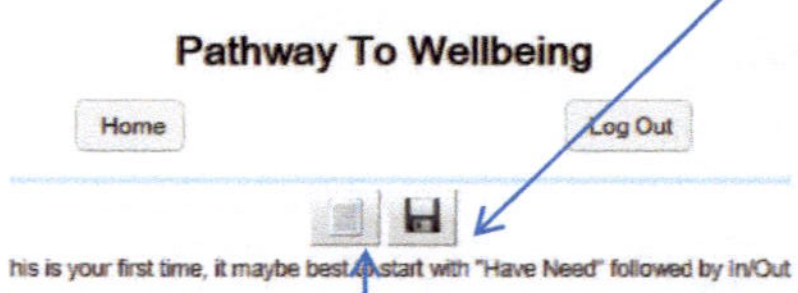

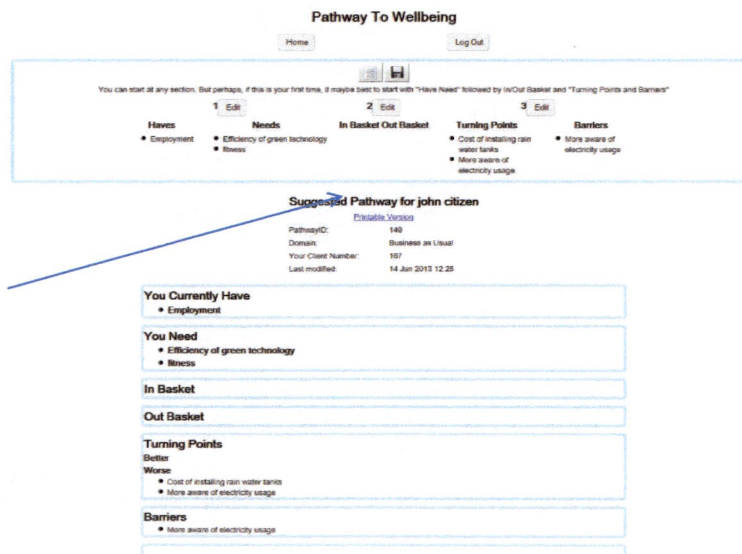

8. Review your report and assess goals over time by clicking the report button.

You should see the screen on the right.

The option also exist for those who wish to obtain a printer friendly version

This information will help local government to plan and deliver services to residents. Thank you for helping us to help the community. The administrators of this site will be able to view data in excel spread sheets.

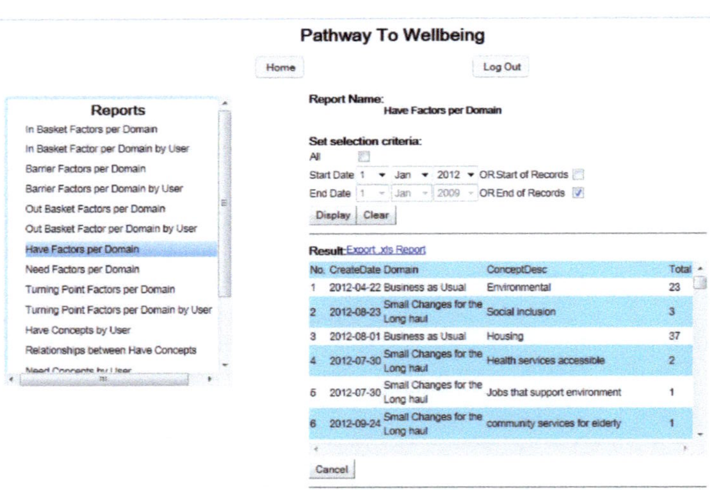

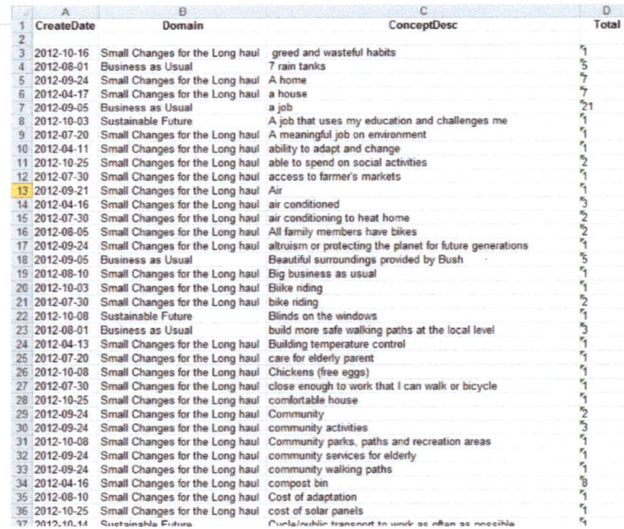

All data that is used will be de-identified so that your privacy is protected. Thank you for helping us helps the community.

References

A frontier-free Europe. 1988. *Commission of the European communities*. Brussels and Luxembourg CEC.
Aarhus Convention. 1998. On access to information. Public participation and access to justice in environmental matters. Denmark, 25 June. http://aarhusclearinghouse.unece.org/resources.cfm?c=1000069.
Abbott, A. 2007. Against narrative: A preface to lyrical sociology. *Social Theory* 25 (1): 67–99.
Abegunrin, O. 2002. 'Truth and reconciliation' the South African truth commission by Kenneth Christie; Looking back, reaching forward: Reflections on the truth and reconciliation commission of South Africa by Charles Villa-Vicencio; Wilhelm Verwoerd; Truth v. Justice: The morality of truth commissions by Robert I. Rotberg; Dennis Thompson. *African Studies Review* 45 (3): 31–34. (Dec 2002). http://www.jstor.org/stable/01.
Adkins, L. 2005. The new economy, property and personhood. *Theory, Culture and Society* 22 (1): 111–130.
Agamben, G.1998. *Homer sacer: Sovereign power and bare life*. Stanford: Stanford University Press.
Ainsworth, M. D., and J. Bowlby. 1991. An ethological approach to personality development. *American Psychologist* 46:333–341.
Archibugi, D. 2008. The architecture of cosmopolitan democracy. *The global commonwealth of citizens: Towards cosmopolitan democracy*. Princeton: Princeton University Press.
Archibugi, D. 2010. The architecture of cosmopolitan democracy. In *Cosmopolitan Reader*, eds. G. W. Brown, and D. Held. Cambridge: Polity Press.
Arendt, H. 1959. *The human condition*. New York: Doubleday Anchor.
Arendt, H. 1963. *Eichmann in Jerusalem: A report on the banality of evil*. New York: Viking Press.
Arendt, H. 1967. *The origins of totalitarianism*. London: Allen and Unwin.
Arendt, H. 1972. *Crises of the Republic*. Orlando: Harcourt Brace. (First published in 1969).
Arendt, H. 2006. *Between past and future*. Harmonsworth: Penguin.
Armitage, C. 2012. Final frontier of climate policy—remake humans. *Sydney Morning Herald* 6 April.
Arnstein, S. 1969. A ladder of citizen participation. *Journal of American Institute of Planners* 35 (4): 216–224.
Arrowsmith-Young, B. 2012. *The woman who changed her brain*. New York: Harper Collins.
Ashby, W. R. 1956. *An introduction to cybernetics*. London: Chapman and Hall.
Aspinal, E., and G. Fealy, eds. 2003. *Local power and politics in Indonesia. Decentralisation and democratization*. Indonesia update series. Research School of Pacific and Asian Studies.
Atkinson, J. 2002. *Trauma trails, recreating song lines: The transgenerational effects of trauma in indigenous Australia*. Melbourne: Spinifex.
AusAid. 2009. Disaster risk reduction. Investing in a safer future. Published by the Australian Agency for International Development (AusAID), Canberra, June

J. McIntyre-Mills, *Transformation from Wall Street to Wellbeing*, Contemporary Systems Thinking, DOI 10.1007/978-1-4899-7466-2,

Australian Government Department of Infrastructure and Transport. 2011. Our cities our future. A national urban policy for a productive, sustainable and liveable future. Department of Infrastructure and Transport. GPO Box 594, Canberra ACT 2601, Australia ISBN 978-1-921769-26-9INFRA-1118/May 2011c Commonwealth of Australia 2011.

Australian Government State of Australian Cities, Department of Infrastructure and Transport. 2011. Major cities Unit, GPO Box 594, Canberra ACT 2601, Australia. http://www.majorcities.gov.au. Accessed 23 July 2014.

Australian Public Service Commission. 2007. Tackling wicked problems. http://www.apsc.gov.au/publications. Accessed 8 Jan 2013.

Axel, B. 2002. *Historical anthropology and its futures. From the margins*. London: Duke University Press.

Bakker, K. 2007. The commons versus the Commodity. *Antipode* 39 (3): 430–458.

Balibar, E. 2006. Strangers as enemies. Further reflections on the aporias of transnational citizenship. Globalization and autonomy. Online Compendium http://www.globalautonomy.ca/global1/article.jsp?index. Accessed 29 March 2011"

Bammer, G. 2005. Integration and implementation sciences: Building a new specialisation. *Ecology and Society* 10 (2): 6.

Banathy, B. 1996. *Designing social systems in a changing world*. London: Plenum.

Banathy, B. 2000. *Guided evolution of society: A systems view*. London: Kluwer/Plenum.

Barber, B. 2005. Global governance from below. In *Debating globalization,* ed. D. Held, et al. Cambridge: Polity Press.

Bartley, T. 2011. Transnational governance as layering of rules: Intersections of public and private standards. *Theoretical Inquiries in Law* 12 (2): Article 6.

Baruma, I., and A. Margalit. 2004. *Occidentalism: The west in the eyes of its enemies*. New York: Penguin.

Bateson, G. 1972. *Steps to an ecology of mind*. New York: Ballantine.

Baubock, R. 2006. Who are the citizens of Europe? http://eudocitizenship.eu. Rainer.Baubock(at)eui.eu.

Baudrillard, J. 1981. *Simulacra and simulation*. Ann Arbor (translator): University of Michigan Press.

Baudrillard, J. 1994. *Simulacra and simulation*. Ann Arbor: University of Michigan Press.

Bauman, Z. 2011. From agora to the market place, and where to from here? *Journal of Globalisation Studies* 2 (1): 3–14.

Bausch, K. 2006. Be your enemy: The contributions of west churchman to doing better governance and international relations. In *Rescuing the enlightenment from itself: Critical and systemic implications for democracy,* ed. J. McIntyre-Mills. (C. West Churchman Series, vol. 1). New York: Springer.

Bausch, K. 2001. *The emerging consensus in social systems theory*. London: Kluwer/Plenum.

Bausch, K. 2010. *Body wisdom. Ongoing emergence*. Online publisher. http://www.books.google.com/books/about/Body_Wisdom.html?id.

Bausch, K. 2011. Visions, hallucinations, and dreams in the context of body wisdom and chaos theory. *Neuro Quantology* 9 (1): 129–134.

Beardsworth, R. 2011. *Cosmopolitanism and international relations theory*. Cambridge: Polity Press.

Beck, U. 1992. *Risk society towards a new modernity*. London: Sage.

Beck, U. 1998. *Democracy without enemies*. Cambridge: Polity Press.

Beck, U. 2005. *World risk society*. Cambridge: Polity Press.

Beck, U. 2009. *World at risk*. Cambridge: Polity Press.

Beck, U. 2010. Climate for change, or how to create a green modernity. *Theory, Culture and Society* 27 (2–3): 254–266.

Beck, U., and N. Sznaider. 2006. Unpacking cosmopolitanism for the social sciences: A research agenda. *The British Journal of Sociology* 57:1–23.

Beer, S. 1974. *Designing freedom*. London: Wiley.

Beer, S. 1975. *Platform for change*. New York: Wiley.

Beer, S. 1994. Governance or government. In *Beyond dispute: The invention of team syntegrity*. London: Wiley.

Beer, A., A. Maude, and B. Pritchard. 2003. *Developing Australia's regions: Theory and Practice*. Sydney: University of New South Wales.

Behrendt, L. 2005. The abolition of ATSIC: Implications for democracy. Democratic audit of Australia. http://democratic.audit.anu.edu.au/. Accessed 4 Jan 2006.

Bell, G. 2009. *Getting connected, staying connected*. South Australia: Department of Premier and Cabinet.

Benhabib, S. 2002. *The claims of culture: Equality and diversity in the global era*. Princeton: Princeton University Press.

Benhabib, S. 2004. On the existential question that moves her scholarly and political life. http://www.globetrotter.berkleu.edu/people4/Benhabib/. Accessed 27 July 2012.

Benhabib, S. 2004. *The rights of others: Aliens, residents and citizens*. Cambridge: Cambridge University Press.

Benhabib, S. 2007. Twilight of sovereignty or the emergence of cosmopolitan norms? Rethinking citizenship in volatile times. *Citizenship Studies* 11 (1): 19–36.

Benhabib, S. 2008. On the public sphere, deliberation, journalism and dignity. http://www.resetdoc.org/Benhabib-interview-media.php. Accessed 27 July 2012.

Benjamin, C. 2012. Ghastly garnishee abuse exposed. *Mail and Guardian* (Business), 30 Nov 2012, 2.

Berger, P., and K. Heinsfield. 1974. *The homeless mind. Modernity and consciousness*. Harmondworth: Penguin.

Bergin, A., and A. Yates. 2009. http://apo.org.au/research/hardening-australia-climate-changeand-national-disaster-resilience.

Berlin, I. 1953. *The hedgehog and the fox: An essay on Tolstoy's view of history*. London: Weidenfeld & Nicolson.

Berlin, I., and H. Hardy. 1979. *Against the current: Essays in the history of ideas*. London: Hogarth.

Binkley, S. 2000. Kitsch as a repetitive system. *Journal of Material Culture* 5 (2): 131–152.

Bird, J., and S. Clarke. 2000. Racism, hatred and discrimination. *Journal of Psycho-Analysis of Culture and Society* 4 (2): 332–335.

Bogue, R. 1989. *Deleuze and Guattari*. London: Routledge.

Bohman, J. 2004. Republican cosmopolitanism. *The Journal of Political Philosophy* 12 (3): 336–352.

Bohman, J. 2004. *Expanding dialogue: The internet, the public sphere and prospects for transnational democracy*. (Editorial Board of the Sociological Review). Oxford: Blackwell.

Bohman, J. 2005. The democratic minimum: Is democracy a means to global justice? *Ethics and International Affairs* 19 (1): 101–115.

Bohmann, J., and Lutz-Bachman, eds. 1997. *Perpetual peace: Essays on Kant's cosmopolitan ideal*. Cambridge: MIT Press.

Bonanno, G. 2004. Loss trauma, and human resilience'. *American Psychologist* 59 (1): 20–28.

Borland, S. 2011. Humans will not get any smarter. Advertiser citing the London Daily Mail. 2 Aug, 28.

Borradori, G. 2003. *Philosophy in a time of terror. Dialogues with Habermas and Derrida*. Chicago: University of Chicago Press.

Bostrom, N. 2011. Existential risk prevention as the most important task for humanity. Faculty of philosophy & Oxford Martin School University of Oxford. http://www.existential-risk.org.

Boulding, K. 1956. General systems theory—The skeleton of science. *Management Science* 2:197–208.

Bourdieu, P. 1977. *Outline of a theory of practice*. Cambridge: Cambridge University Press.

Bourdieu, P. 1986. The forms of capital. In *Handbook of theory and research,* ed. J. C. Richardson, 241–258. Westport: Greenwood.

Bourgon, J. 2008. The future of public service: A search for a new balance. *The Australian Journal of Public Administration* 67 (4): 390–404.

Bowden, B. 2006. Civil society, the state, and the limits to global civil society. *Global Society* 20 (2): 155–178.
Bradbury, H., and P. Reason. 2001. *Action learning and action research handbook. Participative Inquiry and Practice*. London: Sage.
Brassett, J., and D. Bulley. Ethics in world politics: Cosmopolitanism and Beyond? *International politics* 44:1–18.
Braun, K., S. L. Herrmann, S. Konninger, and A. Moore. 2010. Ethical reflection must always be measured. *Science, Technology and Human Values* 34 (6): 839–864.
Brewer, M., and M. Hewstone, eds. 2004. *Social cognition*. Oxford: Blackwell.
Brook Lyndhurst. 2004. Liveability and sustainable development: Bad habits and hard choices. Final report for ODPM, London: Brook Lyndhurst.
Brown, A. J., ed. 2008. Whistleblowing in the Australian public sector. ANU E-Press.
Brown, B. 2012. Global democracy alone will save us from ourselves. Forum *The Saturday Age,* 31 March, 20.
Brown, L. D., and J. Fox. 2001. Transnational civil society coalitions and the world bank: Lessons from project and policy influence campaigns. In *Global citizen action,* eds. M. Edwards, and J. Gaventa. Boulder: Lynne Rienner.
Brown, G. W., and D. Held, eds. 2010. *Cosmopolitan reader*. Cambridge: Polity Press.
Brundtland, G. 1987. The report "Our common future". http://www.worldinbalance.net/agreements/1987-brundtland.html.
Buettner, D. 2013. Live slow, die old. *The Australian Magazine,* 2–3rd Feb.
Burns, D. 2007. *Systemic action research. A strategy for whole system change*. Bristol: Policy Press.
Burroway, M. 1982. The written and the repressed in Gouldner's industrial sociology. *Journal Theory and Society* 11 (6): 831–851.
Butler, J. 2005. *Giving an account of oneself.* New York: Fordham University Press.
Butler, J. 2011. Precarious life: The obligations of proximity. 28 May 2011. The Neale Wheeler Watson Lecture 2011, given by Professor Judith Butler. Nobel Museum: Svenska. http://www.youtube.com/watch?v=KJT69AQtDtg.
Caldwell, C. 2011. Debt fuels Finn anger at European free loaders. *Weekend Australian,* 16–17.
Calland, R. 2013. *The Zuma years: South Africa's challenging face of power*. Cape Town: Zebra Press.
Cameron, F. 2004. *The future of Europe: Integration and enlargement*. London: Routledge.
Caney, S. 2008. Global distributive justice and the state. *Political Studies* 56 (3): 487–518.
Capra, F. 1996. *The web of life: A new synthesis of mind and matter*. New York: Harper Collins.
Carens, J. 1995. Aliens and citizens: The case for open borders. In *The rights of minority cultures,* ed. W. Kymlicka. Oxford: Oxford University Press.
Carrington, D. 2013. Global carbon dioxide in atmosphere passes milestone. *Guardian Weekly,* 17 May 2013, 13.
Cashdan, B. 2002. Local government and poverty in South Africa. In *Democratising local government. The South African experiment,* eds. S. Parnell, E. Pieterse, M. Swilling, and D. Wooldridge. Lansdowne: University of Cape Town Press.
Castells, M. 1998. *The information age: Economy, society and identity*. Malden Mass: Blackwell.
Charlton, A. 2011. Man-made world: Choosing between progress and the planet. *Quarterly Essay,* Issue 44.
Charmaz, K. 2000. Grounded theory: Objectivist and constructivist methods. In *Handbook of Qualitative Research.* 2nd ed. eds. N. Denzin, and Y. Lincoln. London: Sage.
Chalmers, D. 1995. Facing up to the problem of consciousness. *Journal of Consciousness Studies* 2 (3/1): 200–219.
Chase-Dunn, C. 2010. Globalisation from below. *Journal of Globalisation Studies* 146–157.
Checkland, P., and J. Scholes. 1990. *Soft systems methodology in action*. Chichester: Wiley.
Chevalier, J. M. 2009. *The new energy crisis: Climate, economics and geopolitics*. London: Palgrave Macmillan.

Chomsky, N. 2003. *Hegemony or survival: America's quest for global dominance*. Crow's Nest: Allen and Unwin.

Christakis, A. 2004. Wisdom of the people. *Systems research and behavioural science* 21 (5): 479–488.

Christakis, A. 2006. A retrospective structural inquiry into the predicament of humankind: Prospectus of the club of Rome. In *Rescuing the enlightenment from itself. Critical and systemic implications of democracy,* vol. 1. ed. J. McIntyre-Mills. (C. West Churchman and Related Works Series editor J. Van Gigch). London: Springer.

Christakis, A., and K. Bausch. 2006. *How people harness their collective wisdom and power to construct the future in co-laboratories of democracy*. Greenwich: Information Age Publishing.

Christakis, A., and T. Flanagan. 2010. *The talking point: A collaboration project of 21st century Agoras*. Greenwich: Information Age Publishing.

Churchman, C. West. 1971. *The design of inquiring systems*. New York: Basic Books.

Churchman, C. West. 1979. *The systems approach and its enemies*. New York: Basic Books.

Churchman, C. West. 1982. *Thought and wisdom*. California: Intersystems Publications.

Coates, R. 2011. *Covert racism, identity, experiences, issues and theory*. London: Oxford University Press (in press).

Cobbett, E., and R. Germain. 2012. 'Occupy wall street' and IPE: Insights and Implications. *Journal of Critical Globalisation Studies* (5): 110–113.

Collins, R. 1981. 'Microfoundations of macro sociology', University of Chicago Press. *The American Journal of Sociology*. http://www.jstor.org/stable/2778745. Accessed 05 June 2011.

Collins, P. 2000. *Black feminist thought: Knowledge, consciousness and the politics of empowerment*. New York: Routledge.

Collins, R. 2004. *Interaction ritual chains*. Princeton: Princeton University Press.

Collins, R. 2008. *Violence: A micro-sociological theory*. Princeton: Princeton University Press.

Collins. R. 2010. Geopolitical conditions of internationalism, human rights and world law. *Journal of Globalisation Studies* 1:29–45.

Comaroff, J. 2011. '*Theory from the South: Or how Europe is evolving towards Africa'*. Key note address at Knowledge and value in a Globalising world. Disentangling dichotomies, querying unities. University of Western Australia, Perth, 5–5th July.

Condon, P. M. 2008. *Design charrettes for sustainable communities*. Washington: Island Press.

Conrad, P. 2013. A less perfect union. December–January. *The Monthly*.

Connell, L. 2012. Human Trafficking for sexual exploitation in Australia: The deafening silence of demand. Thesis submitted for PhD, University of Victoria, Australia.

Cook, N. 2012. Canadian development workers, transnational encounters and cultures of cosmopolitanism. *International Sociology* 2 (1): 3–21.

Cooke, B. 2004. Rules of thumb for participatory change agents. In *Participation: From Tyranny to transformation*? New York: Zed Books.

Cox, E. 1995. *A truly civil society. Boyer Lectures*. Sydney: ABC Books.

Crish, J., and B. Fayne. 2009. Invisible crisis: Urban food security in Southern Africa. *Food Security Network*. No. 1.

Crish, J., and B. Fayne. 2010. Pathways to insecurity: Urban food supply and access in Southern African cities. *Food Security Network*. No. 3.

Crocker, D. 1995. Functioning and capability: The foundations of Sen's and Nussbaum's development ethic, Part 2. In *Women, culture and development: A study of human capabilities,* eds. M. Nussbaum and J. Glover. Oxford: Clarendon Press.

Crossen, T., and V. Niessen. 2007. NGO standing in the European Court of Justice—Does the Aarhus regulation open the door? *RECEIL* 16 (3): 332–338. ISSN 09628797 at 332.

Crowder, G. 2003. Hedgehog and fox. *Australian Journal of Political Science* 38 (2): 333–377.

Crowder, G. 2003. Pluralism, relativism and liberalism in Isaiah Berlin. Refereed paper presented to the Australasian political studies association conference University of Tasmania, Hobart. 29 Sept–1 Oct.

Crowder, G. 2004. *Isaiah Berlin. Liberty and pluralism*. Cambridge: Polity Press.

Crowley, M. 2011. An Obama doctrine? What drives the president's decisions during the historic convulsions of the 2011 Arab Spring? White House Memo. *Time,* 11 April.

Cruddas, J. 2013. Filling labour's 'One nation' policy blanks | Politics |. *The Guardian.* http://www.guardian.co.uk/politics/2013/may/16/jon-cruddas-labour-policy.

Cruz, I., A. Stahel, and M. Max-Neef. 2009. Towards a systemic development approach: Building on the human scale development paradigm. *Ecological Economics* 68:2021–2030.

Csikszentmihalyi, M. 1991. *The psychology of optimal experience*. New York: Harper and Row.

Dahl, R. 1967. The city in the future of democracy. *The American Political Science Review* 61 (4): 953–970.

Davies, M. 2008. *Asking the law question*. 3rd ed. Sydney: Thomson Law Book Co.

Davies, J. B., and World Institute. 2008. *Personal wealth*. OXford: Oxford University Press.

Dawkins, R. 1976. *The selfish gene*. Oxford: Oxford University Press.

Dawkins, R. 2006. *The god delusion*. Berkshire: Black Swan.

De Tocqueville, A. 1945. *Democracy in America*. New York: Knopf.

De Waal, F. 2006. Morally evolved: Primate social instincts, human morality, and the rise and fall of Veneer Theory. In *Primates and philosophers: How morality evolved,* eds. S. Macedo, and J. Ober. Princeton: Princeton University Press, Princeton Science Library.

De Waal, F. 2009. *The age of empathy: Nature's lessons for a kinder society*. Easton: Harmony.

Dean, J. 2009. *Democracy and other neo-liberal fantasies: Communicative capitalism and left politics*. London: Duke University Press.

Dean, J. 2012. *The communist horizon*. London: Verso.

Derrida, J. 2005. *The politics of friendship*. London: Verso.

Derrida, J. The principle of hospitality. *Parallax* 11 (1)

Desai, M. 2005. Social democracy as world panacea. In *Debating globalization,* eds. D. Held, et al. Cambridge: Polity Press.

Douglas, M. 1978. *Purity and danger. An analysis of the concepts of pollution and taboo*. London: Routledge and Kegan Paul.

Drahos, P. 2005. An alternative framework for the global regulation of intellectual property rights. Working paper forthcoming Austrian Journal of Development Studies. http://cgkd.anu.edu.au/menus/workingpapers.

Dryzek, J. 1999. *Democratising rationality in discursive democracys*. Cambridge: Cambridge University Press.

Dryzek, J. 2000. *Deliberative democracy and beyond*. Oxford: Oxford University Press.

Dryzek. J. 2005. *The politics of the earth. Environmental discourses*, 156–157. 2nd ed. New York: Oxford University Press.

Dryzek, J. 2010. *Green democracy*. Cunningham Lecture Series, ANU, Occasional Paper.

Du Gay, P. 2005. Bureaucracy and liberty: State, authority and freedom. In *The values of democracy*. Oxford University Press.

Dyson, F. 2013. http://www.edge.org/3rd_culture/dyson_ad/dyson_ad_index.html. Downloaded 11 March 2013.

Eckers, M, and A. Loftus. 2008. The power of water. *Environment and Planning: Society and Space* 26:698–718.

Eder, K. 1996. Part 3: The politics of the environment: Exhaustion or renewal. The institutionalisation of environmentalism: Ecological discourse and the second transformation of the public sphere. In *Risk, environment and modernity. Towards a New Ecology,* eds. S. Lash, B. Szerzynski, and B. Wynne. London: Sage.

Edgar, D. 2001. *The patchwork nation: Rethinking government-rebuilding community*. Sydney: Harper.

Edwards, M., and J. Gaventa. 2001. *Global citizen action*. Boulder: Lynne Rienner.

Eisenbergerger, N. I., and M. D. Lieberman. 2004. Why rejection hurts. *Trends in Cognitive Science* 8:294–300.

Elias, N., and P. Lichterman. 2003. Culture in interaction. *The American Journal of Sociology* 108 (4): 735–794.

Elkington, J. 1994. Globalisation's reality checks. In *Debating globalization,* eds. H. Held, et al. Cambridge: Polity Press.

Elkington, J. 1997. *Cannibals with forks*. Oxford: Capstone.

Elliot, A. 2002. Beck's sociology of risk: A critical assessment. *Sociology* 36:293–315.

Elliot, A. 2012. Life on the move: Mobilities in a global age. Public Lecture, Flinders University 19th June. Victoria Square.

Elliot, A., and J. Urry. 2010. *Mobile lives*. New York: Routledge.

Etzioni, A. 2004. *From empire to community: A new approach to international relations*. New York: Palgrave Macmillan.

Etzioni, A. 2010. Unmanned aircraft systems: The moral and legal case. JJFQFQ/issue 57, 2nd quarter, 77–71.

Etzioni, A. 2012. The domestic sources of global adhocracy. *Social Change Review* 10 (2).

Evans, M. 2013. Confronting insecure employment. *Advocate* 20 (3): 28.

Evatt, H. V. 1984. *'Introduction' The Eureka stockade*. 1st ed. By Carboni, R. 1855. Melbourne: Atkinson and Co.

Eyerman, R. 1981. False consciousness and ideology in Marxist theory. Acta Sociologica. On behalf of the Nordic Sociological Association. Downloaded Flinders University 31 July 2001. http://www.sagepublications.com.

Faist, T. 2009. The transnational social question. *International Sociology* 24:17–36.

Farrell, H. 2012. The consequences of the internet for politics. *Annual Review of Political Science* 15:35–5 (online).

Fenby, J. 2013. Scandals undermine Chinas regime. *The Guardian Weekly,* 17 May 2013, 20.

Flanagan, T., and K. Bausch. 2011. *A democratic approach to sustainable futures. A workbook for addressing the global problematique*. Riverdale: Ongoing Emergence Press.

Flannery, T. 2005. *The weather makers. The history and future impact of climate change*. Melbourne: Text Publishing.

Flannery, T. 2010. *Here on earth. An argument for hope.* Melbourne: Text Publishing.

Flannery, T. 2012. After the future: Australia's new extinction crisis. *Quarterly Essay* Issue 48.

Flood, R., and E. Carson. 1993. *Dealing with complexity: An introduction to the theory and application of systems science*. 2nd ed. London: Plenum.

Flood, R., and N. Romm. 1996. *Diversity management: Triple loop learning*. Chichester: Wiley.

Florini, A. 2003. *The coming democracy*. Washington DC: Island Press.

Flyvberg, B. 1998. Habermas and Foucault. *British Journal of Society* 49 (2): 200–232.

Folke, C. 2006. Resilience: The emergence of a perspective for social-ecological systems analyses. *Global Environmental Change* 16:253–267.

Follesdal, A. 2006. Subsidiarity, democracy and human rights in Europe. *Journal of Social Philosophy* 37 (1): 61–80.

Foucault, M., and Gordon, C., eds. 1980. *Power/Knowledge*. Brighton: Harvester.

Fougere, G. 2007. *Wellbeing is an idea whose time has come. New opportunities for health impact assessment in New Zealand public policy and planning*. Wellington: The Public Health Advisory Committee.

Fourade, M., and J. Savelsburg. 2006. Global processes, national institutions, local bricolage: Shaping law in an era of globalisation. *Law and Social Inquiry* 31 (3): 515–519.

Fowler, J. H., and N. Christakis. 2010. Cooperative behavior cascades in human social networks. *Proceedings of the National Academy of Sciences* 107 (9): 5334–5338.

Fox, D. 2011. The limits of intelligence: The laws of physics may well prevent the human brain from evolving into an ever more powerful thinking machine. *Scientific American*. (Online 14 June). http://www.scientificamerican.com/article.cfm?id=the-limits-of-intelligence/. Accessed 29 Aug 2013.

Frank, R. H. 2007. *Falling behind: How rising inequality harms the middle class*. Berkley: California Press.

Frankl, V. 1955. *The doctor and the soul: From psychotherapy to logotherapy*. New York: Vintage.

Freire, P. 1973. Creating alternative research methods: Learning to do it by doing it. In Creating knowledge: A monopoly? eds B. Hall, A Gillette, R. Tandon (pp. 29 -37). Khanpur, New Delhi: Society for Participatory Research in Asia.

Friere, P. 1985. *The politics of education*. Westport: Begin and Garvey, Inc.

Freire, P. 1997. *Pedagogy of the heart*. New York: Continuum.

Fukuyama, F. 2002. *Our post human future*. New York: Farrar, Struas and Giroux.

Fukuyma, F. 2004. *State building: Governance and world order in the 21st century*. Ithaca: Cornell University Press.

Gadamar, H. G. 2001. Education is self-education. *Journal of Philosophy of Education* 35 (4): 529–538.

Gallhofer, S., and A. Chew. 2000. Introduction: Accounting and indigenous peoples. *Accounting, Auditing and Accountability Journal* 13 (3): 256–267.

Galtung, J. 1990. Cultural violence. *Journal of Peace Research* 27 (3): 291–305. (Sage).

Gamble, A. 2000. Economic governance. In *Debating governance: Authority, steering and democracy*. 1st ed. ed. J. Pierre. Oxford: Oxford University Press.

Gandhi, L. 1966. Affective communities: Anti-colonial thought, fin-de-siècle radicalism and the politics of friendship. Durham: Duke University Press.

Garnaut, J. 2009. Crowd vents fury at police after bloodshed. *Sydney Morning Herald,* 8 July.

Garnaut, R. 2011. *The Garnaut review: Australia in the global response to climate change*. Melbourne: Cambridge University Press.

Garnaut, J. 2013. China muscles US in the Pacific. *The Age,* 1.

Gaventa, J. 2001a. Global citizen action: Lessons and challenges. In *Global citizen action,* eds. M. Edwards, and J. Gaventa. Boulder: Lynne Rienner.

Geertz, C. 1973. Thick description: Towards an interpretive theory of culture. In *The interpretation of cultures. Selected essays,* ed. C. Geertz, 3–32. New York: Basic books.

Geertz, C. 1980. *Negara: The theatre state in nineteenth century Bali*. Princeton: Princeton University Press.

Geertz, C. 2004. What is a state if it is not sovereign? Reflections on politics in complicated places. *Current Anthropology* 45:577–593.

Getano Lui. 1993. *Voices from the Land*. Boyer lecture Series.

Gibbons, M., C. Limoges, H. Nowotny, S. Schwartzman, P. Scott, and M. Trow. 1994. *The new production of knowledge: The dynamics of science and research in contemporary societies*. London: Sage.

Giddens, A. 2009. *The politics of climate change*. Cambridge: Polity Press.

Goldsmith, J., and E. Posner. 2005. *The limits of international law*. Oxford: Oxford University Press.

Gore, A. 2007. *Assault on reason*. London: Bloomsbury.

Gould, C. 2007. Transnational solidarities. *Journal of Social Philosophy* 38 (1): 148–164.

Gouldner, A. W. 1971. *The coming crisis of western sociology*. London: Heinemann.

Graham, C. 2009. The economics of happiness. http://www.brookings.edu/.

Graham, C. 2011. *The pursuit of happiness: An economy of well-being*. Washington: Brookings Institution Press.

Graver, M. 2007. *Stoicism and emotion*. Chicago: University of Chicago Press.

Greenberg, G., and E. Tobach. 1987. *Cognition, language and consciousness: Integrative levels*. Vol. 2. Hillsdale New Jersey.

Greenfield, S. 2000. *The private life of the brain: Emotions, consciousness and the secret of the self*. New York: Wiley.

Greenfield. 2003. *Tomorrow's people how 21st century technology is changing the way we think and feel*. Baltimore: Penguin.

Greenfield, S. 2008. *ID: The quest for meaning in the 21st century*. London: Sceptre, Hodder and Stoughton.

Greenwald, G. 2012. New York's top court highlights the meaninglessness and menace of the term 'terrorism'. http://www.guardian.co.uk/commentisfree/2012/dec/16/court-terrorism-morales-gangs-meaningless.

Guddemi, P. 2006. Human views of ecological nature. *Cybernetics and Human Knowing* 12 (1): 86–90.
Habermas, J. 1984. *The theory of communicative action: Reason and the rationalization of society*. Beacon: Boston.
Habermas, J. 1989. *The structured transformation of the public sphere*. Cambridge: Polity Press.
Habermas, J. 2001. *The postnational constellation. Political essays*. Cambridge: Polity Press.
Habermas, J. 2008. *Between naturalism and religion*. Cambridge: Polity Press.
Habermas, J., and J. Derrida. 2003. February 15, or what binds Europeans together: A plea for a common foreign policy, beginning in the core of europe. *Constellations* 10 (3): 291–297.
Habermas, J., J. Derrida, and G. Borradori. 2003. *Philosophy in a time of terror dialogues with Jurgen Habermas and Jacques Derrida*. Chicago: University of Chicago Press.
Hammadi, S., and A. Kelly. 2013. Bangladesh's stark lesson for buyers. *Guardian Weekly,* 17 May 2013, p. 44.
Harris, J. 2013. Can labour transform for 2015? *Guardian Weekly,* 17 May 2013, p. 21.
Hua-Ching, N. 1989. *The complete works of Lao Tzu, Tao The Ching and Hua Hu Ching*. LA: College of Tao and Traditional Chinese Healing.
Haraway, D. 1991. *The reinvention of nature*. London: Free Association Books.
Haraway, D. 1992. The promises of monsters: A regenerative politics for inappropriated others. In *Cultural Studies*, eds. L. Grossberg, C. Nelson, P. A. Treichler, 295–337. New York: Routledge.
Haraway, D. 2010. Speculative fabulations for technoculture's generations: Taking care of unexpected country. *Australian University E press*. http://epress.anu.edu.au/guidelines/author_guidelines.html.
Hardin, G. 1968. The tragedy of the commons. *Science* 162:1243–1248.
Harris, L. D., and J. Wasilewski. 2004. Indigenous wisdom of the people's forum. *Systems Research and Behavioural Science* 21:505–514.
Harrison, K. 2002. Policy perspectives: Social capital. In *Democratising local government. The South African experiment,*s eds. S. Parnell, M. Swilling, and D. Wooldridge. Landsdowne: University of Cape Town Press.
Hassan, R. 2008. *Inside Muslim minds*. Melbourne: Melbourne University Press.
Hayden, P. 2010. The environment, global justice and world environmental citizenship. In *Cosmopolitanism,* eds. G. W. Brown, and D. Held. Cambridge: Polity Press.
Hegel, G. W. F. 1977. *Phenomenology of the spirit* (trans: Miller, A. V.). Oxford: Oxford University Press.
Held, D. 2004. Global covenant: The social democratic alternative to the Washington consensus. Polity Press.
Held, D. et al. 2005. *Debating globalization*. Cambridge: Polity Press.
Held, D., McGrew, A., Goldblatt, D., and Perraton. 1999. *Global transformations. Politics economics and culture*. Stanford: Stanford University Press.
Heller, P. 2001. Moving the state: The politics of democratic decentralisation in Kerela, South Africa, and Porto Alegra. *Politics and Society* 29 (1): 131–163.
Heycox, J., P. Meadows, and B. Vernon. 1997. Environment and energy statistics section Australian bureau of statistics. Measuring environmental expenditures and revenues in Local Government. Australian Centre for Regional & Local Government Studies Working Paper No 2. University of Canberra.
Hickey, S., and G. Mohan eds. 2004. *Participation: From tyranny to transformation?* New York: Zed Books.
Hil, R. 2013. Beyond the cyber cell. *Advocate* 20 (3): 28–29.
Hill Collins, P. 2000. *Blacks feminist thought: Knowledge, consciousness and the politics of Empowerment*. New York: Routledge.
Hinnells, J. R. 1984. *A handbook of living religions*. London: Penguin.
Hirschman, A. O. 1970. Exit, voice, and loyalty: Responses to decline in firms, organizations, and states. Cambridge: Harvard University Press.

HM Government. 2005. Securing the future: Delivering UK sustainable development. Strategy presented to parliament by the secretary of state for environment, food and rural affairs by command of Her Majesty, March 2005. HMSO: St Clements House, 2–16 Colegate, Norwich.
Hobbes, T. Leviathan. http://ebooks.adelaide.edu.au/h/hobbes/thomas/h68l/index.html. Accessed 25 June 2012.
Hobson-West, P. 2007. Beasts and boundaries: An introduction to animals in sociology. Science and Society. *Qualitative Sociology Review* 3 (1): 23–41.
Hoggett, P. 2010. *Politics, identity and emotion*. Boulder: Paradigm.
Hoggett, P., and S. Thomson. 2002. Towards a democracy of emotions. *Constellations* 9 (1): 102–126.
Holloway, J. 2011. The economic platform of the Australian greens, philosophy, policy and electoral appeal. Flinders University Honours Thesiss.
Hooks, B. 1989. *Talking back*. Boston: South End.
Horvath, Z., and B. Odor. *The union after Lisbon. The treaty reform of the EU*. Hungary: HVG-ORAC Publishing. http://www.eurozine.com/articles/2006-12-23-baubock-en.html. Accessed 19 Dec 2012.
Hulme, M. 2009. *Why we disagree about climate change*. Cambridge: Cambridge University Press.
Hulme, M. 2010. Cosmopolitan climates. Hybridity, foresight and meaning. *Theory, Culture and Society* 27 (2–3): 267–276.
Hulme, M. 2011. Climate change and four narratives of growth. AHTC workshop. University of Cambridge. http://climatehistories.innerasiaresearch.org/wp-content/uploads/2011/01/Mike-Hulme.pdf. Accessed 8 Feb 2011.
Huntington, S.1996. *The clash of cultures and the remaking of the world order*. New York: Simon and Schuster.
Husserl, E. 1970. *The crisis of European sciences*. (trans: Carr, David). Evanston: Northwestern University Press.
icps.gwu.edu/. The good life: An international perspective. There's a future: Visions for a better world. https://docs.google.com/viewer?a=v&q=cache:8rnWNHvfIcAJ:icps.gwu.edu/files/2013/02/The-Good-Life-An-International-Perspective.pdf+the+good+life++an+international+perspective+%2B+etzioni&hl=en&gl=au&pid=bl&srcid=ADGEESgpk7jXTiA7uWJH2nWGJm4gOc8rGDjuAHm-oeyW7IQl.
Ingold, T. 1993. The temporality of the landscape (Conceptions of time and ancient society). *World Archeology* 25 (2): 152–174.
International Commission on the Future of Food and Agriculture. 2007. Manifesto on the future of seeds. www.future-food.org.
Irvine, L. 2007. The question of animal selves: Implications for sociological knowledge and practice. *Qualitative Sociology Review* 3 (1): 5–22.
Irvin, R., and J. Stansbury. 2002. Citizen participation in decision making. *Public Administrative Review* 64 (1): 55–65.
Irwin, T. 1985. *Aristotle Nicomachean ethics* (trans). Cambridge: Cambridge University Press.
Ison, R. 2005. Geoffrey Vickers: Contemporary applications and changing appreciative settings. *Systems Research and Behavioural Science* 22 (4): 277–284 (July–Aug).
Jackson, M. 1991. *Systems methodology for the management sciences*. London: Plenum.
Jamieson, D. 2008. *Ethics and the environment: An introduction*. Cambridge: Cambridge University Press.
Jamrozik, A. 2001. *Social policy in the post welfare state: Australians on the threshold of the 21st century*. NSW: Longman.
Jasonoff, S. 2003. Technologies of humility: Citizen participation in governing science. *Minerva* 41:223–244.
Jessop, S. 2009. Children's participation: An Arendtian criticism. *Educational Philosophy and Theory* 43 (9). Article first published online: 8 Nov 2009. doi:10.1111/j1469–5812.2009.00560.x.
Judt, T. 2010. *Ill fares the land*. London: Penguin.

Kabeer, N., and R. Subrahmanian. 1996. Institutions, relations and outcomes: Framework and tools for gender-aware planning. Institute of Development Studies Discussion Paper, No. 357, Brighton, UK.

Kahane, A. 1992. The Mont Fleur scenarios: What will South Africa be like in the year 2002?' *Deeper News*, Vol. 7 Number 1 republication of The Weekly Mail and Guardian Weekly.

Kaldor, M. 2003. *Global civil society: An answer to war*. Cambridge: Polity Press.

Kaldor, M. 2004. *What is human security? Debating globalisation. Open Democracy Debate*. Cambridge: Polity Press.

Kanai, R., B. Bahrami, R. Roylance, and G. Rees. 2011 Online social network size is reflected in human brain structure. Proceedings of Royal Biological Society B. (Published online 19 Oct 2011).

Kant, I. 1976. *The moral law* (trans Paton, H.J.). Oxford: Hutchinson.

Karni, A., ed. 2006. *A celebration of democracy*. Yogyakarta: Wahid Institute and Asia Foundation.

Kauffman, L. 2006. Virtual boundaries. *Cybernetics and Human Knowing* 13 (2): 94–104.

Keane, J. 2009a. *The life and death of democracy*. London: Simon and Schuster.

Keane, J. 2009b. Democracy failure: The root of the global economic crisis is political. http://scholar.google.com.au/scholar?cites=16220241904322824583&as_sdt=2005&sciodt=0,5&hl=en. Accessed 31 March 2011.

Khisty, C. J. 2006. A fresh look at the systems approach and an agenda for action: Peeking through the lens of Churchman's aphorisms. *Systemic Practice and Action Research* 19 (1): 3–25.

Kickert, W. J. M., E. H. Klijn, and J. F. M. Koppenjan. 1999. *Managing complex networks: Strategies for the public sector*. London: Sage.

Kirby, M. 2011. Animals deserve our protection. *Weekend Australian,* Oct 1–2:22.

Kivisto, P., and T. Faist. 2007. Citizenship, discourse, theory, and transnational prospects. Oxford: Blackwell.

Kolben, K. 2011. Transnational labor regulation and the limits of governance. *Theoretical Inquiries in Law* 12 (2) Article no 2.

Korsgaard, C. 2006. Morality and the distinctiveness of human Action. In *Primates and philosophers: How morality evolved,* eds. S. Macedo, and J. Ober. Princeton: Princeton University Press.

Koskenniemi, M. 2005. International law in Europe: Between tradition and renewal. *The European Journal of International Law* 16 (1): 113–124.

Kundera, M. 1984. *The unbearable lightness of being*. New York: Harper and Row.

Kymlicka, W. 2001. Politics in the vernacular: Nationalism, multiculturalism and citizenship. Oxford: Oxford University Press.

Kymlicka, W. 2010. Citizenship in an era of globalization. In *Cosmopolitan reader,* eds. G. W. Brown, and D. Held. Cambridge: Polity Press.

La Forgia, R. 2009. The politics of international law: Twenty years later: A reply to Martti Koskenniemi. *The European Journal of International Law* 20 (4): 979–984, at 993.

Lane, R. J. 2000. *Jean Baudrillard*. London: Routledge.

Laszlo, A. 2000. *The epistemological foundations of evolutionary systems design*. In Proceedings of the world congress of the systems sciences and ISSS 2000 international society for the systems sciences 44th annual meeting, (ed. Allen J. K, Wilby, J.). Toronto, Canada.

Lawn, P. 2010. Ecological economics: The impact of unsustainable growth. In *Routledge handbook of climate change and society,* ed. C. Lever-Tracey, 453–472.

Layard, R. 2005. *Happiness*. London: Allen Lane.

Leonard, A. 1994. The very model of a modern system-general. In *Beyond dispute*, ed. S. Beer. Sussex: Wiley.

Leonard, A. 2011. Governance in the relative When. *Systems Research and Behavioural Science* 28:431–436.

Lever-Tracey, C. 2008. Global warming and sociology. *Current Sociology* 56 (3): 445–466.

Lever-Tracey, C. 2010. Alternative scenarios: Varieties of capitalism. In *Routledge handbook of climate change and society*, ed. C. Lever-Tracey, 274–279.

Lever-Tracey, C. 2011. Globalisation, climate change and bio-diversity. Sociology Seminar, Flinders University. Wednesday 10 Aug.

Lin, A. 2009. Geo-engineering governance issues in legal scholarship. Vol. 8, Issue 3. In *Balancing the risks: Managing technology and dangerous climate change,* 1–24. Berkeley: The Berkeley Electronic Press.

Lindblom, C. E. 1959. The science of muddling through. *Public Administration Review* 19 (2): 79–88.

Linklater, A. 1999. The evolving spheres of international justice. *International Affairs* 75 (3): 473–482.

Lloyd, G. 2012. King Coal still reigns. *The Australian Inquirer* April 28–29 p. 15.

Lovelock, J. 2006. *The revenge of Gaia: Why the earth is fighting back—and how we can still save humanity*. Santa Barbara: Allen Lane.

Lovelock, J. 2009. *The vanishing face of Gaia: A final warning: Enjoy it while you can*. Santa Barbara: Allen Lane.

Luhmann, P. 1995. *Social systems*. Stanford: Stanford University Press.

Lynch, J. 2011. Live cattle exports to resume with Darwin shipment by elders. *The Saturday Age,* 30 July p. 3.

Macedo, S., and J. Ober, eds. 2006. *Primates and philosophers: How morality evolved*. Princeton: Princeton Science Library, Princeton University Press.

Maguire, J. 1996. The tears inside the stone: Reflections on the ecology of fear. In *Risk, environment and modernity. Towards a New Ecology,* eds. S. Lash, B. Szerzynski, and B. Wynne. London: Sage.

Maloney, W. G. Jordan, and A. McLaughlin. 1994. Interest groups and public policy. *Journal of Public Policy* 14:17–38.

Manne, R. 2011. Robert Manne on Julian Assange: Essay (March, 17–35) See also the video line at the monthly.com. http://www.themonthly.com.au/wikileaks-free-speech-and-assanges-message-australia-3016.

March, C., I. Smyth, and M. Mukopadhyay. 1999. *A guide to gender-analysis frameworks*. Oxford: Oxfam.

Marx, K. 1843. A contribution to the critique of Hegel's philosophy of right in the Deutsch-Französische Jahrbücher, as published in Paris on the 7 & 10 Feb.

Mathews, F.1991. *The ecological self.* London: Routledge.

Mathews, F. 2010. Planet beehive. *Australian Humanities Review* 50:159–178.

Maturana, H., and F. Verela. 1980. *Autopoeisis and cognition: The realization of living*. Boston: Reidel.

Maturana, H. R., and F. J. Varela. 1987. *The tree of knowledge: The biological roots of human understanding*. London: New Science Library, Shambhala.

Max-Neef, M. 1991. *Human scale development*. London: Apex.

Mbabela, Z., and M. Kimberley. 2012. Rotten to the core: Why Eastern cape education is in crisis. *The Herald*, 26 Nov.

Mbigi, L., and J. Maree. 1995. *Ubuntu. The spirit of African transformation management*. Randburg: Knowledge Resources.

McCallum, I. 2005. *Ecological intelligence: Rediscovering ourselves in nature*. Cape Town: Africa Geographic.

McIntyre-Mills, J. 2000. *Global citizenship and social movements: Creating transcultural webs of meaning for the new millennium*. The Netherlands: Harwood.

McIntyre-Mills, J. 2003. *Critical systemic praxis. The Contemporary Systems Series*. London: Kluwer.

McIntyre-Mills, J., ed. 2006a. *Rescuing the enlightenment from itself: Critical and systemic implications for democracy*. C.West Churchman Series, vol. 1. London: Springer. ISBN:10 0-387 27587-8, ISBN:10: 0387-27589-4(e book).

McIntyre-Mills, J. 2006b. *Systemic governance and accountability: Working and re-working the conceptual and spatial boundaries of international relations and governance*. C.West Churchman Series, vol. 3. London: Springer.

McIntyre-Mills, J. 2008a. Ethics, energy and climate change. Systemic ethics: Social, economic and environmental implications of eating our yellow cake in South Australia. *Systems Research and Behavioural Science* 25 (2): 225–248. ISSN:1092–7026.
McIntyre-Mills, J. 2008b. Möbius bands and Mandelbrot sets as metaphors for systemic praxis. *Systems Research and Behavioral Science* 25 (2): 323–330.
McIntyre-Mills, J. 2009a. *User-centric design to meet complex needs,* 1–450. N.Y.: Nova Science. ISBN:1604566833.
McIntyre-Mills, J. 2009b. Ethics, boundaries and sustainable futures. In *Systemic development: Local solutions in a global environment,* ed. J. Sheffield. ISCE Publishing, and Litchfield.
McIntyre-Mills, J. 2010a. Representation, accountability and sustainability. *Cybernetics and Human Knowing* 17 (4): 51–80.
McIntyre-Mills, J. 2010b. Wellbeing, mindfulness and the global commons. *Journal of Consciousness Studies* 17 (7–8): 44–72.
McIntyre-Mills, J. 2011a. The food, energy and water crisis: The liberative potential of the Aarhus convention and transboundary governance to protect the global commons and the collective good. In Democratic participation in employment and societal regulation, ed. I. De Costa. Proceedings of the International Conference. At Ecole Normale Superieure de Cachan. Paris 27–30 June.
McIntyre-Mills, J. 2011b. The way forward? Controlling consumption through governance and participatory democracy: Learning less is more when living elegantly and ethically. Paper delivered in the session entitled: Democratic participation in Employment and Societal Regulation. Proceedings of the International Conference. At Ecole Normale Superieure de Cachan. Paris 27–30 June.
McIntyre-Mills, J. 2012a. Anthropocentricism and wellbeing: A way out of the lobster pot? *Systems Research and Behavioural Science*. Published online in Wiley Online Library. (wileyonlinelibrary.com) doi:10.1002/sres.2131.
McIntyre-Mills, J. 2012b. Wellbeing and existential risk. CASS research conference sustainable environmental policy and global governance, Beijing, 18–19 Sept (unpublished).
McIntyre-Mills, J. 2012c. Beyond containerism. UKSS conference, St Anne's College, Oxford.
McIntyre-Mills, J., and D. de Vries. 2009. How lemmings on wheels can make a U-turn through social inclusion and democracy. (Published online: 30 April 2009). *Systems Practice and Action Research* 22:173–200. doi:10.1007/s11213-009-9121-4.
McIntyre-Mills, J., and D. De Vries. 2010. Addressing complex needs. *International Journal of Interdisciplinary Social Sciences* 5 (5): 11–32.
McIntyre-Mills, J., and D. De Vries. 2011. *Identity, democracy and sustainability. Emergence,* 380. ISCE, USA, Litchfield.
McIntyre-Mills, J., and D. de Vries. 2012. Transformation from Wall Street to well-being. *Systems Research and Behavioural Science* First published online: 10 oct 2012. doi:10.1002/sres.2133.
McIntyre-Mills, J., D. De Vries, and J. Deakin. 2008a. Participatory democracy based on user-centric policy design to address complex needs. In *Citizenship in the 21st century,* eds. L. Kane, and M. Poweller, 1–54. New York: Nova Science. ISBN:10 1604564016.
McIntyre-Mills, J., K. Bausch, A. Christakis, and De Vries. 2008b. How can we break the mould? Democracy, semiotics and regional governance. *Systems Research and Behavioural Science* 25:305–321.
McLuhan, M., and B. R. Powers. 1989. *The global village: Transformations in world life in the 21st century*. Oxford: Oxford University Press.
Mead, G. H. 1982. *The individual and the social self.* London: Hogarth.
Meadowcroft, J. 2002. Politics and scale: Some implications for environmental governance. *Landscape and Urban Planning* 61:169–179. http://www.elsevier.com/locate/landurbplan.
Meadows, D., and J. Randers. 1992. *Beyond the limits. Global collapse of a sustainable future*. London: Earthscan.
Meagher, G., and S. Wilson. 2002. Complexity and practical knowledge in the social sciences. *British Journal of Sociology* 53 (4): 659–666.

Michels, R. 1915. *Political parties: A sociological study of the oligarchical tendencies of modern democracy* (trans: Eden and Paul, C. 2001). Kitchener: Batoche Books.

Midgley, G. 2000. *Systemic intervention: Philosophy, methodology, and practice*. New York: Kluwer.

Miller McPherson, L., L. Smith-Lovin, and J. M. Cook. 2001. Birds of a feather: Homophily in social networks. *Annual Review of Sociology* 27:415–444.

Miller, D. 1999. Bounded citizenship. In *Cosmopolitan citizenship*, eds. K. Hutchinson, and Dannreuther. London: Macmillan.

Ministry of Environmental Affairs and Tourism, South Africa. 2004. Enviropaedia. May. Government Publication.

Monbiot, G. 2013. Money just makes the rich suffer. *Guardian Weekly*, 17 May 2013, 9.

Mugabushaka, J. 2012. Life chances of women and children in the failed state of the Congo. PhD thesis, Flinders University.

Mukta, P. 2005. Food and water: Dams, development and transnational struggles. *Global Networks*, 5 (3): 301–306 (Oxford).

Mukta, P. 2012. Who or what do we care about in the 21st century? *International Sociology* 27 (4): 446–463.

Murray, J. et al. 2006. Systems for social sustainability: Global connectedness and the Tuvalu test. Tuvalu at the common wealth games. Melbourne. Photograph by Geoff Ludbrook www.isa.org.usyd.edu.au/publications/documents/ Tuvalu_Test.pdf.

Murray, J., C. Dey, and M. Lenzen. 2007. Systems for social sustainability: Global connectedness and the Tuvalu test. *Cybernetics and Human Knowing* 14 (1): 87–105.

Nagel, T. 2010. The problem of global justice. In *Cosmopolitan reader*, eds. G. W. Brown, and D. Held. Cambridge: Polity Press.

Nagoya Summit. 2010. http://www.cbd.int/2011–2020/. Accessed 19 Dec 2011.

Nakamori, Y., A. Wierzbicki, and Z. Zhu. 2011. A theory of knowledge construction. *Systems Research and Behavioural Science* 28:15–39.

Nathan, D., and S. Sarkar. 2010. Blood on your mobile? *Economic and Political Weekly* xiv (43).

Nathan, L. 2012. Solidarity trumps rule of law. *Mail and Guardian* p. 21.

Nazarea, V. 2006. Local knowledge and memory in biodiversity conservation. *Annual Review of Anthropology* 36:317–335.

Needham, K. 2011. Concern at rising number of detainees self-harming. *The Saturday Age*, 30 July p. 6.

Newton, T., and G. Harte. 1997. Green business: Technicist kitsch? *Journal of Management Studies* 75–98.

Ng, C. 2011. National resilience: Developing a whole-of-society response: A more robust society begins with clarity about shared priorities, risks, constraints and capabilities. *Ethos* 10:21–29.

Nguyen, N., O. Bosch, and K. Maani. 2011. Learning laboratories for sustainable development in biospheres. *Systems Research and Behavioural Science* 28:51–62.

Nietzsche, F. W. 1967. *On the genealogy of morals* (trans: Kauffman Walter). New York: Vintage.

Northrop, FSC and M. Gross. 1961. *Alfred north whitehead: An anthology*. New York: Macmillan.

Nussbaum, M. 1986. *The fragility of goodness: Luck and ethics in Greek tragedy and philosophy*. Cambridge University Press.

Nussbaum, M. 2001. *Upheavals of thought: The intelligence of emotions*. Cambridge University Press.

Nussbaum, M. 2006. *Frontiers of justice*. London: Harvard University Press.

Nussbaum, M., and A. Sen. 1993. *Quality of life*. New York: Clarendon Press.

Nussbaum, M., and J. Glover. 1995. *Women, culture and development: A study of human capabilities*. Oxford: Clarendon Press.

Nye, J. 1990. *Bound to lead: The changing nature of American power*. New York: Basic Books.

Nye, J. 2008. Public diplomacy and soft power. *Annals of the American Academy of Political Power and Social Science* 616:94–109.

Nye, J. Soft power. http://www.abc.net.au/tv/bigideas/stories/2012/05/07/3494634.htm.

O' Neill, B. 2011. New spectre of technocracy is haunting Europe. *The Weekend Australian*. http://www.theaustralian.com.au/national-affairs/opinion/new-spectre-of-technocracy-is-haunting-europe/story-e6frgd0x-1226199444149. Accessed 22 Nov 2011.

O'Connor, M. and W.J. Lines. 2010. *Overloading Australia. How governments and media dither and deny on population*. Canterbury: Envirobook.

O'Hara, M. 1985. Of myths and monkeys: A critical look at a theory of critical mass. *Journal of Humanistic Psychology* 25:61.

Ockwell, D., S. O'Neill, and L. Whitmarsh. 2010. Behavioural insights: Motivating individual emissions cuts through communication, *Routledge Handbook of Climate Change and Society*. ed. Lever-Tracey, 341–350.

Odum, H.T. 1996. *Environmental accounting: Energy and environmental decision making*. New York: Wiley.

Official Journal of the European Union. 2009. C115, Volume 51. http://europa.eu. Accessed 9 July 2009.

Olayiwola, A. 2002. Truth and reconciliation. *African Studies Review*45 (3): 31–34. New York: Organization, Basic Books.

Orwell, G. 1984. Machine-readable version and checking: O. Dag. Last modified on April 23, 2002. MSKOrwell.

Osborn, D. 1997a. A rationale and approach for applying environmental accounting frameworks in local government. *Australian Centre for Regional and Local Government Studies,* University of Canberra, Working Paper No 1.

Osborn, D. 1997b. Interpreting measures of local government's environmental protection payments and revenues. *Australian Centre for Regional and Local government studies, University of Canberra,* Working Paper No 3.

Osler, A and H. Starkeyb. 2005. Violence in schools and representations of young people: A critique of government policies in France and England. *Oxford Review of Education* 31 (2): 195–215.

Ozbekan, H. 1970. On some of the fundamental problems in planning. *Technological Forecasting* 1 (3): 235–240.

Palombi, L. 2007. Trips, bilateralism and patents: How they are failing both the developed and the developing world and what to do about it. *Electronic Journal in Communication, Information and Innovation in Health* 1 (1): 71–81

Pape, R. A. 2005. *Dying to win: The strategic logic of suicide terrorism*. New York: Random House.

Parker, J. 2012. Transdisciplinary systems approach to paradigm change in sustainable economy. In *The Systemist* 34 (3): 138–149.

Parry, M., C. Rosenzweig, A. Iglesias, G. Fischer, and M. Livermore. 1999. Climate change and world food security: A new assessment. *Global Environmental Change*. S51–S67. Elsevier. Available online 25 October. Accessed 7th Feb 2011.

Paskal, C. 2007. How climate change is pushing the boundaries of security and foreign policy. Chatham house. http://www.chathamhouse.org.uk/files/9250_bp0607climatecp.pdf. (Consulted June 2011).

Perls, F. S., R. Hefferline, and P. Goodman. 1951. *Gestalt therapy*. New York: Delta.

Pert, C. 1997. *Molecules of emotion*. New York: Scriber.

Pichler, F. 2012. Cosmopolitanism in a global perspective: An international comparison of open-minded orientations and identity in relation to globalization. *International Sociology* 2 (1): 21–50.

Pierre, J. ed. 2000. *Debating governance: Authority, steering and democracy*. Oxford: University Press.

Pilger, J. 2002. *The new rulers of the world*. London: Verso.

Planet Ark. 2007. *The recycling olympic report*. Sydney: Planet Ark Environmental Foundation.

Pretty, J. 2013. The consumption of a finite planet: Well-being, convergence, divergence and the Nascent green economy. *Environmental and Resource Economics*. doi:10.1007/s10640-013-9680-9.

Poe, D. 2010. Subsidiarity and the bias for the local, *Journal of Globalisation Studies* 1:131–140.

Pogge, T. W. 2001. *Global justice*. Malden: Blackwell.
Pogge, T. 1992. 'Cosmopolitanism and sovereignty. *Ethics* 103:48–75.
Pogge, T. 2002. *World poverty and human rights: Cosmopolitan responsibilities and reforms*. Cambridge: Polity Press.
Poger, A., J. Wanna, J. Ma, and T. Su. Putting the citizens at the centre. *Australian Journal of Public Administration* 71 (2): 101–110.
Polanyi, M. 1962 *Personal knowledge*, London: Routledge and Kegan Paul.
Popper, K. 1968 *The logic of scientific discovery*. London: Hutchinson.
Precht, R. D. 2007. *Who am I? And if so how many? A philosophical journey*. Munchen: Random House. (trans S. Frisch, and published by Scrib. Melbourne in 2011).
Preston, N. 2001. *Understanding ethics*. Annadale: The Federation Press.
Putnam, R. 1995. Bowling alone. *Journal of Democracy* 6 (1): 65–78.
Putnam, R. 2000. *Bowling alone: The collapse and revival of American community*. New York: Simon & Schuster.
Putnam, R. and D. E. Campbell. 2010. *American grace: How religion divides and unites us*. London: Simon and Schuster.
Ramphela, M. 2012. *Conversations with my sons and daughters*. New York: Penguin.
Rawls, J. 1999. *The law of peoples with the idea of public reason revisited*. London: Harvard University Press.
Rayner, A. 2012. *Natures scope*. Earth Books.
Rayner, A. D. M. 2008. From emptiness to openness: How inclusional awareness transforms abstract pride and prejudice into natural sense and sensibility. http://www.inclusional-research.org/furtherreading/inclusionalessays.pdf.
Rayner, A. D. M. 2010b. Sustainability of the fitting—bringing the philosophical principles of natural inclusion into the educational enrichment of our human neighbourhood. http://www.bestthinking.com.
Rayner, A. D. M. 2011. 'Space cannot be cut: Why self-identity naturally includes neighbourhood. *Integrative Psychological and Behavioural Science* 45:161–184
Rayner, A. 2011. http://www.bestthinking.com/articles/society_and_humanities/philosophy/metaphysics_and_epistemology/a-summary-of-natural-inclusionality.
Reason, P. 1988. *Human inquiry in action*. London: Sage.
Reason, P. 1991. Power and conflict in multidisciplinary collaboration. *Complementary Medical Research* 5 (3).
Reason, P.1994. 'Three approaches to participative inquiry', In *Handbook of Qualitative Research*, eds. Denzin and Lincoln. Sage.
Reason, P. 2002. The practice of co-operative inquiry. *Systemic Practice and Action Research* 15 (3): 169–176
Reason, P. 2002. Justice, sustainability and participation. *Concepts and Transformations*, 7 (1): 7–29.
Reason, P. and H. Bradbury. 2001. Handbook of action research: Participative inquiry and practice. London: Sage.
Reason, P. and W. Torbet. 2001. *Concepts and transformations* 6:1–37.
Reddy, A., R Williams, and T. Johansson. 1997. *Energy after Rio: Prospects and challenges*. New York: UNDP.
Reinharz, S. 1979. *On becoming a social scientist*. San Francoisco: Jossey Bass.
Reinharz, S. 1992. *Feminist methods in social research*. New York: Oxford University Press.
Report No 10. University of Western Australia, *Crime research centre* 141.
Rhodes, R.A.W. 1997. *Understanding governance. Policy networks, governance, reflexivity and accountability*. Maidenhead: Open University Press.
Rhys, E. ed. 1910. *The moral discourses of Epictetus: Mrs. Carter's translation everyman's library*. New York: J M Dent.
Richards, B. 2007. *Emotional governance*. Basingstoke: Macmillan.
Rittel, H. and M. Webber. 1984. *Planning problems are wicked problems. Developments in design methodology*. New York: Wiley.

Rizzolatti, G. and C. Sinigaglia. 2008. *Mirrors in the brain: How our minds share actions, emotions and experience*. (trans Frances Anderson). New York: Oxford University Press.

Rockström, J., W. Steffen, and K. Noone. 2009. A safe operating space for humanity. Nature 461:472–475.

Rodenhoff, V. 2002. The Aarhus convention and its implications. *RECIEL* 11 (3).

Romm, N. 2001. *Accountability in social research: issues and debates*. London: Kluwer.

Romm, N. 2002. A trusting constructivist view of systems thinking in a knowledge age. In *Systems theory and practice in a knowledge age*. eds. Ragsdell et al. New York: Plenum.

Romm, N. 2010. *The new racism*. London: Springer.

Rorive, I. 2009. Religious symbols in the public space: In search of a European answer. *Cardoza Law Review* 30 (6): 2669–2698. http://www.cardozolawreview.com/content/30-6/RORIVE.30-6.pdf. Accessed June 2011.

Rorty, R. 1989. *Contingency, irony and solidarity*. Cambridge: Cambridge University Press.

Rorty, R. 2000. *Philosophy and social hope*. New York: Penguin.

Rosen, R. 1991. *Life itself: A comprehensive inquiry into the nature, origin and fabrication of life*. New York: Columbia University Press.

Rose, D. B. 2004. *Reports form a wild country*. Sydney: University of New South Wales Press.

Rose, D. B. 2005. Dislocating the frontier. http://epress.anu.edu.au/dtf/html/frames.php. See http://epress.anu.edu.au.

Rose, D. B. and T. van Dooren. 2010. *Introduction Australian University E press*. http://epress.anu.edu.au/guidelines/author_guidelines.html.

Rosenberg, S. W. 2002. *The not so common sense: Differences in how people judge social and political life*. New Haven: Yale University Press.

Roszak, T. 1993. *The voice of the earth*. London: Bantam.

Rule, P. 2011. Bakhtin and Freire: Dialogue, dialectic and boundary learning. *Educational Philosophy and Theory* 43 (9).

Russell, B. 1957. Why I am not a Christian and other essays on religion and related subjects.

Sagan, E. 1994. *The Honey and the Hemlock*. Princeton: Princeton University Press.

Satre, J.1976. *Critique of dialectical reason*. London: New Left Review.

Saul, B., S. Sherwood, J. McAdam, T. Stephens, and J. Slezak. 2012. *Climate change and Australia: Warming to the global challenge*. Leichhardt: The Federation Press

Schaffer, K., and S. Smith. 2004. *Human rights and narrated lives*. New York: Palgrave.

Schein, E. H. 1996. Kurt Lewin's change theory in the field and in the classroom: Notes towards a model of managed learning'. *Systemic Practice* 9 (1): 27–47.

Schneider, H. 2013. World bank opens floodgates: Hydropower projects are back in favour as greener energy solution. *Guardian Weekly*, 17 May 2013, 14.

Schlozman, K. L., S. Verbena, and H. Brady. 2010. Weapon of the strong? Participatory inequality and the internet. *American Political Science Association* 8 (2): 487–509.

Schumacher, F. F. 1973. *Small is beautiful. Economics as if people mattered*. New York: Harper and Row.

Schweber, H. 2012. Stakeholder, shareholder and citizen: A different approach to the analysis and critique of democratic governance. *Public Lecture Series,* Fulbright Distinguished Chair of American Political Science. 29 May. Victoria Square: Flinders University.

Scott-Hoy, K. 2001. Eye of the other within: Artistic auto ethnographic evocations of the experience of cross-cultural health work in Vanuatu. Doctor of Philosophy, Division of Education, Arts and Social Sciences. University of South Australia.

Scruton, R. 2005. Delusions of internationalism. In *Debating globalization,* eds. D. Held, et al. Cambridge: Polity Press.

Sen, A. 2000. *Development as freedom*. New York: Knopf.

Sen, A. 2009. *The idea of justice*. Cambridge: The Belknap Press.

Seyfarth, R. and D. L. Cheney. 1984. Grooming, alliances and reciprocal altruism in Vervet monkeys. *Nature* 308:541.

Shanor, K. and J. Kanwal. *Bats sing, mice giggle: Revealing the secret lives of animals*. London: Icon.

Sharpe, L. 2005. *Creatures like us*. Exeter: Imprint Academic.

Sheng, A. 2012. Green grids for life, not grid lock. Jakarta Post 3rd March.

Sherburne, D. 1966. *A key to Whitehead's process and reality*. London: Indiana University Press.

Shiva, V. 1989. *Staying alive: Women, ecology and survival in India*. London: Zed Books.

Shiva, V 2002. *Water wars: Privatization, pollution and profit*. London: Pluto Press.

Shiva, V. 2011. Earth democracy. Portland University. http://www.youtube.com/watch?v=UOfM7QD7-kk/.

Shrivastava, A. 2008. Stiglitz and Sen on profit and pain. Hard News. http://hardnewsmedia.com/2008/08/2301.

Siljander, P., A. Kivelä, and A. Sutinen,eds. 2012. *Theories of Bildung and growth: connections and controversies between continental educational thinking and American pragmatism*. Rotterdam: Sense Publishers.

Singer, P. 2002. *One world: the ethics of globalisation*. Melbourne: Text Publishers.

Somerville, M. 2006. *The ethical imagination: Journeys of the human spirit*. Melbourne: Text Publishers.

Sorensen, H., and T. Watson. 2011. Graziers dispute call for live export ban. http://www.brisbanetimes.com.au/environment/animals/graziers-dispute-call-for-live-export-ban-20110601-1ffad.html#ixzz1nypxkilt. Accessed 1 June 2011.

Spivak, G. C. 1998. Can the Subaltern speak, In *Marxism and the interpretation of culture,* eds. C. Nelson, and L. Gossberg. Illinois: University of Illinois Press.

Stanescu, J. 2012. Species trouble: Judith Butler, mourning, and the precarious lives of animals. *Hypatia* 27:563–582.

Steffen, W., A. Burbridge, L. Hughes, R. Kitching, D. Lindenmayer, W. Musgrave, M. Stafford-Smith, and P. Werner. 2009. Australia's biodiversity and climate change. Australian Government. Melbourne: CSIRO Publishing.

Steinberg, F. 2007. Environmental problems and sustainability'. *Habitat International* 31:354–365.

Steketee, M. 2011. Ideology not cause of debt: Blaming social democratic governments for European crisis makes no sense. *The Weekend Australian* Nov 19–20. http://www.theaustralian.com.au/news/opinion/ideology-not-cause-of-debt/story-e6frg7ax-1226199439960. Accessed 22 Nov 2011.

Stern, N. 2006/2007. *The economics of climate change*. Cambridge: Cambridge University Press.

Stewart, C. 2012. Law of the sea versus the dictates of Canberra: There are daunting obstacles to a policy of turning back asylum seeker boats. *Weekend Australian* March 11–12:19.

Stiglitz, J. 2010. 'From measuring production to measuring wellbeing. Australian Productivity Commission Review of Government Service Provision. http://www.pc.gov/lectures/stiglitz. Accessed 29 Jul 2010.

Stiglitz, J. E. 2012. *The price of inequality: how today's divided society endangers our future*. New York: WW Norton.

Stiglitz, J., A. Sen, and J. P. Fitoussi. 2010. *Mis-measuring our lives: Why the GDP doesn't add up*. New York: The New Press.

Stoker, G. 2002. International trends in local government transformation. In *Democratising local government. The South African experiment,* eds. S. Parnell, E. Pieterse, M. Swilling, and D. Wooldridge. Lansdowne: University of Cape Town Press.

Sunker, H. 2006. Knowledge, society/knowledge capitalism and education. *Policy Futures in Education* 4 (3): 217–219.

Surowieki, J. 2005. *The wisdom of crowds*. New Yorks: Random House.

Swann, W. 2012. The 0.01 Percent: The rising influence of vested interests in Australia. *The Monthly Essays*. http://www.themonthly.com.au/. Accessed 03 Dec 2013.

Szell, G. 2004. Environmental Kaizen: environmental protection as a process. In *Environmental challenges for Japan and Germany—interdisciplinary and inter cultural perspectives,* 253–268, eds G. Szell, and K. Tominaga. Frankfurt: Peter Lang.

Szell, G. 2004. Environmental Kaizen: Environmental protection as a process. In *Environmental challenges for Japan and Germany—interdisciplinary and intercultural perspectives,* 253–268, eds. G. Szell, and K. Tominaga. Frankfurt: Peter Lang.

Szell, G. 2010. How to develop further the European social model. In *The ambivalent character of participation,* 699–707. Frankfurt: Peter Lang.

Talpin, J and S. Wojcik. 2010. Deliberating environmental policy issues: Comparing the learning potential of online and face-to-face discussion on climate change. Policy and Internet. Policy Studies Organization.

Tausch, A. 2010. 'Towards yet another age of creative destruction? *Journal of Globalisation Studies* 1 (1): 104–130.

Thom, B. 2010. *Assessing regional sustainability and land use change*. Impacts of Climate Change on Future Urban Societies. Shanghai, China, August 3–4.

Thompson, G. 1967. *Travels and adventures in Southern Africa*. Cape Town: Van Riebeck Society.

Thompson, G. 2005. The limits to globalization: Questions for Held and Wolf. In *Debating globalization,* eds. D. Held. et al. Cambridge: Polity Press.

Thurok, N. 2012. *The universe within*. London: Allen and Unwin. (Based on the CBC Massy Lectures).

Treaty of Maastricht. 1992. *Article 5 on Subsidiarity*.

Triandis, H. C. 1995. *Individualism and collectivism*. Boulder: Oxford.

Turner, V. 1969. *The ritual process: Structure and anti-structure*. London: Routledge.

Turner, V. and International African Institute. 1968. *The drums of affliction: A study of religious processes among the Ndembu of Zambia,* (by V. W. Turner). Oxford: Clarendon Press. International African Institute.

Turner, R. and C. Whitehead. 2008. How collective representations can change the structure of the brain. *Journal of Consciousness Studies* 15 (10–11): 43–57.

Ulrich, W. 1983. Critical heuristics of social planning: A new approach to practical philosophy. New York: Wiley.

Ulrich, W. 2001. The quest for competence in systemic research and practice. *Systems Research and Behavioural Science* 18:3–28.

UNESCO. 2007. Biosphere reserves: Dialogue in biosphere reserves. References, practices and experiences. ISSN:2071–1468. Paris: UNESCO.

United Nations.1993. Integrated environmental and economic accounting: Handbook of national accounting: studies in methods, Series F (61). Department for Economic and Social Information and Policy Analysis, Statistical Division. New York: United Nations.

United Nations Economic and Social Development Local Agenda 21 1992.

United Nations. 2011. The millennium goals report. http://www.aidsdatahub.org/en/whats-new/287-all-data-alerts/728-the-millennium-development-goals-report-2011-united-nations-2011. Accessed 19 July 2011.

Urry, J. 2007. *Mobilities*. Cambridge: Polity Press.

Urry, J. 2010. Consuming the planet to excess. *Theory, Culture and Society* 27:191–212.

Uslaner, E. 1999. Democracy and social capital. In *Democracy and trust,* ed. M. Warren. Cambridge: Cambridge University Press.

Van Gigch, J. 2003. Metadecisions: Rehabilitating epistemology. London: Kluwer/Plenum.

Van Gigch, J. in collaboration with McIntyre-Mills, J. 2006. *Wisdom, knowledge and management*. London: Springer.

Van Onselen, P. 2011. Treasurer will stand or fall on his message. *Weekend Australian* May 5–6, 22.

Vaske, J. and K. Kobrin. 2001. Place attachment and environmentally responsible behavior. *Journal of Environmental Education* 32 (4): 16–21.

Veblen, T. 1899. *The theory of the leisure class,* 64–70. New York: Macmillan. Posting Date: August 6, 2008 [EBook #833] Release Date: March, 1997 [Last updated: January 21, 2011].

Vickers, G. 1983 *Human systems are different*. London: Harper and Row.

Vickers, G. 1968. *Value systems and social process*. London: Tavistock Publications.

Vickers, A. 2005. *A history if modern Indonesia*. Cambridge: Cambridge University Press.

Vidal, J. 2013. Toxic e-waste dumped in poor nations, warns UN. *Guardian Weekly,* 20 Dec 2013.

Von Foerster, H. 1995. *Cybernetics of cybernetics*. Second edition. Minneapolis: Future Systems, Inc.

Wadsworth, Y. 1997. *Do it yourself social research*. London: Allen and Unwin, Alexander.

Wadsworth, Y. 2000. The mirror, the magnifying glass, the compass and the map: facilitating participatory action research. *Handbook of Action Research*. London: Sage.

Wadsworth, Y. 2008. Is it safe to talk about systems again yet? Self-organizing processes for complex living systems and the dynamics of human inquiry. *Systemic Practice and Action Research* 21 (2): 153–170.

Wadsworth, Y. 2010. Building in research and evaluation. Human inquiry for living systems. Sydney: Allen and Unwin.

Walsh, F. 2002. *Planning for country*. Alice Springs: IAD Press.

Walzer, M. 2004. Emergency ethics in arguing about war. New Haven: Yale University Press.

Ward, P., F. Verity, P. Carter, G. Tsourtos, J. Coveney, and K. C. Wong. 2012. Food stress in Adelaide. *Journal of Environmental and Public Health*. http://dx.doi.org/10.1155/2013/968078.

Warren, E. 1999. *Democratic theory and trust*. Cambridge: Cambridge University Press.

Watson, P and A. Jones. 2006. Former World Bank economist predicts global crash. http://www.prisonplanet.con/articles/october2006/301006globalcrash.htm. Accessed 30 Oct 2006.

Wear, A. 2012. Collaborative approaches to regional governance—lessons from Victoria. *Australian Journal of Public Administration* 71 (4): 469–474.

Weber, M. 2003. Keeping it real? Kant and systematic approaches to IR—a response to Harrison. *Review of International Studies* 29:145–50.

Weil, S. 1998. Reflexive turns in paradigm dialogues; tensions and challenges in transcending different domains for knowledge generation. 14th World Congress of Sociology, Montreal.

Xiang, W-N. 2012. Editorial: Working with wicked problems in socio-ecological systems: Awareness, acceptance, and adaptation. *Landscape and Urban Planning* 110:1–4.

Weir, A. 2012. Collaborative approaches to regional governance. *Australian Journal of Public Administration* 71 (4): 469–474.

Wenger, E, N. White, and J. Smith. 2009. *Digital habitats: Stewarding technology for communities*. Portland: CP Square.

Wenger, E. 1998. *Communities of practice*. Cambridge: Cambridge University Press.

West, M. 2009. *White women writing white: Identity and representation in post-apartheid literatures of South Africa*. Claremont: David Philip.

Wheatley, M. 2009. *Turning to one another: Simple conversations to restore hope to the future*. San Franciso: Barett-Koehler.

White, H. 2013. Papering the cracks: The nation reviewed. *The Monthly* Dec-Jan.

Whitehead, C. 2001. Social mirrors and shared experiential worlds. *Journal of Consciousness Studies*, 8 (4): 3–36.

Wilde, O. 1892. *Lady Windermere's Fan*, Act 3.

Wilkinson, R. and K. Pickett. 2009. *The spirit level. Why more equal societies almost always do better*. London: Allen Lane.

Wilson, P. 2011. Moments of madness amid calculated rage, The *Weekend Australian* August 13–14:21

Wilson, P. 2011. Our union boss joins the Arab uprising Europe correspondent. *The Australian*. http://www.theaustralian.com.au/news/world/our-union-boss-joins-the-arab-uprising/story-e6frg6so-1226027935768. Accessed 26 Mar 2011.

Wilson, P. 2012. Bitter pill Europeans won't take. *Weekend Australian* May 5–6:16.

Wynne, B. 1996. May the sheep safely graze? A reflexive view of the expert—lay knowledge divide. In *Risk, environment and modernity: Towards a new ecology*, eds. L. S. Szerszynski and B. Wynne. London: Sage.

Yeatman, A. 2003. Global ethics, Australian citizenship and the 'boat people': A symposium. *Journal of Sociology* 39 (1): 15–22.

Young, I. M. 1990. *Justice and the politics of difference*. Princeton: Princeton University Press. (2011. First published in 1990).

Young, I. M. 2000. *Inclusion and democracy*. Oxford: Oxford University Press.

Young, I. M. 2001. Activist challenges to deliberative democracy. *Political Theory* 29 (5): 670–690. (Published by: Sage Publications, Inc. Article Stable). http://www.jstor.org/stable/307253410.2307/3072534.

Index

J. McIntyre-Mills, *Transformation from Wall Street to Wellbeing*, Contemporary Systems Thinking, DOI 10.1007/978-1-4899-7466-2,

MIX
Papier aus verantwortungsvollen Quellen
Paper from responsible sources
FSC® C105338

If you have any concerns about our products,
you can contact us on
ProductSafety@springernature.com

In case Publisher is established outside the EU,
the EU authorized representative is:
Springer Nature Customer Service Center GmbH
Europaplatz 3, 69115 Heidelberg, Germany

Printed by Libri Plureos GmbH
in Hamburg, Germany